INTERPERSONAL PROCESSES
IN PSYCHOLOGICAL PROBLEMS

Interpersonal Processes in Psychological Problems

CHRIS SEGRIN

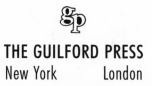

THE GUILFORD PRESS
New York   London

©2001 The Guilford Press
A Division of Guilford Publications, Inc.
72 Spring Street, New York, NY 10012
www.guilford.com

Printed in the United States of America

This book is printed on acid-free paper.

Last digit is print number: 9 8 7 6 5 4 3 2 1

Library of Congress Cataloging-in-Publication Data

Segrin, Chris.
    Interpersonal processes in psychological problems / Chris Segrin.
        p. cm.
    Includes bibliographical references and index.
    ISBN 1-57230-679-3
        1. Interpersonal relations. 2. Mental illness. I. Title.

RC455.4.I58 S44 2001

2001033504

About the Author

Chris Segrin, PhD, is Associate Professor of Communication at the University of Arizona, where he also holds adjunct appointments in the Departments of Psychology and Family Studies. His research focuses on the role of interpersonal relationships and social skills in psychosocial problems such as depression, loneliness, and anxiety. Current research interests also include family communication and predictors of relational and marital distress. Dr. Segrin's work can be found in such journals as *Human Communication Research*, *Journal of Abnormal Psychology*, *Communication Monographs*, *Journal of Social and Clinical Psychology*, and *Journal of Social and Personal Relationships*.

Preface

At any point in time, millions of people throughout the world are afflicted with psychological problems. For many, these problems persist for years, and in some cases for a lifetime. Consider, for example, the results of recent epidemiological investigations indicating that in any given year 28% of the adults in the United States have some form of psychological disorder (Regier et al., 1993) and that 48% of the U.S. population will have a diagnosable psychological disorder at some time in their lives (Kessler et al., 1994). Given the pervasiveness of mental health problems in society, it is likely that most people will have a relationship (be it romantic, family, friendly, occupational, or professional) with someone suffering from a mental health problem and/or will experience a mental health problem themselves.

As scientists, therapists, students, educators, physicians, and the lay public alike seek a better understanding of psychological problems, it has become evident that these problems influence, and are influenced by, the interpersonal context in which they are situated. Regardless of whether a particular disorder is thought to be caused by biological, cognitive, or behavioral factors, a sufficient understanding of that problem simply cannot be attained without careful attention to the interpersonal communication and relationships of those afflicted with the disorder. Obviously this perspective focuses attention not just on those who seek help for psychological problems, but also on the significant people in their lives, such as spouses, parents, children, coworkers, friends, and dating partners.

Human beings are social creatures. Perhaps this is why psychological disturbances often follow disruptions in interpersonal relationships and problems with interpersonal communication. Mental well-being is inherently tied to social or interpersonal well-being. Findings reviewed in this book show that many mental health problems are as much relationship/communication problems as they are psychological problems. This is why problems such as depression, alcoholism, and social anxiety are often characterized as "psychosocial"problems. Empirical evidence indicates that some mental health problems can actually be precipitated by disrupted or distressed interpersonal relationships. In other cases, mental health problems have a corrosive effect on interpersonal relationships. This often happens as a result of interpersonal communication problems that coexist with many mental health problems. In still other cases, a mental health problem and a distressed interpersonal relationship appear to constitute a vicious cycle where one perpetuates the other. In such instances, where depression, alcoholism, or schizophrenia may be involved, the consequences can be both psychologically and socially disastrous.

The major premise of this book is that mental health problems and interpersonal problems are so entwined that an adequate understanding of one set of problems requires thorough consideration of and attention to the other. Even in cases where a psychological problem can clearly be traced to a biological etiology, for example, there are often interpersonal ramifications associated with the disorder that can have a profound impact on its course and consequences, and possibly even on the biology of the disorder. It should be emphasized, however, that the point of this book is not to present the interpersonal paradigm in mental health as a competitor to other dominant paradigms, such as the cognitive-behavioral, psychodynamic, or biological paradigms. Rather, the interpersonal perspective is presented as another immensely significant piece of the puzzle that scientists and practitioners refer to as "psychopathology."

Interpersonal Processes in Psychological Problems is designed to expose readers to a diverse array of research findings, theories, and hypotheses pertinent to an equally diverse array of psychological problems. Despite the variety inherent in these studies and the problems that they are designed to address, readers will find many interpersonal themes recurring in discussions of the different problems. Because most researchers and theorists tend to focus their efforts on an individual psychological problem, the identification of these "universal" interpersonal problems in mental health has rarely been addressed or undertaken. However, a great deal can be learned about psychopathology and interpersonal relations by understanding that different problems can have common interpersonal antecedents and consequences. At the same time, different interpersonal antecedents may each be sufficient to contribute to the development of the same psychological problem.

Some of the primary goals of science are to explain, predict, and control phenomena. *Interpersonal Processes in Psychological Problems* is written in respectively descending service of those goals. It is virtually impossible to predict or control a phenomenon in the absence of any understanding and explanation of how and why it exists and behaves. Once explanation has been reasonably satisfied, prediction and control become more manageable endeavors. In the area of psychological problems, the goal of controlling a phenomenon centers on therapy and prevention efforts. For the most part, these issues are beyond the scope of this book. Although interpersonally oriented therapy regimens are becoming more common in the treatment of mental health problems, such programs clearly need to be informed by current scientific findings and explanations for why the disorders developed in the first place. This is where in-depth explanation, along with the blueprints for prediction, becomes exceptionally important. The material reviewed in this book is one step toward providing such an explanation and forecast from an interpersonal perspective.

Chapter 1 begins with a historical analysis of the quest to understand psychopathology, and of the various paradigms developed in the pursuit of that quest. The origins and rudiments of an interpersonal paradigm in psychopathology are then presented in more detail. Chapters 2–9 are organized around different psychological problems. Each chapter examines the scientific inquiry into a different problem from an interpersonal perspective. Although the problems are different, readers will notice remarkable consistency in some of the interpersonal motifs emerging from the literatures on distinct disorders. The book concludes in Chapter 10 with a more formal presentation of the interpersonal paradigm of psychopathology, distilled from the interpersonal findings on different psychological problems.

A number of scientists, students, and editors have made significant contributions to this book. I would like to thank Dick Bootzin, Kathryn Dindia, and Peter Wissoker for their suggestions to write this book and input on getting the process started; Michelle Givertz, Nathan Miczo, and Heather Powell for their outstanding editorial assistance; Seymour Weingarten, Editor-in-Chief of The Guilford Press, and his editorial and production staffs for their helpful guidance throughout the entire course of preparation and production; and Thomas Joiner and Mark Leary for their valuable feedback and suggestions, as well as their major contributions to our understanding of the psychosocial problems described herein.

Contents

1

Origins and Overview of Interpersonal Approaches to Mental Health Problems

Interpersonal approaches to psychological problems assume that people's social relationships are intimately tied to their well-being and mental health. When interpersonal relationships become distressed and dissatisfying, they become sources of stress with remarkable power to disrupt psychological well being. Sometimes this disruption is brought about by problems with the ability and/or motivation to engage effectively in interpersonal communication. At other times it occurs because of problematic interactions and relations with other people who are themselves distressed, or likely to behave in ways that are interpersonally destructive. In either case, interpersonal problems are strongly connected to psychological problems, since interpersonal relationship quality is one of the most important aspects of human existence. Research findings and evidence for this interpersonal perspective are rapidly developing and expanding. Despite its newness and its relatively recent recognition, the interpersonal perspective on psychological problems can be traced back at least 100 years, and it shares assumptions with many other modern-day paradigms in psychopathology.

Throughout recorded history, human beings have sought to develop explanations for psychopathology. Although they bear little resemblance to modern scientific theories, hypotheses and explanations for deviant behavior and thinking can be traced back thousands of years. For example, as far back as 1000–2000 B.C., psychological problems were explained by some through demonology. According to this perspective, an autonomous evil being would inhabit a person's body and cause odd and destructive behavior that the person could not control. As preposterous as such a "theory" of mental illness may appear to most of us today, demonology persevered as a common explanation for psychopathology well into the 17th century. However, diverse schools of thought on psychopathology were still evident before modern scientific thinking. For example, Hippocrates advocated a somatogenic explanation for aberrant behavior, arguing that many mental health problems originate in physiological disturbances. Proponents of modern-day biological theories of psychopathology will recognize some basic similarities with concepts outlined by Hippocrates, dating back to approximately 300 B.C.

MODERN PARADIGMS IN MENTAL HEALTH

The 20th century witnessed a great proliferation of paradigms developed to explain psychological problems. Many of these paradigms continue to be very influential to this day, generating hundreds of research studies and dictating a variety of approaches to the treatment of psychopathology. It is instructive to compare and contrast these paradigms briefly, as many of their elements have found their way into modern interpersonal approaches.

The *psychoanalytic*, or *psychodynamic*, school of thought has its origins in the work of Sigmund Freud. Many recognize this paradigm for its tripartite approach to the human psyche in the form of the id, ego, and superego. These theoretical functions of the human mind are thought to operate and be influenced by unconscious desires and their interface with perceived realities. Although sometimes not recognized as such, interpersonal relations figure prominently in the psychodynamic school. For example, various complexes (e.g., the Oedipus and Electra complexes), certain defense mechanisms (e.g., projection), and the therapeutic processes of transference and countertransference are all inherently interpersonal in nature. Viewed from this perspective, psychological problems are thought to be best treated by psychotherapy that seeks to help the client understand and make sense of early relationships with parents as well as significant others, and their impact on present-day psychological and social functioning. Modern-day approaches that are strongly rooted in the psychodynamic school, such as object relations theory (Greenberg & Mitchell, 1983), are even more acutely focused on interpersonal issues. Indeed, the very concept of *object relations* refers to patterns of interpersonal functioning and relationships (Westen, 1990). Perhaps it is not surprising then that the contemporary interpersonal paradigm in mental health has something of an ancestry in the psychoanalytic approach, despite bearing little resemblance to it today.

In a radical departure from psychoanalytic thinking, John Watson developed the *behavioral* paradigm in the early 20th century. Unlike psychodynamic theorists, behavioral scientists focus largely on observable behavior and eschew appeals to the unobservable and often hypothetical functions of the mind for explaining psychopathology. According to this school of thought, behaviors that are reinforced will persevere, whereas those that are not reinforced or are punished will tend to disappear from the behavioral repertoire. Proponents of the behavioral paradigm seek to treat psychological problems by teaching and directing clients to engage in behaviors that are rewarding and to avoid those that lead to punishing responses. In some cases, behavior therapists may attempt to teach clients to associate reward with behaviors that previously were associated with punishing sensations. A number of landmark scientific theories were developed in the behavioral tradition, some of which continue to be essential to our understanding of mental health problems today. For example, the processes of operant conditioning and classical conditioning figure prominently in some hypotheses developed to explain such problems as substance misuse, eating disorders, and anxiety disorders. It is also important to note that behavioral principles have clearly found their way into interpersonal approaches to mental health problems. For instance, Lewinsohn's (1974, 1975) behavioral theory of depression is an interesting mix of behavioral and interpersonal approaches that views other people in the social environment as the source of rewards and punishments.

The behavioral tradition was itself met with steadfast critics who reacted to the "black box" view of the human mind—that is, the view of behavior as simply a product of stimulus–response patterns, with little intervening thought of any complex nature. Out of this reaction grew the *cognitive* paradigm, which conceptualizes mental health problems as derivatives of distorted and illogical ways of thinking about the self and surrounding environment, as well as the past and the future. In the last third of the 20th century, the cognitive paradigm proliferated so rapidly that it was often characterized as a "revolution." Problems such as marital distress,* depression, anxiety, alcoholism, and loneliness are all understood within this paradigm as the by-products of maladaptive cognitive patterns. These cognitions include attributions for various events,

---

*The term *family of orientation* (see below) refers to the relationships of adult couples in the families formed by adults (of course). These relationships are not restricted to legal marriage. Most research on such couples has been done on married couples, however. For this reason, as well as for ease of reference, I use such terms as *marital*, *spouses*, and the like in much of this book to refer to adult couples in families of orientation.

memories of past situations and encounters, and expectations for the future. Adherents of the cognitive paradigm treat psychological problems with psychotherapy that attempts to challenge and correct maladaptive cognitions, in order to help a client see the self and world in a more realistic (and, ideally, more positive) light. Cognitive approaches still figure very prominently in our understanding of many mental health problems and in the ways they are treated.

In the past several decades, several theories and models of mental health problems have been developed that draw heavily on both interpersonal and cognitive paradigms (Peplau & Caldwell, 1978; Sacco, 1999). These cognitive–interpersonal integrations illustrate how cognitive patterns may play an instrumental role in shaping the interpersonal relationships and interactions that have teleological significance in the development and maintenance of mental health problems. For example, attributional accounts of loneliness argue that lonely people often blame themselves for interpersonal failures, thus reducing their motivation to remedy their undesirable interpersonal situation. This attributional tendency, combined with negative expectations and evaluations of other people, serves to maintain an unfortunate interpersonal life for a lonely person.

It is also possible to identify threads of the cognitive paradigm woven into interpersonal hypotheses for certain problems such as alcoholism and eating disorders. As the cognitive perspective itself was combined with elements of the behavioral paradigm, resulting in the amalgam known as *cognitive-behavioral theory*, interpersonally oriented hypotheses were quick to emerge. For instance, the process of *modeling*, a pillar in the cognitive-behavioral school, has been implicated in the development of both eating disorders and alcoholism. In each case, exposure to an individual who models the problematic behavior, and is rewarded for doing so, can lead to the acquisition of the problem behavior by an observer (e.g., the child of a parent with the problematic behavior). The observer is thought to hold cognitive representations of the behavior in his or her mind, which then becomes the eventual stimulus for producing the behavior in the absence of the model. A hypothesis such as this clearly draws on cognitive-behavioral concepts to explain what is essentially the interpersonal transmission of a psychological problem. As might be expected, cognitive-behavioral therapy for psychological problems draws on principles of both cognitive and behavioral therapies—focusing on cognitive patterns, attributional styles, and maladaptive expectations, along with engaging in pleasant activities and learning to disassociate punishing responses with otherwise functional behaviors (e.g., experiencing extreme nervousness when going to a party).

Although some might associate *biological* explanations for mental health problems with recent discoveries, this paradigm is in fact one of the oldest in science. As noted earlier, Hippocrates articulated physiological hypotheses for what are now regarded as forms of psychopathology. Even though he and his followers did not always accurately specify the precise physical bases for psychopathology, relative to modern knowledge, the general idea that psychological problems have a foundation in the physiology of the human body has held up quite well over time. As new technologies such as positron emission tomography (PET), electroencephalography (EEG), magnetic resonance imaging (MRI), and sensitive blood assays have been developed and deployed, scientists have begun to discover and document what appear to be biological bases of psychological disturbances. As a result, advocates of the biological paradigm explain mental health problems with an appeal to such factors as depletion or excess of various neurotransmitters, genetic predispositions and vulnerabilities, disturbed endocrine functioning, and irregular anatomical structures or functions in the brain. Of course, treatment of psychological problems from this vantage point entails agents that have their action on the biological entities thought to be responsible for the problem. For example, those who feel that depression is caused by the depletion of a certain neurotransmitter may treat it with drugs that block the reuptake of that neurotransmitter, so that it can be present in greater quantity and duration to have its desired effect. It is noteworthy that many of the focal processes in the biological paradigm have established links to interpersonal behavior. For instance, the neurotransmitter serotonin appears to play a role in regulating competent social behavior and establishing social dominance in nonhuman primates (Edwards & Kravitz, 1997; Higley et al., 1996). Modern biological explanations for mental health problems enjoy great popularity and promise, perhaps as logical extensions of the medical model that dominates the classification of mental disorders.

DEVELOPMENT OF THE INTERPERSONAL PARADIGM

To this day, it is easy to locate books, chapters, and articles that survey different paradigms or schools of thought in psychopathology without mentioning the interpersonal perspective. On the other hand, surveys that omit cognitive or behavioral approaches are extremely rare. At a minimum, the "References" section of this book attests to the fact that hundreds, if not thousands, of empirical studies document a clear association between problematic interpersonal relationships and mental health problems. However, there are at least three reasons why interpersonal approaches to mental health problems do not always enjoy the same status as cognitive, behavioral, or biological approaches.

First, the interpersonal paradigm has been painfully slow to develop. Whereas the cognitive school emerged so rapidly that it rightfully came to be known as the "cognitive revolution," the interpersonal school of thought has been brewing for at least 100 years, sometimes showing little development from one decade to the next (until the 1970s, when interpersonally oriented theories began to proliferate).

Second, a *paradigm*, of the kind described by Thomas Kuhn (1970), that is uniquely interpersonal has yet to be as formally articulated as other more recognizable paradigms in mental health. Only a few writers have attempted to outline the basic principles of an interpersonal school of thought for understanding and treating mental health problems. Consequently, this paradigm is still emerging in modern conceptualizations of psychological disorders. Nevertheless, within the realm of particular mental health problems such as schizophrenia and depression, there exist some extremely well-articulated and researched interpersonal theories from which one can extrapolate a more general interpersonal paradigm.

Third, the scientists who have developed and who currently practice in the interpersonal school of mental health are not as well organized as those who work in other paradigms. Interpersonally oriented theorists and researchers tend to be situated in the fields of psychology, sociology, psychiatry, interpersonal communication, family studies, nursing, and social work. Perhaps as a consequence, it is not always easy to clearly identify a core group of researchers and theories that typify this paradigm, as they are scattered across numerous academic disciplines.

The connection between mental health problems and interpersonal relationships was recognized decades before scientists began collecting the data that would later empirically verify this association. For example, Freud (1917/1966) spoke of the causes and consequences of mental illness by referring to "the misfortunes of life from which arise deprivation of love, poverty, family quarrels, ill-judged choice of a partner in marriage, [and] unfavorable social circumstances" (p. 432). Even his now well-known psychodynamic theory stresses the importance of early interpersonal relationships, particularly with parents, in determining later mental health or illness. The neo-Freudians, such as Karen Horney and Frieda Fromm-Reichmann, continued to develop the thesis that interpersonal relationships play an important role in the development of mental problems (e.g., Fromm-Reichmann, 1960). However, it was one of their neo-Freudian contemporaries, Harry Stack Sullivan, who most strongly emphasized the role of interpersonal and social forces in the development of self and disruption of mental health (Sullivan, 1953b).

Despite being in close touch with his psychoanalytic roots, Sullivan was himself influenced by a more eclectic range of theorists, including the neurologist Adolf Meyer. Like Meyer, Sullivan felt that mental problems cannot be adequately explained by only biological or only psychological constructs. He recognized the need to take the social milieu into account. In his writings Sullivan unabashedly advocated an interpersonal orientation toward the understanding of mental illness, describing his theoretical intentions in plainly interpersonal terms: "As a psychiatrist, I had come to feel over the years that there was an acute need for a discipline which was determined to study not the individual human organism or the social heritage, but the interpersonal situations through which persons manifest mental health or mental disorder" (Sullivan, 1953b, p. 18). He argued that "the field of psychiatry is neither the mentally sick individual, nor the successful and unsuccessful processes that may be observed in groups and that can be studied in detached objectivity. Psychiatry, instead, is the study of processes that involve or go on between people. The field of psychiatry is the field of interpersonal relations" (Sullivan, 1953a, p. 10).

Obviously, interpersonal relations figured very prominently in Sullivan's thinking about mental disorders. He characterized psychological problems simply as "patterns of inadequate and inappropriate action in interpersonal relations" (Sullivan, 1953b, p. 314). In discussing depression, for example, he noted that "it is a chiefly destructive process. It cuts off impulses to integrate constructive situations with others. Only destructive situations are maintained, and these are extremely stereotyped" (Sullivan, 1953a, p. 102). It would be at least 25 years before researchers started to test such claims empirically. The accumulation of such data clearly indicates that Sullivan was indeed far ahead of his time.

One of Sullivan's more notable contributions involved focusing attention on the importance of same-sex adolescent peer relationships in the developmental process. Sullivan unquestionably endorsed the proposition set forth by Freud that the architecture of our early interpersonal relationships can lead to later mental health problems. However, he definitely broadened the field of vision beyond the traditional psychoanalytic focus on relations with the mother and father.

Another significant development in interpersonal approaches to psychopathology came with the publication of Timothy Leary's (1957) *Interpersonal Diagnosis of Personality*. Leary described his well-known "interpersonal circle," whose lineage is clearly traceable to Sullivan's thinking, as a method of defining a range of interpersonal behavior that includes abnormal or disturbed extremes. In so doing, Leary advocated dimensionalizing over categorization. Of course, the prevailing ideology of the time involved labeling abnormal behavior as falling into a particular category (i.e., diagnosis). Instead, Leary felt that normal and abnormal personalities simply occupy different points on the same continuum. It has been argued that Leary's interpersonal circle operationalized concepts originally set forth by Sullivan (Wiggins, 1996). Leary's interpersonal circumplex, defined by the dimensions of dominance–submissiveness and love–hate, has been revised and refined several times since its original appearance (e.g., Kiesler, 1983; Wiggins, 1982) and continues to be a useful tool for understanding interpersonal relations and mental health problems (e.g., Sheffield, Carey, Patenaude, & Lambert, 1995).

There can be no question that Leary's ideas about interpersonal issues in psychopathology, like Sullivan's views, were far ahead of their time. He reminded readers that "what a person does in any social situation is a function of at least two factors: (1) his multilevel personality structure; and (2) the activities and effect of the *other one*, the person with whom he in interacting" (Leary, 1955, p. 147). Students of interpersonal communication will immediately recognize the transactional and dyadic conceptualization inherent in Leary's explanation of behavior in social contexts. This conceptualization moves the locus of attention from purely internal psychological structures to the intersection of the self and the other. Leary also drew attention in his writings to the way in which both verbal and nonverbal behaviors play a role in the communication process.

Some of Leary's discussions of various mental health problems and disrupted interpersonal processes would prove to be quite prophetic. For example, he asserted that "severe neurotics—defined at this level as persons with limited ranges of reflexes—are incredibly and creatively skilled in drawing rejection, nurturance, and so on, from the people with whom they deal. In many cases the 'sicker' the patient is the more likely he is to have abandoned all interpersonal techniques except one, which he can handle with magnificent finesse" (Leary, 1955, p. 157). A review of contemporary research on depression and personality disorders demonstrates just how accurate this statement was and is.

Despite his accomplishments and recognition in the area of interpersonal relations and psychopathology, Leary's career took a decidedly different path not long after the publication of *Interpersonal Diagnosis of Personality*. He drew a great deal of attention for his work with psychoactive drugs (e.g., Leary, 1969) and his public statements about their use. One can only wonder how much faster the interpersonal paradigm would have developed and proliferated had Leary remained in the academic and scientific milieu. As an interesting footnote to his career, which at times bore greater resemblance to vaudeville than to science, in 1994 the American Psychological Association held a symposium in honor of his work in interpersonal psychology. The presentations at this symposium, by a number of prominent interpersonal theorists, were eventually published as a special issue of the *Journal of Personality Assessment* (e.g., Carson, 1996; Strack, 1996; Wiggins, 1996). Leary himself wrote a commentary on the symposium that would appear in print within months of his death. In this final academic publication of his career, Leary (1996) paid homage to the influence of Sullivan, plainly stating that "the interpersonal viewpoint came from the street smarts of Harry Stack Sullivan" (p. 306).

These early interpersonal approaches to understanding mental health problems, advocated by the likes of Sullivan and Leary, have now developed into what has been described as the "social-interactional viewpoint" (Carson, 1983) and the "interpersonal school" (Klerman, 1986). Carson (1983) summarized the foundation of this paradigm by stating that among those seeking psychological treatment, "the underlying problems usually turn out to be interpersonal in nature—frequently having the form, 'I can't (do something interpersonal)' " (p. 147).

Modern-day instantiations of this perspective were developed rapidly in the 1960s and 1970s by those who stressed the import of concurrent, as opposed to early childhood, interpersonal relationships and mental health problems. In departing from some of the tenets of Sullivan's interpersonal theory and expanding the focus to a wider variety of interpersonal relationships, modern interpersonal approaches to psychopathology bear less resemblance to their originators. This era was launched by approaches such as the family communication and double-bind theory of schizophrenia by Bateson and his associates in the 1960s; it continued with Coyne's interactional theory of depression, Lewinsohn's behavioral theory of depression, and the family systems model of alcoholism by Steinglass, all from the 1970s. Each of these approaches is discussed later in this book. Several successors to Leary's position in the interpersonal school have emerged to carry on the tradition of analyzing personality and social behavior with the circumplex model (e.g., Carson, 1969; Wiggins, 1982). Most notably, Lorna Smith Benjamin has developed Leary's interpersonal circle into the Structural Analysis of Social Behavior model (Benjamin, 1974; McLemore & Benjamin, 1979). This model is a more explicit and detailed extension of the original interpersonal circle, and continues to guide research and clinical understanding of psychological disorders to this day (e.g., Benjamin, 1996). These theories, models, and hypotheses have been developed to explain a wide range of disorders, but they all share the postulate that distressed and dysfunctional interpersonal relations are inextricably entwined with psychological distress. The dozens, and in some cases hundreds, of studies that have been spawned by these pioneering efforts are testimony to their heuristic value; this research illustrates that interpersonal approaches to mental health problems have been, are, and will continue to be very influential (Brokaw & McLemore, 1991; Joiner & Coyne, 1999; Kiesler, 1996).

As noted earlier, each paradigm has its own explanation of psychological problems, and different approaches to treatment emerge from these different explanations. The interpersonal approach suggests that treatment of psychological problems will be most effective when the social context is examined and modified. The focus of therapy is not on the individual, but on his or her important relationships with other people. Thus interpersonal therapy may involve the spouse, friends, and family members, in addition to the person who presents with the problem. Sometimes clients need to be taught how to improve their communication with other people, with the goal of building more desirable relationships. This can be achieved through social skills training (Segrin & Givertz, in press). Interpersonal psychotherapy is a very well-developed and useful technique for treating psychological problems (Weissman, Markowitz, & Klerman, 2000), and has been fruitfully applied to problems such as depression and eating disorders (e.g., Rounsaville, Klerman, Weissman, & Chevron, 1985).

INTERPERSONAL "VERSUS" OTHER SCHOOLS OF THOUGHT

The description and promulgation of the interpersonal paradigm in mental health should not be interpreted as an indictment against other paradigms or schools of thought. In the social and behavioral sciences, it is rarely fruitful to compare and contrast theories with an "either/or" mentality. Rather, a more useful approach asks, "When or under what conditions does factor X explain and predict the development, course, and outcome of a given disorder?" There is no justification for attempting to explain mental health problems as the results of a single factor. Often biological, cognitive, behavioral, and interpersonal factors work together to create a disturbance in mental health. Some may even view interpersonal theories as a portion of the cognitive paradigm in which the cognitions are about interpersonal events, or as a portion of the behavioral paradigm in which the behaviors are interpersonal. Notwithstanding the contributions of cognitive, neurochemical, life stress, genetic, and behavioral theories that provide valid accounts of the etiology of numerous psychological problems, this book shows that problematic interpersonal relationships also play a contributory causal role in the development and/or course of these disorders. As such, they can be characterized rightfully as "psychosocial" disorders.

FOCAL POINTS OF THE INTERPERSONAL PARADIGM

One of the important functions of any scientific paradigm is to direct attention to important variables and processes. In the extreme, paradigms dictate what count as "data." The interpersonal paradigm in psychopathology focuses on at least three key variables or processes. First, a great deal of attention is paid to the social behavior of the afflicted individual. How do people with a particular psychosocial problem communicate with others? This focus includes an examination of verbal behaviors (i.e., content of the speech) as well as nonverbal behaviors (e.g., eye contact, speech rate, facial expression, posture, gesture, etc.). The idea behind such an analysis is that people's communication behaviors often provide insights into their psychological state. But even more importantly, communication behaviors are what help to create the interpersonal context in which a mentally distressed person finds him- or herself. As such, most interpersonally oriented researchers assume, at least implicitly, that the person suffering from a psychological problem has an active role in shaping his or her social environment.

A second and closely related area of interest within the interpersonal school consists of other people's reactions and responses to the psychologically troubled person and his or her interpersonal behavior. Scientists have discovered that people often react in consistent and predictable patterns to a person with certain psychological problems. In such cases, it is impossible to overlook the powerful effect of such widespread reactions on the mentally distressed individual. It is most intriguing to learn that other people often exhibit behavior toward the ill individual that is itself sometimes reflective of psychosocial disturbances. Such observations inevitably lead to the question of which came first: the psychopathology, or the harsh, odd, or ambiguous behaviors of others in the social environment?

A third area of attention in the interpersonal paradigm is the architecture of current and past interpersonal relationships with significant others. In some sense, the first and second focal points—the ill person's interpersonal behaviors and other people's interpersonal reactions—are midlevel or even microscopic interpersonal appraisals. The practice of focusing on the relational landscape is a slightly more global perspective. Here the examination focuses on how caring, supportive, abusive, coercive, or neglectful past and present relationships with significant others were and are. There is almost always trouble to be found in the terrain of interpersonal relationships with people who are or will become psychologically distressed. There is clear support for the notion that these troubled relationships somehow contribute to the development and course of the psychopathology.

In Chapters 2–9, research findings on the interpersonal and social aspects of various mental health problems are examined. Although conceptually and empirically distinct, these disorders have a common correlate: disturbed and dysfunctional relationships with other people. Perhaps as a function of their inherently social nature, the well-being of most humans is inextricably entwined with the well-being of their interpersonal relations. When interpersonal relationships sour, when the ability (and/or motivation) to communicate and interact with others fails to develop or deteriorates, and when behavioral reactions from other people become stressful, mental health begins to break down.

In the interpersonal paradigm, a number of motifs cut across the literatures associated with multiple psychological problems. The chapters on particular psychological problems are organized around these motifs. The recurrence of these various themes indicates that interpersonal well-being is interwoven in a most fundamental way with mental health.

As described earlier, one of the focal points of interpersonal research has been on current and past relationships with significant others. This research focus has produced two consistent patterns of results that are absolutely endemic in the psychopathology literature. First, *family-of-origin experiences* play a powerful role in creating and/or maintaining psychological problems. Looking back at the childhoods of people with psychological problems, one often finds poor family cohesion, neglect, abuse, parental overinvolvement or overprotection, hostility and criticism, and even parental modeling of dysfunctional behavior and attitudes. Most of these family processes have been implicated in multiple psychological problems. For example, parental abuse and neglect appear to be relatively common childhood experiences for people who later go on to develop depression, social anxiety, personality disorders, and substance use disorders. Similarly, excessive family cohesion (either too high or too low) can be found in the families of people with social anxiety, eating disorders, and substance use disorders. Obviously, the social environment in which a child develops a sense of self and relations to other people has a immense impact on not just current, but future, psychological well-being. When these family relations decompose into neglect, abuse, overprotectiveness, and excessive hostility and criticism, the probability of a child's developing psychological problems increases dramatically.

A second pattern of findings to emerge from the focus on past and present relationships concerns *family-of-orientation experiences*. Most people eventually leave their families of origin and create their own families of orientation. Unfortunately, some of the problems in a family of origin have a tendency to be recreated in a family of orientation. It is intriguing, for example, that one finds elevated rates of parental neglect, low parental care, and excessive parental criticism in the childhood backgrounds of people with problems such as depression, bipolar disorder, and substance use disorders; yet adults with these same problems exhibit elevated rates of parenting problems with their own children. Sometimes, as in the case of depression, the nature of these parenting problems is reminiscent of those experienced in patients' own childhoods. A further family-of-orientation experience that is prolifically covered in the mental health literature is marital distress. Psychological problems invariably damage the happiness of marriage. Symptoms of these problems are very taxing for spouses—often to such an extent that spouses exhibit psychological problems of their own. At the same time, the deterioration of a marriage can precipitate a number of psychological problems, such as depression, alcoholism, and loneliness. Findings on family-of-orientation experiences again reinforce the notion that psychological problems spill over into immediate family relationships, and appear to be yoked to the quality of these relationships.

A combination of the focus on a psychologically troubled person's relationships with the focus on other people's responses to the person has produced a consistent pattern of results on *general personal relationships*. Although family relationships, past and present, occupy considerable importance for most people, we sometimes overlook the fact that other relationships can be particularly consequential for many people. For those who have already left their homes but have not yet formed their own families, these other relationships are perhaps the most immediately important in their lives. Often these friendships and dating/romantic relationships are quite simply lacking for people afflicted with depression, social anxiety, personality disorders, and eating disorders. One interpersonal phenomenon that may inhibit the development of such relationships is rejection. Numerous studies show that people with psychological problems such as schizophrenia, eating disorders, depression, and social anxiety incite rejection from others. Even when personal relationships are available to an individual with a psychological problem, they are often characterized by turbulence and conflict. Findings on general personal relationships bring badly needed attention beyond past and present family issues for people who are experiencing psychological distress. This evidence shows that the power of these relationships to disrupt and be disrupted by psychological problems must not be underestimated.

Finally, the focus on the social behavior of the afflicted individual has produced a distinct pattern of results on *interpersonal communication*. The most fundamental building blocks of personal relationships, verbal and nonverbal communication behaviors, are seriously altered by psychological distress. In the case of problems such as depression, social anxiety, schizophrenia, bipolar disorder, eating disorders, and substance use disorders, these communication problems are often studied under the rubric of "social skills deficits." Social skills involve the ability to communicate with other people in ways that are appropriate and effective. They involve the knowledge of what behaviors are appropriate, the capability to exhibit these behaviors, and the motivation to mobilize and apply that knowledge and behavioral repertoire. People with psychological problems often exhibit concurrent deficits in social skills. In some cases, these social skills deficits may be causally involved in the development of the disorder; in other cases, they may be secondary to the problem. In some instances, certain trait-like tendencies to engage in particular forms of communication behavior have been linked to various psychological problems. For example, people with depression often engage in excessive reassurance seeking from others. People with personality disorders use interpersonal communication to get attention from others. On the other hand, people with somatoform disorders often shun direct communication with others; rather, they express their symptoms as an "indirect" form of communication. In all of these cases, researchers have documented strong associations between psychological problems and breakdowns in fundamental interpersonal communication behaviors.

Results in the domains of family-of-origin experiences, family-of-orientation experiences, general personal relationships, and interpersonal communication are as compelling as they are clear. People with psychological problems frequently have histories of troubled interpersonal relationships. Often these interpersonal troubles predate the onset of the disorder; in other cases, they seem to follow symptoms of the disorder. One obvious reason why these relationships are troubled has to do with interpersonal communication problems, which covary rather strongly with psychological problems. It is extremely difficult to establish and maintain healthy interpersonal relationships without possessing at least minimal social skills. Yet it is an unfortunate reality that many people who are afflicted with psychological problems do not have the interpersonal savvy to build rewarding relationships and marshal social support from others. For these reasons, it is impossible to fully understand the origins, course, and consequences of psychological problems without careful consideration of the interpersonal context in which they are deeply embedded.

2

Depression

DEFINITION AND SYMPTOMS

Major depressive disorder is a pervasive illness with a lifetime risk of 10–25% for women and 5–12% for men (American Psychiatric Association, 2000; Kessler et al., 1994). Among certain segments of society, such as socially disadvantaged women, lifetime prevalence can be as high as 33% (Boyce et al., 1998). Results of the Epidemiologic Catchment Area study indicate that in any given year approximately 5% of the population, or 8 million people, will be afflicted with major depression (Regier et al., 1993). The disorder is associated with a dangerously high mortality rate, as 4–6% of its victims die by suicide (Inskip, Harris, & Barraclough, 1998; Simon & Von Korff, 1998). According to the text revision of the *Diagnostic and Statistical Manual of Mental Disorders*, fourth edition (DSM-IV-TR), major depressive episodes are marked by the following symptoms: severely depressed mood, diminished interest in any activities, significant weight loss or gain, sleep disturbance, psychomotor agitation or retardation, fatigue, feelings of worthlessness and guilt, difficulty concentrating, and recurrent thoughts of death or suicidal ideation (American Psychiatric Association, 2000). For a formal diagnosis, these symptoms must be evident for a period of at least 2 weeks, but for many people with depression they may last months or even years.

Joiner, Coyne, and Blalock (1999) have recently stated that "regardless of what other factors may be involved, the interpersonal context affects greatly whether a person becomes depressed, the person's subjective experience while depressed, and the behavioral manifestations and resolution of the disorder. Consideration of the interpersonal context is simply a necessity for an adequate account of the disorder" (p. 3). In fact, the interpersonal context of depression has drawn a great deal of empirical attention from researchers since the mid-1970s. It was at this time that two prominent theories of depression were developed, each having very strong interpersonal components: Lewinsohn's (1974, 1975) behavioral theory of depression, and Coyne's (1976a, 1976b) interactional theory of depression. These theories and their attendant research collectively explain how a depressed person's interpersonal behaviors, and the pursuant reactions of other people to those behaviors, can lead to and perpetuate symptoms of depression.

PREVIEW

Interpersonal problems in both the past and present are abundantly evident in the lives of people with depression. In the domain of *interpersonal communication*, research shows that people with depression often exhibit problems with social skills. These problems are evident in a number of microcommunication behaviors, as well as in more global evaluations of depressed people's communication behavior. One particular type of interpersonal communication problem that is pervasive in depression is excessive reassurance seeking. At the intersection of the interpersonal communication domain and the domain of *general personal relationships*, people with depression tend to elicit interpersonal rejection, perhaps because of emotional contagion (i.e., they make other people feel sad, depressed, and hostile). The general personal relationships of people with depression are often lacking or distressed, contributing to a high comorbidity with loneliness. The *family-of-origin experiences* of people with depression are marked by relatively high rates of neglect, abuse, low parental care, and even signs of rejection from parents. The *family-of-orientation experiences* associated with depression are characterized by very high rates of marital distress and parenting problems. Again, there is remarkable comorbidity between depression and loneliness.

INTERPERSONAL COMMUNICATION IN DEPRESSION: SOCIAL SKILLS DEFICITS

An early interpersonally oriented approach to depression appeared in the form of Lewinsohn's (1974, 1975) behavioral theory of depression. A key component of this theory was the concept of *social skills*. Lewinsohn stressed that depressed people often exhibit disrupted social skills, which make it difficult for them to obtain positive reinforcement from their relationships with other people. At the same time, their poor social skills make it difficult to avoid negative outcomes in social relationships. The inability to produce positive, and avoid negative, social outcomes is thought to precipitate episodes of depression. A considerable body of literature generally supports the notion that depressed people have social skills problems that can create relational difficulties (for reviews, see McCann & LaLonde, 1993; Segrin, 1990, 2000; and Segrin & Abramson, 1994). Particularly impressive is the fact that differences between depressed and nondepressed persons in social skills are apparent across a wide range of operationalizations of the social skills construct.

Self-Descriptions of Social Skills

One of the most common and straightforward ways of measuring social skills is through self-report inventories. These have the advantage of assessing feelings and tendencies over a wide range of often unobservable social behaviors and situations. People with depression consistently evaluate their own social skills on such inventories more negatively than nondepressed people do (e.g., Cole, Lazarick, & Howard, 1987; Lewinsohn, Mischel, Chaplin, & Barton, 1980; Segrin & Dillard, 1993; Vanger, 1987; Youngren & Lewinsohn, 1980). This pattern appears when both state (e.g., Dow & Craighead, 1987; Edison & Adams, 1992) and trait (e.g., Gotlib, 1982) operationalizations of social skills are employed, and it is evident among both adults (Meyer & Hokanson, 1985) and children (Garland & Fitzgerald, 1998).

Students of depression are unlikely to be surprised by the finding that depressed people evaluate their social skills negatively. Depressed people evaluate themselves negatively on a number of different variables, not just their social skills. Some studies revealed differences between depressed and nondepressed persons in self-reports, but not behavioral indicators of social skills (e.g., Dow & Craighead, 1987; Ducharme & Bachelor, 1993; Segrin & Dillard, 1993). Consequently, it has been suggested that depressed people's negative views of their social skills may be part of a more generalized negative self-evaluation bias (cf. Gotlib, 1983; Grabow & Burkhart, 1986). A key assumption of Beck's cognitive theory of depression, for example, is that depressed people hold negative views of themselves and distort feedback from the environment in ways that are unfavorable to themselves (Beck, Rush, Shaw, & Emery, 1979). Although self-ratings of social skills are undoubtedly contaminated by this bias, depressed people's general tendency to evaluate themselves negatively does not fully account for the self-reported social skills deficits often noted to be associated with the disorder (Dykman, Horowitz, Abramson, & Usher, 1991). Dykman et al. (1991) convincingly demonstrated that depressed people's negative evaluations of their social skills are an amalgamation of negative schematic processing biases and actual performance deficits. Furthermore, results from studies of observer ratings and behavioral indicators of social skills are also suggestive of deficits associated with depression.

A related issue to emerge in the literature on depressed people's evaluations of their own social skills concerns their agreement with observers. Although depressed people are often judged by others as having poorer social skills than nondepressed people, the depressed people's judgments are in closer agreement with observers' judgments (Edison & Adams, 1992; Lewinsohn et al., 1980). In the Lewinsohn et al. study, nondepressed people actually overestimated their social skills relative to observers who also made judgments of the subjects' social skills. This pattern is consistent with the *depressive realism* effect (Alloy & Abramson, 1979, 1988). The depressive realism effect is the tendency for depressed people to interpret feedback accurately, in contrast to nondepressed people, who are often unrealistically optimistic in their interpretation of incoming information.

Results from a meta-analysis (a study that analyzes the data from numerous past studies) of the literature on depression and social skills indicated effect sizes of $r = .30-.61^*$ for the differences between depressed and nondepressed people's ratings of their own social skills (Segrin, 1990). Whether the indicator of social skills was self-reports, observer ratings, or social behaviors, depressed subjects scored lower than nondepressed subjects. Using the statistical technique of confirmatory factor analysis, Cole et al. (1987) demonstrated that most studies have traditionally underestimated the strength of this effect, due to imprecise measurement. In fact, "true" depressed–nondepressed differences in self-reported social skills can be as high as $r = .85$.

Partner and Observer Ratings of Social Skills

When observers or conversational partners are asked to evaluate depressed people's social skills, they often give them lower ratings than they give nondepressed controls (Dalley, Bolocofsky, & Karlin, 1994; Edison & Adams, 1992; Lewinsohn et al., 1980; McNamara & Hackett, 1986; Segrin, 1992). However, interpretation of these findings must be tempered by some notable instances where observers' ratings did not discriminate between the two groups (e.g., Ducharme & Bachelor, 1993; Gotlib & Meltzer, 1987; Haley, 1985). When summed across multiple studies, the effect for depressed–nondepressed differences in partner or observer ratings of their social skills is $r = .22$ (Segrin, 1990)—consider-

---

$^*r$ is used in Hunterian meta-analysis for effect size.

ably weaker than that associated with self-reports, but still suggestive of a perceived deficit in social skills.

Behavioral Indicators of Social Skills

One useful method for measuring social skills involves behavioral assessment, in which researchers examine the social and communication behaviors of depressed and nondepressed people as they interact with others. This line of research further illustrates some of the interpersonal behavioral problems associated with depression.

Paralinguistic Behaviors

Paralinguistic behaviors involve the noncontent portions of human speech, such as rate, volume, pitch, and pause duration. People use and vary these behaviors to give their discourse interest and liveliness. Numerous studies indicate that people with depression do not use paralinguistic behaviors with the same degree of "skill" as nondepressed people. Studies of the temporal aspects of paralanguage indicate that people who are depressed speak more slowly (Pope, Blass, Siegman, & Raher, 1970; Siegman, 1987; Weintraub & Aronson, 1967; Youngren & Lewinsohn, 1980), speak less (Breznitz & Sherman, 1987; Edison & Adams, 1992; Ellgring, Wagner, & Clark, 1980; Fossi, Faravelli, & Paoli, 1984; Hale, Jansen, Bouhuys, Jenner, & van der Hoofdakker, 1997; Hinchliffe, Lancashire, & Roberts, 1971a; Williams, Barlow, & Agras, 1972), exhibit longer pauses (Ellgring & Scherer, 1996), and take longer to respond to the speech behaviors of others (Breznitz & Sherman, 1987; Mandal, Srivastava, & Singh, 1990; Talavera, Saiz-Ruiz, & Garcia-Toro, 1994) than nondepressed people do. In fact, pause duration is so powerfully linked to depression that many have argued for it as an indicator of an individual's degree of depression (Greden & Carroll, 1980; Hardy, Jouvent, & Widlocher, 1984; Hoffman, Gonze, & Mendlewicz, 1985; Szabadi, Bradshaw, & Besson, 1976; Teasdale, Fogarty, & Williams, 1980).

Investigations of speech production indicate that people with depression generally speak more quietly (Darby, Simmons, & Berger, 1984; Gotlib, 1982), and with more silences (Greden, Albala, Smokler, Gardner, & Carroll, 1981; Natale, 1977a; Nilsonne, 1988; Pope et al., 1970; Rutter & Stephenson, 1972; Vanger, Summerfield, Rosen, & Watson, 1992) and hesitancies, than nondepressed persons. When prompted by a topic, people with depression have more difficulty producing speech than nondepressed controls do (Calev, Nigal, & Chazan, 1989).

There is evidence to suggest that people with depression speak in a monotonous tone and with a lower pitch than nondepressed persons do (Darby et al., 1984; Kuny & Stassen, 1993; Nilsonne, 1988; Talavera et al., 1994; see Scherer, 1987, for a review). The voices of depressed people are often perceived by others as sad and/or tense (Tolkmitt, Helfrich, Standke, & Scherer, 1982). In one investigation, there was a greater presence of *spirantization* in voice samples of depressed elderly patients versus nondepressed elderly controls (Flint, Black, Campbell-Taylor, Gailey, & Levinton, 1993). Spirantization is the presence of voice-related noise during what would normally be total closure of the vocal tract.

Studies on subjective perceptions of the voices of depressed speakers show that they are rated as less clear in their communication (Lewinsohn et al., 1980) and more difficult to hear and understand (Dow & Craighead, 1987) than nondepressed speakers. In one particular investigation, depressed subjects were asked to speak about happy, sad, and angry experiences they had had (Levin, Hall, Knight, & Alpert, 1985). The vocal qualities of the depressed persons did not differentiate between happy and angry experiences. Levin et al. (1985) concluded that depressed people communicate only sad affect effectively and appropriately through their voices. Depressed people appear to be very "skilled" at communicating sadness and despair paralinguistically. However, they may be less concerned about cultural display rules that often proscribe the outward display of such emotional states. Alternatively, depressed people may be unable to mask their negative affect paralinguistically, since vocal cues such as pitch, speech rate, and intonation are difficult to control consciously.

Speech Content

Studies of speech content and depression have generally focused on topics and themes that emerge in the discourse of people with depression. A married couple with a depressed partner is more likely than a nondepressed couple to express dysphoric feelings and negative well-being verbally, to talk more about well-being, to ask questions about well-being, and (in the case of the depressed partner) to engage in negative self-evaluation (Hautzinger, Linden, & Hoffman, 1982). Depressed spouses have also reported being more verbally aggressive and less constructive in problem solving—a view corroborated by their nondepressed spouses—when engaged in marital interaction (Kahn, Coyne, & Margolin, 1985; see also Segrin & Fitzpatrick, 1992).

When depressed students were asked to get acquainted with another student, they emitted fewer statements that reflected a positive appraisal of their partner, and made more directly negative statements than their nondepressed peers (Gotlib & Robinson, 1982). Similar findings of negative verbal content among depressed speakers were obtained in studies of interactions with strangers (Coyne, 1976b), unstructured interviews (Hinchliffe, Lancashire, & Roberts, 1971b), 10-minute monologues (Weintraub & Aronson, 1967), telephone conversations with confidants (Belsher & Costello, 1991), and psychotherapy sessions (Weissman & Klerman, 1973). Likewise, Blumberg and Hokanson (1983) demonstrated that depressed individuals communicate self-devaluation, sadness, and general negativity to their interpersonal partners.

It now appears that negative verbal content is especially pronounced in interactions between depressed people and intimate others (Hautzinger et al., 1982; Ruscher & Gotlib, 1988). Segrin and Flora (1998) coded the linguistic behavior of depressed and nondepressed students discussing the "events of the day" with either a friend or a stranger. An interaction between depression and relationship with the partner indicated that the depressed speakers withheld their negativity when talking with a stranger, but were more inclined to introduce negative topics into the conversation (e.g., criticize, disagree, engage in negative self-disclosure) when talking with a friend.

On a related point, negative self-disclosures appear more generally to be a problem area for depressive speech behaviors (Gibbons, 1987; Gurtman, 1987; Jacobson & Anderson, 1982). In one study, people with depression emitted negative statements about the self at a higher rate than their nondepressed counterparts did (Jacobson & Anderson, 1982). In addition, depressed subjects in this study were more inclined to emit unsolicited self-disclosures, and were more likely to self-disclose following a partner self-disclosure, than were the nondepressed subjects. This indicates not only that depressed subjects self-disclose more than their nondepressed counterparts do, but that their timing of these disclosures is often inappropriate and the content is often negative. The timing of disclosures tends to be inappropriate because they are often provided in the absence of any utterance from the partner that solicits such information (e.g., "How have you been?"). This finding is noteworthy, in that self-disclosures have been shown to be a key ingredient in the rejection of depressed persons by others (Gurtman, 1987).

Not only do people with depression exhibit more negative verbal content behaviorally, but they also appear inclined to evaluate such topics of conversation as more appropriate than nondepressed people do. In an examination of depressed people's views of topics for self-disclosure, Kuiper and McCabe (1985) gave depressed and nondepressed respondents items to rate from a self-disclosure scale. A separate panel of judges labeled items as "positive" if they thought that they would feel comfortable or good discussing it with another person, and that a positive social interaction would follow in the pursuit of the topic. Items labeled negative were those that judges thought would make them unhappy and uncomfortable, and would lead to negative social interaction.

As might be expected, the depressed subjects rated the negative topics as more appropriate for discussion than the nondepressed subjects did (see also Breznitz, 1992; Wenzlaff & Beevers, 1998). There were no group differences for the positive topics.

Facial Expression

Human beings use facial expression, both consciously and unconsciously, to send information to others about their emotional states and attitudes. Most available evidence indicates that depressed people are less facially animated than nondepressed people, except when it comes to conveying sadness through the face. This trend is evident in two studies conducted by Schwartz, Fair, Salt, Mandel, and Klerman (1976a, 1976b), in which participants were connected to electromyographic (EMG) electrodes that measured subtle facial activity in the form of electrical discharge produced by muscle movements. In the first investigation, depressed subjects evidenced an attenuated EMG response while trying to imagine happy situations and images, and an exaggerated reaction (relative to controls) while trying to imagine sad situations and feelings. In a second and similar investigation, both depressed subjects and nondepressed controls evidenced similar abilities to self-regulate a happy facial state when requested to do so; however, when no instructions were offered, the controls spontaneously assumed a happy expression, while the depressed subjects showed no evidence of a happy expression (cf. Oliveau & Willmuth, 1979; Schwartz et al., 1978).

In a related investigation, depressed and nondepressed people had their facial expressions recorded while having a hand and arm immersed in ice water (Ganchrow, Steiner, Kleiner, & Edelstein, 1978). Under this physical pain condition, there were no differences between the two groups. However, at rest the depressed group had higher incidences of corrugated brow, squinting or closed eyes, and turned-down mouth, and were more frequently judged as looking "depressed." Correlations between depressed mood and corrugator (brow region) EMG activity have been noted by other investigators (Greden, Genero, Price, Feinberg, & Levine, 1986; Teasdale & Bancroft, 1977), including Jones and Pansa (1979), who found depressed patients less likely to have their brows raised than controls. Other inquiries revealed differences as a function of depression in facial expression of pleasantness and arousal (Youngren & Lewinsohn, 1980), smiles (Ellgring, 1986; Williams et al., 1972), expressions of anger (Berenbaum, 1992), and facial expressions of happiness, sadness, fear, surprise, and interest (less in the depressed group; Fossi et al., 1984).

To determine how well judges could read the nonverbal expressions of depressed people, Prkachin, Craig, Papageorgis, and Reith (1977) videotaped clinically depressed women as they viewed a series of interesting pictures, heard loud sounds, or were presented with nothing. Judges then had to guess from the videotaped record which of the three conditions each stimulus person was in. Depressed people proved to be significantly more difficult to judge accurately than their nondepressed peers.

Generally, depressed people exhibit diminished animation of involuntary facial expression of emotion (Gaebel & Wolwer, 1992). As their emotional state improves, increases in smiles and general facial activity become evident (Ellgring, 1986). Although results clearly converge to suggest a deficit in the encoding of facial expressions, depression shows no such association with performance on decoding tasks. When asked to decode emotional facial expressions, depressed individuals perform similarly to nondepressed persons (Gaebal & Wolwer, 1992; Rubinow & Post, 1992; but see Persad & Polivy, 1993). This finding is consistent with a larger body of literature indicating few impairments in social perception or decoding associated with depression (e.g., Segrin, 1993c).

Despite the generally accurate decoding of facial expression by people with depression, there is evidence to suggest that depressed people with a certain profile of inaccuracy at decoding facial expressions may be particularly at risk. Bouhuys, Geerts, Mersch, and Jenner (1996) presented depressed patients with ambiguous faces to judge. Those patients who perceived less sadness, rejection, and anger in the faces were less likely to improve after 6 weeks. In this study the perception of facial expressions explained 14% of the variance in improvement of symptoms over 6 weeks, and 42% of the variance in improvement over 30 weeks. These authors concluded that those depressed patients who are hyposensitive to negative emotions are at risk for an unfavorable course of depression. They offered two potential explanations for this effect. First, hyposensitivity to negative emotions in others may influence patients' interpersonal behavior in such a way as to promote greater interpersonal rejection. People who are unaware of negative affective states in others may continue to engage in aversive behaviors, such as excessive reassurance seeking. This may serve only to further produce rejection from others, making the reassurance increasingly difficult to obtain, and thereby perpetuating depressive symptoms. Second, hyposensitivity may be a consequence of protracted depression. If depressed people elicit rejection from others over a period of time, some may develop hyposensitivity as a means of preserving social interaction and avoiding social isolation. Thus some depressed people may learn to ignore signs of negative affect in others. These may be the cases of depression that are the most intractable.

Eye Contact

Eye contact, or gaze, is an important indicator of interest and attention in conversation and is an important component of social skill (Cherulnik, Neely, Flanagan, & Zachau, 1978). Numerous interaction analyses indicate that depressed persons engage in less eye contact with others than nondepressed interactants do (Dow & Craighead, 1987; Ellgring et al., 1980; Fossi et al., 1984; Hinchliffe, Lancashire, & Roberts, 1970, 1971b; Jones & Pansa, 1979; Kazdin, Sherick, Esveldt-Dawson, & Rancurello, 1985; Natale, 1977b; Segrin, 1992; Troisi & Moles, 1999; Waxer, 1974; Youngren & Lewinsohn, 1980). Rutter and Stephenson (1972) discovered an interaction between depression and the presence or absence of speech, such that depressed subjects were less likely than controls to be looking while speaking. Because looking while speaking is a behavior associated with confidence and status (Exline, Ellyson, & Long, 1975), it is likely that depressed people's negative feelings about themselves precipitate this gaze avoidance.

The majority of studies that have documented negative associations between depression and eye contact with others have provided subjects with a topic to discuss or instructions for a role-play interaction (e.g., Edison & Adams, 1992; Gotlib, 1982; Shean & Heefner, 1995). These subjects almost always knew that they were being observed and/or videotaped. Differences in eye contact between depressed and nondepressed people are much more pronounced in unstructured situations, with unobtrusive recording and observation, than they are in the more standard laboratory interactions where instructions are given (Segrin, 1992). Consequently, in "real-life" interactions, depressed people may exhibit even less eye contact with others than what is suggested by much of the scientific research. Undoubtedly, this lack of eye contact does not give other people a positive impression.

Posture and Gesture

People's postures and their use of gesture can indicate interest, boredom, agreement, disagreement, and other attitudes and emotional states (Bull, 1987). Some researchers have noted certain patterns or tendencies in gesture and posture that are associated with the experience of depression (Dittmann, 1987; Ekman & Friesen, 1974; Miller, Ranelli, & Levine, 1977). For example, depressed patients have been observed to engage in significantly less gesturing and head nodding than controls do (Fossi et al., 1984; Troisi & Moles, 1999). Similarly, depressed children appear to have a diminished tendency to use *illustrators*, which are gestures that accompany speech (Kazdin et al., 1985). Ekman and Friesen (1972) found that the tendency to use illustrators increased dramatically in depressed individuals as symptoms lifted (see also Ekman & Friesen, 1974).

Depressed subjects engage in more body contact (self-touching, including rubbing and scratching) than nondepressed subjects do (Jones & Pansa, 1979; Ranelli & Miller, 1981). Depressed individuals are also more likely to hold their head in a downward position than nondepressed persons (Waxer, 1974). It appears that the tendency for depressed people to engage in head movements indicative of eagerness (e.g., head nods indicating "yes" and minimal head shakes indicating "no") is much greater when they are interacting with strangers than with close friends (Hale et al., 1997). This finding is reminiscent of those for depressive language use, in which depressed people are inclined to withhold their negativity from strangers.

Most of depressed persons' tendencies in the use of posture and gesture are the same cues that indicate sadness, anxiety, and lack of interest. Since this pattern has been absent in some samples (e.g., Gotlib, 1982; Segrin, 1992; Youngren & Lewinsohn, 1980), tentativeness is warranted until these findings are better replicated.

Summary

A review of the findings on interpersonal behaviors of depressed people suggests a pattern of social withdrawal (Troisi & Moles, 1999). Many of the things that people normally do to indicate interest, attention, and enthusiasm in conversation, such as smiling, making eye contact, speaking in an animated tone, and using gestures, are often lacking in the interpersonal communication of depressed people. The inhibited use of these behaviors, which are often treated as microindicators of social skills, is consistent with the self-reports and observer ratings of depressed people's social skills. The extent to which the inhibited interpersonal behavior of depressed people reflects true skills deficits (i.e., inability to use these skills) or a lack of motivation has yet to be precisely determined. It is clear that people with depression are less motivated to communicate with other people (Segrin, 1992). This may at least partially explain why depression is associated with restricted communication behavior. It is worth noting that some of these behaviors may have actual prognostic value. An intriguing study from the Netherlands indicates that depressed patients' failure to converge or match nonverbal behaviors with those of an interviewer is predictive of a poor prognosis (Geerts, Bouhuys, & Van den Hoofdakker, 1996). Over the course of conversation, people normally begin to match their nonverbal behaviors (e.g., speech rate, eye contact). In the Geerts et al. (1996) study, this phenomenon was not evident among patients who ultimately showed no improvements in their symptoms of depression. Evidence from vastly divergent sources converges to suggest that many people with depression have documentable problems with social skills.

Theoretical Associations between Poor Social Skills and Depression

Elsewhere (Segrin, 2000), I have argued that there is at least some evidence to support three different potential relationships between social skills and depression. First, social skills deficits may be a causal antecedent to depression. This is consistent with the hypothesis outlined in the original version of Lewinsohn's (1974, 1975) behavioral theory of depression. According to this theory, poor social skills make it difficult to secure positive reinforcement through social interaction, and equally difficult to avoid punishing responses in social contexts. People with poor social skills have a difficult time making a good impression on others, and instead often come across as inept, uninterested, and dull. The resultant abundance of punishing social response and absence of positive social reinforcement are thought to contribute to eventual depression.

A series of longitudinal studies conducted by Wierzbicki and his associates provides some evidence for the causal role of social skills deficits in depression (Wierzbicki, 1984; Wierzbicki & McCabe, 1988, study 1 and study 2). In all three studies, social skills at time 1 were found to predict changes in depression over 1- to 2-month intervals, such that lower social skills scores at time 1 predicted a worsening of depressive symptoms. These results are clearly consistent with Lewinsohn's social skills deficits hypothesis of depression. However, other longitudinal investigations using diagnostic interviews for the assessment of depression (Hokanson, Rubert, Welker, Hollander, & Hedeen, 1989; Lewinsohn et al., 1994), multiple indicators of social skills (Segrin, 1996), longer interwave time intervals of 4–12 months (Hokanson et al., 1989; Lewinsohn et al., 1994; Segrin, 1993b, 1996), very large samples (Lewinsohn, Hoberman, & Rosenbaum, 1988; Lewinsohn et al., 1994), and three waves of assessment (Segrin, 1999) have not been able to establish poor social skills as a predictor of subsequent worsening of depression. This suggests that the covariation between poor social skills and depression may be explained by other possible relationships.

A second possibility (Segrin, 2000) is that poor social skills are a consequence of depression—a hypothesis once proposed by Lewinsohn, Hoberman, Teri, and Hautzinger (1985). Many of the symptoms of depression have implications for inhibited production of skilled social behavior. For example, depression is generally accompanied by a number of psychomotor symptoms that entail slowed and delayed motor behaviors (Sobin & Sackeim, 1997; Williams et al., 1972). These psychomotor tendencies include slowed speech, long response latencies, diminished eye contact, and increased nervous gesturing (i.e., *adaptors*, or body-focused gestures). These are the same behaviors that are considered indicative of poor social skills.

To date, several empirical studies have been conducted to examine the hypothesis that depression at one point in time will predict decrements in social skills at a later point in time. In a test of the *scar hypothesis* (i.e., the view that people are permanently changed by an episode of depression), Rohde, Lewinsohn, and Seeley (1990) demonstrated that the self-rated social skills of once-depressed people remained lower than those of never-depressed controls, even 1–2 years after the depressive episode had lifted. A pair of studies reported by Cole and Milstead (1989) provided mixed support for the hypothesis. Their first investigation, with university students, indicated a significant effect for depression's leading to lowered social skills. However, their second study, with third- and sixth-grade students, revealed a weak and nonsignificant effect for depression's leading to a worsening of social skills over time. Here again, not all of the evidence conclusively supports the hypothesis that poor social skills follow depression, but enough evidence exists to suggest that it is a likely explanation for at least some cases.

A third possible relationship linking poor social skills and depression is that poor social skills may be a distal contributory cause, or vulnerability factor, in the development of depression (Segrin, 1996; Segrin & Flora, 2000; Vanger, 1987). Such a relationship could account for some of the mixed findings from past research. In the tradition of diathesis–stress models of psychopathology, Segrin proposed that poor social skills may serve as a diathesis in the development of depression (Segrin, 1996; Segrin & Flora, 2000). It is possible that some people with poor social skills who live alone in an isolated area or work by themselves in a laboratory, for example, may be satisfied with the state of their lives, and may not experience the kinds of stressors and cognitions that may precipitate depression. Only those people who have poor social skills, *and* who experience events and outcomes that they perceive as stressful, are predicted to develop depressive symptoms. It is therefore the combination of poor social skills and negative life events that is thought to produce depressive distress. The reasoning behind this model is that people with good social skills can marshal the kind and quantity of social support that will be effective for coping with stressful events. On the other hand people with poor social skills are expected to (1) experience more stressors (e.g., Segrin, 2001), and (2) be less able to secure assistance and social support for dealing with those stressors when they do occur.

In an empirical test of this vulnerability model for social skills deficits, Segrin and Flora (2000) studied a sample of people undergoing stressful life events: incoming college freshmen who had moved at least 200 miles from their hometowns to come to school. These students were assessed at the very end of their senior year in high school, and once again at the end of their first semester of college. Results indicated that the relationship between stressful life events and depression was strongest among those with the poorest social skills. On the other hand, those with high social skills scores exhibited a relationship near zero between stressful life events and depression. In other words, poor social skills made these students vulnerable to the development of depression when faced with stressors, whereas good social skills produced a prophylactic effect in the face of stressors. Similar results were obtained by Cummins (1990), using a measure of social insecurity that is similar to many commonly used measures of social skills. Collectively, these studies indicate that poor social skills on their own may not always produce strong prospective main effects for predicting depression. Only when poor social skills are combined with stressful life events should one expect prediction of subsequent depressive symptoms.

A diverse collection of research findings shows that people with depression often have concomitant problems with social skills. Three theoretical explanations for this association have been offered: (1) Poor social skills are a causal antecedent to depression, (2) depression leads to a deterioration of social skills, and/or (3) poor social skills create a vulnerability to depression. The evidence associated with these hypotheses is just beginning to emerge, and thus far there is at least some supportive evidence for each. These findings highlight the complexity of the relationship between social skills and depression. There is every reason to believe that the nature of this relationship is not the same for all people with depression.

THE COMMUNICATION–RELATIONSHIPS INTERSECTION: INTERPERSONAL REACTIONS TO DEPRESSION

One of the principal interpersonal problems for people afflicted with depression is *rejection* from other people (e.g., Amstutz & Kaplan, 1987; Gotlib & Beatty, 1985; Gurtman, 1987; Siegel & Alloy, 1990). Much of the research on this phenomenon has been guided by Coyne's interactional perspective on depression (Coyne, 1976a, 1976b). According to this perspective, depressed people are hypothesized to induce a negative mood in their interactional partners through a process of emotional contagion. This hypothesis is predicated on the assumption that it is an irritating, negative experience to interact with a depressed person. Coyne explained that this is because of the depressed person's excessive reassurance-seeking behaviors. Initially others are thought to react to these with supportiveness, but as their irritation with the depressed person grows, they respond with increasingly nongenuine support and reassurance. As a consequence of the negative mood induced through interaction with the depressed person, other people eventually respond with outright rejection and avoidance. Interested readers may wish to consult Coyne (1990), Coyne, Burchill, and Stiles (1990), Coyne, Kahn, and Gotlib (1987), McCann (1990), and Segrin and Dillard (1992) for additional reviews of this literature.

This provocative theoretical statement by Coyne led to numerous empirical investigations of various hypotheses and ideas embedded within his interpersonal conceptualization of depression. Perhaps the chief hypothesis—namely, that depressed people experience a great deal of rejection from others—has been studied and supported conclusively (e.g., Amstutz & Kaplan, 1987; Elliott, MacNair, Herrick, Yoder, & Byrme, 1991; Gurtman, 1987; Segrin & Dillard, 1992), and it holds up across different cultures (Vanger, Summerfield, Rosen, & Watson, 1991) and age groups (Connolly, Geller, Marton, & Kutcher, 1992; Peterson, Mullins, & Ridley-Johnson, 1985; Rudolph, Hammen, & Burge, 1994). The interpersonal rejection of depressed people has thus been characterized as a reliable and robust phenomenon (Segrin & Abramson, 1994).

This interpersonal rejection effect associated with depression appears to be moderated by a number of different variables. For example, depressed males elicit more rejection from others, especially other females, than do depressed females (Hammen & Peters, 1977, 1978; Joiner, 1996; Joiner, Alfano, & Metalsky, 1992). Some evidence also indicates that friends are less rejecting of depressed persons than strangers (Segrin, 1993a; but see Sacco, Milana, & Dunn, 1985); that other people who assume a "helper" role are less rejecting (Marks & Hammen, 1982); and that those who rely on advice giving, and joking with the depressed person, are more rejecting (Notarius & Herrick, 1988). Other findings on moderators of the depression–rejection effect indicate that physically attractive depressed targets elicit less rejection from others (Amstutz & Kaplan, 1987), and that depressed people who are low in self-esteem and seek reassurance from their partners are especially likely to elicit rejection (Joiner et al., 1992).

Depressed people may actually seek and elicit negative reactions from other people. *Self-verification* theory holds that people are motivated to preserve self-views to enhance their sense of prediction and control (Swann, 1990). For depressed persons, self-confirming feedback would take the form of negative appraisals from others, or rejection, since depressed people generally hold negative self-views. Indeed, a sizable body of research indicates that depressed people actually seek and desire negative feedback from other people (Giesler & Swann, 1999). In a sample of child and adolescent psychiatric inpatients, symptoms of depression, but not anxiety, were positively associated with interest in receiving negative feedback from others (Joiner, Katz, & Lew, 1997). Giesler and Swann (1999) note that the quest for self-verification can perpetuate a state of depression: "Eventually, a depressogenic cycle may develop: The receipt of negative feedback will induce increased levels of depressive affect and related symptoms, which in turn will increase self-focus and the salience of negative self-views, thereby perpetuating the cycle" (p. 203). As psychologically damaging as interpersonal rejection may be, this type of feedback may actually be sought after by depressed persons.

Self-verification theory is not the only tenable explanation for depressed people's desire for negative feedback. A related possibility is that people who are depressed and/or have low self-esteem may find security in associating with others who have a less than flattering view of them. Being viewed favorably could create a sense of tension and anxiety in such a person, because others would be expected eventually to discover the person's "true" self, and presumably would be let down. This may create a fear of rejection. On the other hand, being in a relationship with those who view the self negatively may be reassuring, since there is no need to worry about leaving a bad impression and being discovered as undesirable.

Coyne's (1976a) interactional perspective on depression also suggests that depressed people induce a negative mood in others through interpersonal interactions. This has come to be known as the *emotional contagion* hypothesis. Several experiments designed to test this hypothesis have failed to document this negative mood induction effect (e.g., Gotlib & Robinson, 1982; McNiel, Arkowitz, & Pritchard, 1987; but see Coyne, 1976b), although it may become more evident over repeated interactions with a depressed target person (Hokanson & Butler, 1992). A meta-analysis of this literature (Segrin & Dillard, 1992) indicated rather modest support for the emotional contagion hypothesis. However, a more recent meta-analysis that included a number of studies published since Segrin and Dillard's original 1992 meta-analysis provides somewhat stronger support for the hypothesis that depressed people induce a negative mood in others through social interaction (Joiner & Katz, 1999).

Joiner and Katz (1999) have noted some evidence suggesting that depressed people may actually produce symptoms of depression, not just a negative mood state, in other people with whom they have relationships (e.g., roommates, spouses, etc.). Indeed it is common to observe significant associations between dating partners' (Katz, Beach, & Joiner, 1999), roommates' (Joiner, 1994), and spouses' (Segrin & Fitzpatrick, 1992) symptoms of depression. However, as Katz et al. (1999) rightfully note, findings such as these must be interpreted with caution, as they could be the results of *assortative mating* (i.e., depressed people seeking out other depressed people to form a relationship with) or reactions to common stressors. For example, through structural equation modeling with longitudinal data, Westman and Vinokur (1998) showed that the experience of common stressors can explain the relationship between partners' levels of depression better than the direct effect from one partner's depression to the other's can. In terms of assortative mating, there is substantial evidence indicating that people have a preference for mates with psychological distress similar to their own (du Fort, Kovess, & Boivin, 1994; Maes et al., 1998). Studies on depression in particular suggest that depressed people tend to marry other depressed people (Merikangas, 1984). Compelling evidence for this phenomenon came from a study showing not only that depressed people were married to other depressed people, but that the first-order relatives of these depressed spouses also exhibited increased prevalence of mood disorders (Merikangas & Spiker, 1982). This implies that depression ran in the families of these people, and thus it is likely that each spouse brought depression into such a marriage, rather than becoming depressed as a result of marriage to a depressed spouse.

With these important caveats in mind, it should be noted that some scientific evidence shows what appears to be the direct transmission of depression from one person to another. In one of the few studies with a design appropriate for demonstrating a causal relationship between interaction with a depressed person and contagion of depressive symptoms, Joiner (1994) demonstrated that over the course of 3 weeks, roommates of depressed students became more depressed themselves. This study provides tantalizing evidence to suggest that depressed people's ill effects on others may reach far beyond simple negative mood induction, and may perhaps extend to the induction of depression itself.

Another hypothesis contained in Coyne's interactional perspective on depression is that depressed people excessively seek reassurance from others, and that this *reassurance seeking* is irritating to others. A substantial body of data now exists to suggest that reassurance seeking is common in depressed people and can have corrosive relational effects (e.g., Joiner, 1995; Katz & Beach, 1997). The tendency for depressed people to seek reassurance from others may be driven by their increased experience of negative life events and low self-esteem (Joiner, Katz, & Lew, 1999). The consequences of excessive reassurance seeking from others include an increase in the experience of minor stressors, which in turn predicts increases in subsequent depressive symptoms (Potthoff, Holahan, & Joiner, 1995), consistent with Coyne's interactional model. More recently, Joiner and his associates have argued that excessive reassurance seeking is *the* interpersonal linchpin in depression—responsible for both the contagion of depression and interpersonal rejection from others (Joiner, Metalsky, Katz, & Beach, 1999).

A final component of Coyne's (1976a) interactional perspective on depression to receive empirical attention is the key assumption that rejection from others serves to create, maintain, or worsen a state of depression in the recipient of that rejection. It had been demonstrated that depressed people are acutely aware of other people's reactions toward them (Segrin, 1993a), and that negative interpersonal feedback can exacerbate their negative mood state (Segrin & Dillard, 1991). It was subsequently demonstrated that increased depressive symptoms following partner devaluation were particularly pronounced among dating women who had either low self-esteem or tendencies toward excessive reassurance seeking (Katz, Beach, & Joiner, 1998; Nezlek, Kowlaski, Leary, Blevins, & Holgate, 1997). Finally, in an unusually clever study, Lane and DePaulo (1999) showed that depressed people were quite astute at detecting insincere positive feedback from others. Collectively, these studies show that depressed people are most likely aware of the reactions that others exhibit toward them, and that these negative reactions can exacerbate feelings and symptoms of depression.

GENERAL PERSONAL RELATIONSHIPS IN DEPRESSION

The general personal relationships of depressed people are characterized by dissatisfaction (Burns, Sayers, & Moras, 1994), lower influence and intimacy (Nezlek, Imbrie, & Shean, 1994; Patterson & Bettini, 1993), and reduced activity and involvement (Gotlib & Lee, 1989). Some evidence indicates that the *quality* of social interaction with others is more strongly associated with depression than the sheer *quantity* (e.g., Rotenberg & Hamel, 1988). As might be expected, the availability of a confidant with whom one can self-disclose and engage in rewarding conversation is negatively associated with depression. It is the case, however, that many depressed people lack an intimate relationship altogether (Brown & Harris, 1978; Costello, 1982; Mulder, Joyce, Sullivan, & Oakley-Browne, 1996). This finding is particularly important, in that the lack of a close and confiding relationship appears to create a heightened vulnerability to experiencing depression (Brown & Harris, 1978). Research on the personal relationships of depressed persons leads one to question the worth of their relational partners. For example, in Fiske and Peterson's (1991) investigation, depressed participants complained of dissatisfaction and anger with their dating/romantic partners, as well as increased quarreling relative to nondepressed participants. These same respondents reported being hurt or upset by their romantic partners more frequently than did nondepressed controls, despite (or perhaps as a cause of) their greater desire for more love in the relationship. Depressed people also perceive their intimate partners as more hostile than nondepressed persons do (Thompson, Whiffen, & Blain, 1995). One recently studied group of depressed women reported that they received less social support from their confidants than did a group of nondepressed controls (Belsher & Costello, 1991). The confidants of these depressed women exhibited more depressogenic speech (e.g., "I can't do anything right any more," "I'm never going to find a job") than confidants of either nondepressed or psychiatric controls. One might speculate that these friends may actually contribute to the depressed person's aversive psychological experience. Findings such as these are one illustration of how being in dysfunctional, hostile, and unsupportive relationships that are wanting in intimacy may precipitate depression and other undesirable affective states (Coyne & DeLongis, 1986; Coyne, Kessler, et al., 1987).

If it is the case that depressed persons typically find themselves in low-quality interpersonal relationships, it is necessary at least to contemplate the extent to which the relationships may actually be better than the depressed persons make them out to be. Depressed people have a tendency to be overly negative in evaluating their interpersonal relationships (Hokanson, Hummer, & Butler, 1991) and in estimating the frequency with which negative interpersonal events occur (Kuiper & MacDonald, 1983). In addition, depression is associated with perfectionist standards (Hewitt & Flett, 1991a, 1993). Both *self-oriented* perfectionism (excessive motivation to attain perfection) and *socially prescribed* perfectionism (the belief that others expect perfection from the self) are positively correlated with symptoms of depression (Hewitt & Flett, 1991b). Depressed people may therefore hold negative views of personal relationships either because they may fall short of unrealistically high self-oriented perfectionist standards, or because they think that they are failing to meet the perfectionist standards of their relational partners. Undoubtedly, many depressed people are in truly dysfunctional or dissatisfying interpersonal relationships. However, there is reason to suspect that at least some of the variance in these reports of aversive and dissatisfying interpersonal relationships is due to the depressed person's general tendency toward negatively biased assessments of such relationships, and the tendency to hold perfectionist standards.

FAMILY-OF-ORIENTATION EXPERIENCES IN DEPRESSION

Depressed Persons as Spouses

In addition to the experience of disrupted personal relationships, depression is also associated with problems in marital interactions and relationships (for reviews, see Beach, Sandeen, & O'Leary, 1990, and Coyne, Kahn, & Gotlib, 1987). Repeatedly, this research has shown that depression and marital distress go hand in hand (Beach & O'Leary, 1993; Beach et al., 1990; Hinchliffe, Hooper, & Roberts, 1978). For instance, estimates indicate that 50% of all women in distressed marriages are depressed (Beach, Jouriles, & O'Leary, 1985), and 50% of all depressed women are in distressed marriages (Rounsaville, Weissman, Prusoff, & Herceg-Baron, 1979). As depressive symptoms worsen or improve, so too does relationship quality with the spouse (Judd et al., 2000).

The communication between depressed people and their spouses is often negative in tone and tends to generate more negative affect in each spouse than the communication of nondepressed couples does (Gotlib & Whiffen, 1989; Kahn et al., 1985; Ruscher & Gotlib, 1988). This negative affect often takes the form of anger and hostility (Goldman & Haaga, 1995). Biglan and his coworkers suggested that depressed persons and their spouses often find themselves in dysfunctional vicious cycles of interaction (Biglan et al., 1985; Hops et al., 1987). Their findings indicate that depressed persons are often "rewarded" by their spouses for emitting depressive behaviors, in that the depressive behaviors tend to inhibit the spouses' hostile and irritable behaviors (see also Nelson & Beach, 1990). McCabe and Gotlib (1993) showed that over the course of a marital interaction, the verbal behavior of depressed wives becomes increasingly negative. It is therefore not surprising that this study demonstrated that depressed persons and their spouses viewed their marital interactions as more hostile and less friendly than did the nondepressed couples.

In an impressive program of research, Hinchliffe and her colleagues investigated a number of specific marital communication problems experienced by depressed people (e.g., Hinchliffe, Hooper, & Roberts, 1978; Hinchliffe, Hooper, Roberts, & Vaughan, 1978; Hinchliffe, Vaughan, Hooper, & Roberts, 1978; Hooper, Vaughan, Hinchliffe, & Roberts, 1978). These investigations reveal that depressed persons exhibit distorted patterns of responsiveness, such that there is a lack of synchrony between them and their spouses. This is evident through increased self-focus and decreased responsiveness to the nondepressed spouses' states and opinions. In addition, depressed people tend to be most expressive with their spouses when they are discussing issues that are negative in nature. It is interesting to note that in one study, acute depression in one spouse was associated with a tendency to control and influence the other spouse (Hooper et al., 1978). Findings such as these indicate that the marital interactions of depressed persons are not always withdrawn and avoidant; they can take on a hostile and manipulative tone was well.

A recent sequential analysis of depressive marital communication has documented a number of caustic communication processes that unfold over time in such marriages (Johnson & Jacob, 2000). For both husbands and wives, a history of depression is associated with less positive reciprocity in marital interaction. In other words, depressed spouses are less likely to follow their partners' positive communication with positive messages of their own. Johnson and Jacob further discovered that depressed husbands' positive contributions to conversations actually *suppressed* their wives' positivity and *increased* their wives' negativity. That is, when depressed husbands make positive contributions to conversations, their wives respond with negativity. Consistent with the assumptions of systems theory, this pattern illustrates how all members of an interpersonal system may contribute to and maintain a member's depression. Johnson and Jacobs (2000) offer two potential explanations for these differential husband–wife effects. First, it is possible that depressed men may make their positive comments with less conviction than depressed wives do. The men may have a difficult time making positive comments clearly and convincingly. Second, wives may be less responsive to their depressed husbands' efforts to create positivity in the interaction. Wives may get exhausted by their husbands' depression, and after repeated interactions, they may be more guarded in their reactions to the husbands' positivity. If they doubt the positive comments, or are simply overwhelmed and exhausted by their husbands' depression, they may not respond with positive remarks. Johnson and Jacobs (2000) suggest that this may be a long-term relationship pattern for some couples with depressed husbands.

Other investigations of marital interaction find depression to be associated with poor communication during problem-solving interactions (Basco, Prager, Pite, Tamir, & Stephens, 1992), negative self-evaluations and statements of negative well-being (Hautzinger et al., 1982; Linden, Hautzinger, & Hoffman, 1983), verbal aggressiveness (Segrin & Fitzpatrick, 1992), and problems in establishing intimacy (Bullock, Siegel, Weissman, & Paykel, 1972; Basco et al., 1992). Given all of these negative communication behaviors and marital problems, it is easy to understand why depression and martial distress are so powerfully related. Some evidence indicates that these communication problems may be more the results of marital distress than of depression per se (Schmaling & Jacobson, 1990). However, the similarity of these findings to those on depressed persons' other personal relationships points to obvious and pervasive interpersonal problems across a variety of different relational contexts.

In addition to the problems with social skills and negative reactions from others discussed earlier in this chapter, another factor that may link depression with poor marital adjustment is the haste with which young depressed people marry (Gotlib, Lewinsohn, & Seeley, 1998). Results from this extensive longitudinal investigation reveal that depression among adolescents predicts higher rates of marriage among younger women, diminished marital satisfaction, and increased marital disagreements. It is possible that depression may motivate young people to seek out marriage, perhaps indiscriminately, as a solution to problems. Not surprisingly, such marriages are often doomed to failure.

The strong and well-documented association between depression and marital distress has led many to ask, "Which comes first: depression or marital distress?" The answer appears to depend on the sex of the married partner. In a longitudinal study of newlywed couples, wives' depression appeared to follow a decrease in their marital satisfaction, whereas husbands' initial levels of depression led to decreases in their marital satisfaction over time (Fincham, Beach, Harold, & Osborne, 1997). Thus women appear more vulnerable than men to symptoms of depression following declines in marital satisfaction. This patten of findings is consistent with a recent meta-analysis showing that the association between depression and marital distress is stronger for women than it is for men (Whisman, 2001). This suggests that wives' psychological well-being may be more closely tied to the perceived quality of their marriages than husbands' well-being is.

In an even more sophisticated attempt to explore the temporal relationship between depression and marital satisfaction, Karney (2001) assessed the two variables in newlyweds once every 6 months for 4 years. Using sensitive growth curve analyses to take into account individual trajectories in depression and satisfaction, Karney found that trajectories from depression to declines in satisfaction were as strong as trajectories from low satisfaction to increases in depression. Again, these associations were slightly more powerful for wives than for husbands. The findings from both cross-sectional and longitudinal studies generally suggest that depression and marital dysfunction are reciprocal processes that unfold in parallel over time (Davila, 2001).

Spouses of depressed persons experience significant burden, and often experience clinical levels of depression themselves (e.g., Benazon & Coyne, 2000; Coyne, Kessler, et al., 1987). There is reason to believe that spouses' distress may be manifested through expressed emotion (e.g., intrusiveness, negative attitudes toward the illness, low tolerance) that could further perpetuate strained relations with their depressed partners (Benazon, 2000). Living with a depressed person leads to profound family transformations, as spouses and other family members attempt to cope with and understand the symptoms of the disorder (Badger, 1996a, 1996b). A family systems perspective suggests that the effects of depression on spouses are not unidirectional. Rather, spouses may introduce issues of their own into the marriage that agitate or maintain the depression. Coyne, Downey, and Boergers (1992) note that "family systems associated with depression can be characterized by a lack of coherence and agency and a general emotional dysregulation . . . so that negative interactions are not repaired, disagreements are not resolved, negative affect becomes contagious, and there is little chance for negative affect to be transformed into positive affect" (pp. 228, 230). From this perspective, both the depressed individual and his or her spouse are seen as active participants in creating a dysfunctional marriage, each acting on and reacting to the other.

Depressed Persons as Parents

Depressed persons experience as many problems in their parental role as they do in their spousal role. In numerous investigations, depression has been linked to disrupted and dysfunctional parenting behavior (e.g., Hamilton, Jones, & Hammen, 1993; Hammen et al., 1987). Chiariello and Orvaschel (1995) explained that depression interferes with parenting skills by corrupting the parents' capacity to relate to their children. In general, the parenting behavior of depressives is characterized by much the same negativity, hostility, complaining, and poor interpersonal problem solving that are associated with their other relationships. Apparently as a consequence of this disrupted parenting behavior, the children of depressed parents are at a much higher risk for behavioral, cognitive, and emotional dysfunction than are those of nondepressed parents (e.g., Lee & Gotlib, 1991; Whiffen & Gotlib, 1989; for reviews, see Downey & Coyne, 1990; Gelfand & Teti, 1990; and Morrison, 1983). Among the problems experienced by children of depressed mothers is depression itself (Hammen et al., 1987; Warner, Weissman, Fendrich, Wickramaratne, & Moreau, 1992). Although the effects of maternal depression have received much attention in the literature, evidence suggests that paternal depression also has ill effects on children (Forehand & Smith, 1986; Thomas & Forehand, 1991).

Children of depressed mothers typically exhibit a behavioral pattern indicative of rejection. During mother–child interaction, children of depressed mothers express negative affect, are generally tense and irritable, spend less time looking at their mothers, and appear less content than children who interact with their nondepressed mothers (e.g., Cohn, Campbell, Matias, & Hopkins, 1990; Field, 1984).

FAMILY-OF-ORIGIN EXPERIENCES IN DEPRESSION

It is apparent that many depressed people experienced difficulties in their families when they were growing up. People who are depressed typically describe their families of origin as rejecting (Lewinsohn & Rosenbaum, 1987) and uncaring (Gotlib, Mount, Cordy, & Whiffen, 1988; Rodriguez et al., 1996). In a study of psychiatric patients with depression, feelings of being rejected by parents were significantly and linearly associated with symptoms of depression at the time of admission, discharge, and 3 months' follow-up (Richter, Richter, & Eisemann, 1990). Among some individuals with depression, reports of low parental care coupled with overprotection are common (Lizardi et al., 1995; Parker, 1983). Parker (1983) found depressed outpatients to be 3.4 times more likely than matched control subjects to have at least one parent who exhibited low care coupled with high protection, or so called "affectionless control" (see also Gerlsma, Emmelkamp, & Arrindell, 1990). Parker used the tenants of attachment theory to explain these findings, noting that parents who are uncaring tend to create anxious attachment in the child. This predisposes the child to overdependency and insecurity, which culminates in depression when stressed.

Are memories of dysfunctional parenting merely an artifact of being in a state of depression? Gotlib et al. (1988) found for example that both subjects with current depression and those with remitted depression recalled greater parental overprotectiveness than a group of nondepressed subjects. Richter et al. (1990) documented similarly consistent perceptions of parental rejection after symptoms of depression lifted. On the other hand, memories of parental rejection in Lewinsohn and Rosenbaum's (1987) subjects with *remitted* depression were similar to never-depressed controls. Only subjects with current depression in this study recalled rejecting parental behaviors.

A clever study of students with depression and their siblings suggests that perceptions of dysfunctional parenting are not a state-dependent phenomenon (Oliver, Handal, Finn, & Herdy, 1987). In this investigation, students with depression and their nondepressed siblings reported significantly lower family cohesion, expressiveness, and higher conflict than nondepressed student–nondepressed sibling pairs. These collateral data provide compelling evidence of parenting practices that are awry in the family backgrounds of people with depression—a view corroborated by their nondepressed siblings.

In addition to the ill effects of maladaptive parenting, it is also evident that the experience of abuse as a child makes a person likely to experience persistent depression as an adult (Andrews, 1995). As in so many other psychological problems, accounts of physical and sexual abuse and neglect are relatively common in the childhood backgrounds of people with depression (e.g., Lizardi et al., 1995). Childhood maltreatment (i.e., physical abuse, sexual abuse, or neglect) increases the odds of having a depressive disorder by 3.4 to 4.5 times (Brown, Cohen, Johnson, & Smailes, 1999). A recent survey of low-income women revealed a 45.7% rate of depression among those with a history of sexual abuse, compared to 16.4% among those without a history of abuse. In a clinical setting, about half of the children referred for behavioral problems following abuse (physical, sexual, or neglect) exhibited symptoms suggestive of major depression or dysthymia; this is approximately four times the incidence of depression in nonabused children (Stone, 1993). In Stone's (1993) study, the effects of emotional abuse (e.g., repeated name calling, overt rejection, family violence, abandonment of parental responsibilities to relatives outside the home) on depression were stronger than those for physical and sexual abuse.

Considerable attention had been paid to examining the family environments in which children experience abuse. Families in which children are abused, or who permit abuse to occur to their children, often have problems above and beyond the abusive episodes. Could it be the troubled family environment rather than the actual abuse that explains the elevated risk for subsequent depression? Although these family environments surely contribute to depression in their offspring, abuse appears to predict this depression above and beyond the effects attributable to the general atmosphere in the family (Boney-McCoy & Finkelhor, 1996; Zuravin & Fontanella, 1999). Even after controlling for the quality of the parent–child relationship, as assessed from the child's perspective, sexual assault and parental violence were longitudinally predictive of depression in boys and girls followed over a period of 15 months (Boney-McCoy & Finkelhor, 1996). Zuravin and Fontella (1999) found similar effects in a sample of low-income adult mothers, even after controlling for whether the woman lived with her biological mother through age 16, whether her mother was depressed, whether her mother died, history of foster care, availability of social support while growing up, and her history of receiving verbal abuse.

Some interpersonal factors both within and beyond the family of origin may significantly mitigate the deleterious effects of abuse and neglect. On the downside, a child is at greatest risk for depression when experiencing sexual abuse in a family environment that is high in conflict and cohesiveness, and low in control (Yama, Tovey, & Fogas, 1993). Those familiar with the family functioning literature (e.g., Olson, 1993) will immediately recognize this as an extremely volatile and caustic combination of family characteristics, that is almost certain to yield distressed offspring. On a more positive note, the effects of childhood sexual abuse and later depression are substantially minimized when individuals manage to establish and maintain highly intimate relationships as adults (Whiffen, Judd, & Aube, 1999). An intriguing implication of the Whiffen et al. (1999) investigation is that childhood sexual abuse may cause later depression because it sets people up for interpersonal difficulties that interfere with establishing intimacy with others. This is consistent with an attachment theory explanation of the childhood abuse–depression relationship (Downey, Feldman, Khuri, & Friedman, 1994). For those who manage to develop rewarding intimate relationships, despite a history of maltreatment, depression need not be an inevitable consequence of these aversive childhood experiences.

In summary, family-of-origin experiences often portend the psychological distress experienced by people with depression. Parental rejection, overprotectiveness, and emotional unavailability while growing up significantly increase the likelihood of subsequent depression. More caustic behaviors such as physical and sexual abuse, along with neglect, also predispose children to develop depressive disorders that persist into adulthood. Even when such episodes of abuse do not occur in the actual context of the family of origin, there is often something suspect about the qualities of those families whose children incur repeated abuse. In all of the above instances, aversive interpersonal experiences in and around the family of origin appear to set the stage for psychological distress that is often evident many years into the child's future.

COMORBIDITY OF DEPRESSION WITH LONELINESS

Loneliness is a discrepancy between a person's *desired* and *achieved* relationships with other people (Peplau, Russell, & Heim, 1979). Depression and loneliness are two psychosocial problems that are strongly associated. There are a great number of interpersonal, as well as psychological, similarities between the two problems. Problems with social skills are equally evident among depressed persons (Segrin, 2000) and lonely individuals (Jones, Hobbs, & Hockenbury, 1982). Difficulties in establishing and maintaining rewarding and intimate relationships are also very prevalent in loneliness (e.g., Hamid, 1989; Revenson & Johnson, 1984; Vaux, 1988). Both depressed and lonely people often lack structured social support networks (Dill & Anderson, 1999). This may be explained by the fact that lonely people have a difficult time making friends (Medora & Woodward, 1986), communicate poorly with family members (Brage, Meredith, & Woodward, 1993), and experience low social integration (Vaux, 1988).

As in the case of people with depression, there is reason to suspect the family relationships of people who are lonely. Children's loneliness tends to be positively correlated with that of their parents, just as in depression (Henwood & Solano, 1994; Lobdell & Perlman, 1986). What the lonely person appears to long for are meaningful and intimate friendships. Relationships with family members, on the other hand, do little to prevent or ameliorate the experience of loneliness (e.g., Jones & Moore, 1990). In fact, Jones and Moore found that the more social support students had from their family, the *more* lonely they were. Although the increased family social support may have been a result of the students' loneliness, it is clear that these types of relationships do little to help a lonely person's situation. In fact, very close family relationships may set people up for future loneliness (Andersson, Mullins, & Johnson, 1990). Retrospective reports of early childhood experiences indicate that children who had an excessively close, warm, and nurturing relationship with at least one parent were significantly *more* lonely as elderly adults than a group of controls. Andersson et al. (1990) concluded that the effects of overinvolvement from parents can be as noxious as underinvolvement or neglect when it comes to producing lonely children. This is due in part to the fact that parental overinvolvement can create a sense of narcissism in the child. It has also been suggested that extremely close parent–child relationships build great expectations that other relationships chronically fail to meet, and that such relationships may displace the interactions that children would have with peers (Segrin, 1998).

Given the extent of problems with social skills, personal relationships, and family relationships in both depression and loneliness, the exceptionally high rate of comorbidity between these two problems is understandable (e.g., Brage et al., 1993; Rich & Scovel, 1987; Weeks, Michela, Peplau, & Bragg, 1980). Correlations between depression and loneliness typically fall in the $r = .40–.60$ range (Brage et al., 1993; Moore & Schultz, 1983; Rich & Bonner, 1987), with some studies indicating a relationship closer to $r = .70$ (e.g., Moore & Schultz, 1983).

Why is it that these two pervasive problems should coexist with such regularity? Dill and Anderson (1999) argue that in addition to sharing common interpersonal and psychological antecedents, problems such as depression and loneliness are causally related to each other. From an interpersonal standpoint, there are several plausible versions of such relationships. First, people who are depressed often infect others with their negative mood and elicit interpersonal rejection. As this rejection accumulates and personal relationships become scarce, depressed persons would be expected to experience loneliness. If we look at these variables in reverse order, depression may be a more generalized reaction to prolonged loneliness. Momentary or state loneliness may be a painful experience that many can endure without global distress. However, as loneliness persists, people may become emotionally worn down, resulting in a major depressive episode. Human beings are inherently predisposed to find rewards in social relationships. For people who become chronically dissatisfied with the quality of such relationships, depression may be viewed as the inevitable consequence of this extinction of social rewards. Finally, depression and loneliness may each be associated with common interpersonal and psychological variables that contribute to each condition. One such interpersonal variable may by shyness. People who are characteristically shy, and lacking in social support, are particularly vulnerable to developing depression (Joiner, 1997). However, this relationship is partially mediated by the experience of loneliness, which is itself predicted by the interaction of shyness and low social support. Joiner (1997) conceptualized loneliness as a proximal contributor to depression, indicating that its presence is a sign of impending depression.

Presently, there is at least some support for the view of loneliness as a causal factor in depression (Brage & Meredith, 1994; Rich & Scovel, 1987). However, in their structural equation analysis, Weeks et al. (1980) found no such causal relation between the two variables. In this study cross-factor paths for depression and loneliness were ruled out, indicating that neither caused the other. Ultimately, Weeks et al. (1980) concluded that depression and loneliness may share a common causal origin, one of which, as noted, may be shyness (Dill & Anderson, 1999; Joiner, 1997).

Both depression and loneliness have clear links to problems with interpersonal communication and relationships. These include deficits in social skills, and problems with general personal as well as family relationships. Such problems, when sufficiently severe and chronic, surely have the potential to precipitate episodes of either state. However, interpersonal communication problems are certainly not the cause of *all* cases of depression or loneliness.

CONCLUSION

Depression is one of the most common mental health problems. It is clear that many people with depression exhibit deficiencies in their social skills. Inadequate social skills make it difficult to have rewarding interactions and relationships with other people. Depressed people will often rate their own social skills negatively, as do others who observe their interpersonal communication behavior. Many of the verbal and nonverbal behaviors that make communication lively and interesting are not used effectively by depressed people. They often speak in a monotone, exhibit long silences in their speech, fail to make eye contact, have a blank or sad facial expression, speak at a slow rate, and gesture infrequently. People with depression often talk about things with a negative theme, especially with people they know well. These poor social skills may be a cause or consequence of depression, or they may be a predisposing factor that makes people particularly vulnerable to depression when they encounter stress.

People with depression often have a negative impact on others. Depressed people may make others feel sad, angry, or hostile, and they often elicit eventual rejection from other people. This may be due in part to the excessive reassurance seeking that depressed people engage in. There is reason to believe that depressed people are able to detect the rejection that others show toward them, and that this may maintain or worsen their negative psychological state.

The interpersonal relationships of people with depression are generally fraught with problems. Both the dating/romantic relationships and the marriages of depressed people are lacking in intimacy and positivity. Many people with depression also describe problematic relationships with their parents when they were growing up. When depressed people raise children of their own, these children often behave as if they are irritated and agitated by their parent's behavior. Given these troubles with personal relationships, it is perhaps no wonder that depression is highly comorbid with loneliness. Collectively, these findings show that depression has a very powerful relationship with disrupted communication behavior and troubled interpersonal relationships.

3

Social Anxiety

DEFINITION AND SYMPTOMS

The term *social anxiety* refers to "anxiety resulting from the prospect or presence of personal evaluation in real or imagined social situations" (Schlenker & Leary, 1982, p. 642). Anxiety is experienced as an aversive cognitive and affective state accompanied by heightened autonomic arousal that can be extremely debilitating. (However, as discussed later in this chapter, in some cases social anxiety can facilitate behavior and be adaptive). In particularly severe instances, this phenomenon may develop into the clinical syndrome of *social phobia*. According to the DSM-IV-TR people with social phobia have an intense and debilitating fear of social or performance situations in which there will be exposure to unfamiliar others or scrutiny by others (American Psychiatric Association, 2000). To cope with this fear, many people will avoid any social situations in which novelty or scrutiny may be present; this avoidance sometimes culminates in a reclusive lifestyle. The most fear-provoking stimuli include speaking in public, entering a room occupied by others, meeting strangers, eating in public, and writing in public (Faravelli et al., 2000). For those who have social phobia, exposure to such social situations may cause panic attacks. Less severe and/or more circumscribed forms of social anxiety include communication apprehension, public speaking anxiety, and shyness (Jones, Briggs, & Smith, 1986; Leary, 1983a, 1983b; McCroskey, 1982). These concepts overlap considerably with the symptomatology of social phobia (Patterson & Ritts, 1997; Turner, Beidel, & Townsley, 1990). The general concept of *social anxiety* may be manifested as a clinical disorder (e.g., social phobia), as an enduring trait (e.g., shyness), or as a momentary state (e.g., state social anxiety).

Results from the National Comorbidity Survey indicate a lifetime prevalence of 13.3% for social phobia (Kessler et al., 1994). The lifetime prevalence of this disorder is higher in women (15.5%) than in men (11.5%). Social phobia is also more common among those with lower income and less education, as well as among those who are unemployed, unmarried, and/or residing with their parents (Kessler et al., 1994). Inherent in these demographic correlates is a subtext of social dysfunction. Milder versions of social anxiety are far more common than social phobia. Such forms of social anxiety as communication apprehension and heterosocial anxiety are evident in 20–30% of most samples studied (e.g., Arkowitz, Hinton, Perl, & Himadi, 1978; McCroskey, 1977). Social phobia most commonly has its onset during adolescence (Hudson & Rapee, 2000; Lecrubier et al., 2000).

In addition to being especially prevalent in the population, social phobia has a devastating impact on quality of life (Mendlowicz & Stein, 2000). Problems with family relations, educational attainment, employment, marriage and romantic relationships, and friendships are evident in a majority of patients with social phobia (Schneier et al., 1994). As reflected in these domains of psychosocial functioning, this disorder can be exceptionally pervasive, marring numerous aspects of people's social lives. Even those with subthreshold social phobia suffer social consequences similar to those of individuals with diagnosable social phobia (Mendlowicz & Stein, 2000). These findings lend credence to the argument that social phobia is simply a more intense and enduring form of social anxiety (Leary & Kowalski, 1995a).

Social phobia is a rather recent addition to the DSM, not appearing until the publication of DSM-III in 1980. A lack of attention to or awareness of this serious problem led to its characterization as a "neglected anxiety disorder" (Liebowitz, Gorman, Fyer, & Klein, 1985). Recently, some have called for a new name for this problem: *social anxiety disorder* (Liebowitz, Heimberg, Fresco, Travers, & Stein, 2000). These authors assert that *social anxiety disorder* more appropriately connotes the pervasiveness and impairment that is evident among those with the disorder, and also helps to distinguish it from specific phobias (which are often very circumscribed, such as fear of spiders).

Because of its brief history as a recognized psychological disorder, the research literature on social phobia or social anxiety disorder is not as extensive as the literature on such disorders as depression and schizophrenia. However, an understanding of this problem is informed by research on related problems, such as reticence, shyness, communication apprehension, and what many refer to simply as "social anxiety." All of these constructs are associated with apprehensiveness about being judged negatively by others, and a fear that one will not be able to project a desired image. Research on these related constructs essentially examines the behavioral manifestations of social anxiety (Leary, 1983b), and as such contributes to our understanding of this problem.

PREVIEW

In the domain of *interpersonal communication*, people with social anxiety harbor doubts about their ability to make a desired impression on others. Social anxiety is clearly associated with social skills deficits, and socially anxious individuals tend to hold negative expectations about how they will perform in social contexts and how other people will react to them. At the intersection of interpersonal communication and *general personal relationships*, people with social anxiety frequently encounter interpersonal rejection; loneliness and relational distress are other common themes of general personal relationships. Often such relationships are simply lacking. (Indeed, the difficulties experienced by socially anxious people in forming relationships partially accounts for why *family-of-orientation experiences* are not discussed in this chapter, since such people are less likely than others to form stable romantic relationships or marry, and thus to create families of orientation. Another reason is that there simply have not been many research studies on romantic and marital relations among the socially anxious.) Finally, people with social anxiety often have a history of problems associated with *family-of-origin experiences*. Their families of origin often exhibit excessive cohesion and poor adaptability. Socially anxious people frequently have a history of parental abuse, overinvolvement, and parental modeling of maladaptive attitudes and behaviors. Social anxiety is highly comorbid with loneliness and depression.

INTERPERSONAL COMMUNICATION PROBLEMS IN SOCIAL ANXIETY

The Self-Presentational Model of Social Anxiety

One of the best-developed and most widely recognized interpersonal theories of social anxiety has been generated by Mark Leary (Leary & Kowalski, 1995a, 1995b; Schlenker & Leary, 1982) and is built around the concept of self-presentational concerns. Leary argues that social anxiety arises when people are motivated to make a desired impression on others but feel that they may not be successful in doing so. Two components of social anxiety can be distilled from this perspective. First, social anxiety occurs when a person has some *motivation* to leave a desired impression on others. Second, social anxiety involves some *subjective prob-*

ability, reflecting the anxious person's doubt about his or her ability to succeed in making that impression.

Leary argues that some of the components of social anxiety may be functional when one considers the evolutionary basis for the need to belong. The emotional distress that people sense when they feel that they have made undesirable impressions on others can deter them from making such impressions in the first place, make them interrupt what they are doing to make the undesired impression, and/or motivate behaviors to repair the damage caused by their behavior (Leary & Kowalski, 1995a). All of these are functional for humans as social animals who depend on others for their livelihood and survival. Unfortunately, for some people this emotional distress becomes crippling; it has the effect of drastically reducing their social contacts and/or producing exactly the kind of disastrous social behavior that worries them.

Self-presentational concerns are at the heart of all socially oriented anxiety problems (e.g., social anxiety disorder, communication apprehension, shyness, public speaking anxiety, reticence). Therefore, Leary's self-presentational theory contributes to an understanding of all these problems. In the context of an interpersonal paradigm, one must ask these questions: "What leads people to feel that they will not be able to make a desired impression on others? And what are the interpersonal consequences of such feelings?" As in all psychosocial problems, the answers to these questions are multiple; they involve problematic experiences in the family of origin, poor social skills, maladaptive reactions and interpretations of social encounters, rejection from others, and loneliness.

Social Anxiety and Social Skills Deficits

People with social anxiety tend to exhibit deficiencies in social skills. As in the case of depression, a model of social skills deficits has emerged as one of the theoretical paradigms in the explanation of social anxiety and social phobia (Liebowitz et al., 1985; Schlenker & Leary, 1985; Segrin, 1996). According to this perspective, people with poor social skills are expected to experience negative outcomes from their interpersonal encounters. Over time this causes these people to dread social interactions and anticipate negative responses from others. Of course, this anticipation may create a self-fulfilling prophecy. Furthermore, the avoidance of social interaction that often follows social anxiety may lead to an atrophying of social skills, which can only further worsen the circumstances. Thus far, research evidence is generally supportive of the hypothesis that social anxiety is linked to poor social skills, although the causal ordering of these variables has yet to be definitively established.

Global Evaluations of Social Skills

On general measures of social skills, people with social anxiety rate their own social skills more negatively than their nonanxious counterparts do (e.g., Beidel, Turner, & Dancu, 1985; Segrin & Kinney, 1995; Smari, Bjarnadottir, & Bragadottir, 1998; Spence, Donovan, & Brechman-Toussaint, 1999; Twentyman & McFall, 1975). People who know and/ or observe the social behavior of socially anxious people also rate them low in social skills (Beidel et al., 1985; Spence et al., 1999). Even parents rate their socially anxious children's social skills more poorly than the parents of nonanxious children rate their offspring's skills (Chansky & Kendall, 1997). Although socially anxious individuals may exhibit problems with social skills, they tend to perceive these problems more negatively than others do (Rapee & Lim, 1992; Segrin & Kinney, 1995; but see Hope, Sigler, Penn, & Meier, 1998), suggesting that they may be unduly negative in their self-evaluations (Curran, Wallander, & Fischetti, 1980).

Nonverbal Communication Skills

Although a precise behavioral profile of social anxiety has yet to be developed, it is evident that this problem interferes with the skilled use of many nonverbal behaviors. For example, people with social anxiety gaze less, particularly while talking (Beidel et al., 1985; Farabee, Holcom, Ramsey, & Cole, 1993), and talk less (Daly, 1978; Fydrich, Chambless, Perry, Buergener, & Beazley, 1998; Spence et al., 1999) than people who are socially secure. Gaze and talk duration are clear behavioral markers of social skill (Conger & Farrell, 1981). In addition, social anxiety has been associated with poor vocal tone (Fydrich et al., 1998). What is particularly noteworthy about the Fydrich study is that it included both nonanxious and anxious control groups; the investigators found that the nonverbal skills deficits (e.g., gaze, vocal tone, speech duration) were most pronounced among those with *social* anxiety, and were not attributable to anxiety more generally. Socially anxious individuals also interact with others at a greater distance (Patterson, 1977).

One function of nonverbal skill that appears to be particularly disrupted among socially anxious individuals is conversational turn taking (Cappella, 1985a). People use nonverbal behaviors to manage and negotiate conversation. Adherence to the tacit rules of turn taking produces smooth and efficient conversation. The effective use of certain nonverbal behaviors that are critical to the turn-taking function, such as gesture and pausing, appear to be impaired by the increased cognitive load of socially anxious persons in conversational settings. Research evidence from studies of planning, discussion of unfamiliar topics, and responding to difficult questions indicates that increased cognitive load can interfere with the effective use of nonverbal turn-taking behaviors (Cappella, 1985b). This same phenomenon may also be responsible for disrupting the timing, not just the duration, of nonverbal behaviors that serve the turn-taking function (Fischetti, Curran, & Wessberg, 1977). People often think of interruption as a breakdown of turn taking. At the same time, interruptions are a definite sign of enthusiasm and involvement in a conversation. It is therefore understandable that socially anxious people are less likely than socially secure individuals to interrupt their conversational partners (Natale, Entin, & Jaffe, 1979).

Another nonverbal skill that is impaired by social anxiety is deception. Although this may not be the most prosocial nonverbal function, it is generally considered to require considerable skill in the management of nonverbal behaviors (DePaulo & Friedman, 1998). In one study, socially anxious people were less successful than socially secure individuals at deceiving others (Riggio, Tucker, & Throckmorton, 1988). Socially anxious subjects in this study exhibited a deceptive nonverbal demeanor that made them appear to be dishonest, regardless of whether or not they really were.

A recent meta-analysis identified various themes or functions of the nonverbal behaviors of people with social anxiety (Patterson & Ritts, 1997). Some behaviors, such as speech dysfluencies and self-manipulative gestures, are characteristic of *increased arousal* and are very prevalent among socially anxious individuals. Diminished verbal output, and inhibited initiation of conversation are behaviors that signify *diminished behavioral involvement*, which is also characteristic of socially anxious persons. Each of these nonverbal profiles is consistent with poor or problematic social skills.

Verbal Communication Skills

Social skills deficits associated with social anxiety may also extend into the domain of verbal behaviors. In a unique study of social anxiety and verbal behavior, Leary, Knight, and Johnson (1987) demonstrated that socially anxious people tend to make more "safe" utterances such as questions, acknowledgments, and confirmation, and to avoid more "risky" utterances such as those expressing objective information. The functional value of "safe" utterances is that they allow the socially anxious person to be responsive while simultaneously making few bids for the floor during conversation. Consistent with this explanation, social anxiety has also been found to influence people's willingness to self-disclose to others (Snell, 1989). Socially anxious subjects in this study were less likely than nonanxious controls to engage in risky self-disclosures, such as mentioning gender-role-inconsistent information about the self to a same-sex conversational partner.

In the Patterson and Ritt (1997) meta-analysis, social anxiety was found to be positively associated with cautious self-descriptions, expressions of similarity, conformity, and *innocuous sociability,* which is behavior that indicates interest and agreement without getting actively involved in the interaction. This is accomplished though communication behaviors such as asking questions, using back-channel responses (e.g., "uh-huh," "I see," "hmm" while the partner is talking), and not interrupting.

Social Perception Skills

Although behavioral inhibition in social settings may be the hallmark of social anxiety, social perception skills also appear to be negatively associated with social anxiety. This less visible aspect of social skill involves the ability to accurately detect and identify emotional states in other people, the impact one is having on others during conversations, and other people's interest in continued interaction.

When asked to identify interpersonal information from audio–video presentations of dyadic interaction, socially anxious individuals decode more poorly than nonanxious controls (Schroeder, 1995). Socially anxious people perform no better than chance, and considerably worse than control subjects, when asked to detect deceptive communications in videotaped presentations (DePaulo & Tang, 1994). Evidence is also accumulating to indicate that social anxiety influences the interpretation of emotional facial expressions in other people. Socially anxious persons show a negative response bias when judging facial expressions (Winton, Clark, & Edelmann, 1995). Thus they more readily identify negative facial expressions, but are less accurate in identifying neutral facial expressions, with a tendency to characterize them incorrectly as negative. The heightened social vigilance of socially anxious people may make them more accurate at identifying facial expressions of emotion, provided that the situation is nonstressful. However, when they are stressed, their accuracy in identifying facial expressions decreases noticeably (Gard, Gard, Dossett, & Turone, 1982).

The Relationship between Social Anxiety and Social Skills Deficits

Evidence from the domains of nonverbal social behaviors, verbal behaviors, and social perception skills indicates that social skills deficits are evident among people with social anxiety. The evidence is sufficiently pervasive that social skills deficits are now regarded as a potential theoretical explanation for social anxiety (e.g., Schlenker & Leary, 1985; Segrin, 1996). However, this theorizing, and its associated evidence, have yet to determine the precise causal ordering of these two variables.

One plausible account of the relationship between social skills deficits and social anxiety holds that social anxiety may be the result of poor social skills. Accordingly, people with poor social skills are expected to experience negative interpersonal outcomes, and to fail to achieve many positive interpersonal outcomes. Such people may consequently come to fear and avoid interpersonal encounters as a result of such a learning history. Two rare longitudinal studies in this literature provide at least some support for this conceptualization. In one of these studies (Segrin, 1996), university students were followed over a period of 4 months; in the other (Segrin & Flora, 2000), high school students were followed over a 6-month period as they made the transition to college life. In each case, social skills at time one were predictive of residual changes in social anxiety (i.e., time 2 social anxiety with time 1 social anxiety partialed out), such that those with poor social skills at time 1 evidenced increases in social anxiety over the course of the study. These findings demonstrate that poor social skills can in fact lead to a worsening of social anxiety.

The self-presentational model of social anxiety (Schlenker & Leary, 1982) provides an explanation for why poor social skills may lead to social anxiety. People who are aware of their less than adequate social skills may reasonably expect that they will not be able to leave a desired impression on others. This expectation may then create a sense of anxiety in social situations. Unfortunately, the social anxiety that results from this negative expectation is likely to create a self-fulfilling prophecy.

An alternative explanation of the relationship between social skills deficits and social anxiety suggests that social skills deficits may be pursuant to symptoms of social anxiety. According to such a hypothesis, some people may become socially anxious, perhaps due to a traumatic event, and consequently avoid social encounters in an effort to cope with and manage their anxiety. As a result, their social skills are assumed to atrophy from disuse. Although this hypothesis has considerable face validity, it has yet to be extensively investigated and is a prime candidate for immediate research attention.

It should go without saying that it may not be appropriate to pit these two hypothesized causal paths against each other. In all likelihood, there are multiple avenues to both poor social skills and social anxiety. For some poor social skills may be a cause of social anxiety, while for others they may be a consequence.

It is also important to note that the relationship between the "skilled" use of communication behaviors and social anxiety is neither perfect nor straightforward. A number of studies have found no differences between socially anxious and nonanxious subjects in various communication behaviors such as eye contact (e.g., Cappella, 1985a), use of questions and assertions (e.g., Segrin & Kinney, 1995), or performance on a simulated job interview (Strahan & Conger, 1998). Some socially anxious people may do a good job of masking their anxiety, and may develop and exhibit adequate social skills. Similarly, some people with poor social skills may be so socially oblivious and nonchalant that they have no social fears. Finally, some socially anxious people may have social skills that are quite functional from their own point of view. Socially anxious people appear to be very "skilled" at avoiding intense involvement in conversation, listening to others, being socially facilitative, and being attentive (Leary & Kowalski, 1995a).

Negative Expectations and Interpretations

One of the more robust patterns of social cognition associated with social anxiety is the expectation that social encounters will go badly and that others will respond negatively (Leary, Kowalski, & Campbell, 1988; Greenberg, Pyszczynski, & Stine, 1985; Patterson, Churchill, & Powell, 1991; Schlenker & Leary, 1985; Wallace & Alden, 1991). Even children with anxiety disorder expect negative outcomes to result from interaction with other children (Chansky & Kendall, 1997). The particularly harsh self-evaluations of social skills (see above) and expectations of rejection from others are consistent with the self-presentational model of social anxiety, particularly the doubt that one will be able to achieve a desired impression (Leary & Atherton, 1986).

The imagined and expected negative social responses from others that are characteristic of socially anxious individuals appear to be fairly automatic, robust, and not easily challenged. For example, a group of socially anxious female college students who told stories about themselves to partners felt more strongly that their partners perceived them as dishonest and insincere than nonanxious controls felt about their partners (DePaulo, Epstein, & LeMay, 1990). When patients with social phobia were asked to interpret ambiguous social events (e.g., "You are in class and are asked to read a passage out loud. When you finish, you see that two people are staring at you"), they tended to choose negative interpretations, such as "They think you messed up the passage" (Amin, Foa, & Coles, 1998; Stopa & Clark, 2000). However, persons with social phobia did not exhibit this negative interpretation bias for nonsocial scenarios (Amin et al., 1998). When presented with objectively negative social scenarios, such as "You've been talking with someone for a while and it becomes clear that they're not interested in what you're saying," people with social anxiety disorder interpreted these with *catastrophizations*—that is, interpretations such as "I was stupid, boring, incompetent," and "I will lose all my friends, be rejected, lose my job" (Stopa & Clark, 2000).

Even in a study where social interactions had objectively positive outcomes, people with social anxiety disorder overestimated the visibility of their anxiety and underestimated the interest they conveyed to their partner and their overall likability (Alden & Wallace, 1995). However, the socially anxious subjects in this study exhibited a *positive* evaluation bias for their conversational partners, indicating that such negative evaluations and expectations may be specific to the self. Lake and Arkin (1985) found that socially anxious people doubt the authenticity of positive feedback from others. When socially anxious individuals experience objectively positive social outcomes such as enthusiastic and friendly responses from a partner, their expectations for future interaction become even *more* pessimistic (Wallace & Alden, 1995, 1997). This is because they feel that their partners will raise their standards and expect even more in future interactions—an expectation that socially anxious persons "know" they will be unable to meet.

Social anxiety may be associated with expectations for failure, in part, because of heightened self-focused attention. In interpersonal contexts, socially anxious persons will pay less attention to the environment and more attention to themselves and their performance (Daly, Vangelisti, & Lawrence, 1989). Although findings are mixed as to whether this self-focused attention impairs actual performance (e.g., Daly et al., 1989; Woody, 1996), it is likely to taint cognitions. Self-focused attention implies that socially anxious people focus on the somatic and affective anxiety reactions that they experience in social situations, as opposed to focusing on the task at hand, the environment, and the partner. For example, when preparing to give a speech or public presentation, a person with social anxiety may notice such sensations and feelings as rapid heartbeat, sweating, nausea, and rising terror. Socially anxious people use perceptions of their bodily sensations to make more global inferences about their appearance (Mansell & Clark, 1999). This tendency to make negative inferences from signs of autonomic arousal is known as *anxiety sensitivity*, and is a risk factor for developing anxiety (Schmidt, Lerew, & Jackson, 1999; Schmidt, Lerew, & Joiner, 1998). So the conclusion of the hypothetical public speaker with self-focused attention would be "I must look terrible to them." It then becomes a "logical" conclusion that "I will do badly."

Social anxiety is associated with the tendency to expect social failure and negative reactions from other people. For socially anxious individuals, neutral social stimuli are interpreted negatively; negative social outcomes result in catastrophization; and, most interestingly, positive social outcomes prompt even more pessimistic appraisals for future success. Social success appears to have little positive impact on socially anxious persons' self-efficacy expectations. Their negative expectations for social interaction may be fed in part by heightened self-focused attention in social contexts. It is certainly possible that the negative expectations for interpersonal interactions that are characteristic of socially anxious individuals serve also to create a self-fulfilling prophecy. Findings on interpersonal rejection show that, unfortunately, these negative expectations are not baseless.

THE COMMUNICATION–RELATIONSHIPS INTERSECTION: INTERPERSONAL REJECTION IN SOCIAL ANXIETY

As noted in Chapter 2, one of the principal interpersonal theories of depression emphasizes the role of interpersonal rejection in maintaining the disorder (Coyne, 1976a, 1976b). This interpersonal phenomenon is evidently not specific to depression, as people with social anxiety disorder are also likely to experience interpersonal rejection. Of course, it is possible that in at least some cases, the relationship between anxiety and rejection is secondary to the relationship between depression and rejection. Notwithstanding this possibility, the anxiety–rejection relationship appears robust. Evidence for this rejection effect comes from a variety of populations and interpersonal contexts. For example, a group of socially anxious male high school students who interacted with female confederates received less desirable ratings as potential dates by those confederates (Johnson & Glass, 1989). Friends and family members of socially anxious people view them as less likable and more difficult to talk to, in comparison to their nonanxious peers (Jones & Carpenter, 1986). Socially anxious high school students in one study indicated that they received less support and less acceptance from their classmates (La Greca & Lopez, 1998). However, there was no relationship in this study between social anxiety and support from parents or teachers, indicating that this rejection effect is most evident from peers.

Younger children with social anxiety also experience interpersonal rejection. For example, Spence et al. (1999) observed 7- to 14-year-olds interacting with peers, and observed the quality (positive, negative, or neutral) of peer responses to interaction with the target child. Children with social anxiety disorder received fewer positive responses from their peers during the observed interactions than nonanxious children did.

Another sample of children aged 6–11 with social anxiety disorder indicated that they did not feel socially accepted and that they had more negative interactions with peers (e.g., being teased, made fun of, having enemies) than nonanxious controls did. Children with anxiety disorders tend to be disliked by their peers (Strauss, Lahey, Frick, Frame, & Hynd (1988). In a study of over 1,000 children aged 6–11, Walters and Inderbitzen (1998) classified students as "cooperative," "friendly–dominant," "hostile–dominant," or "submissive," based on peer nominations. As might be expected, social anxiety was highest among the submissive group. When students were asked who they "liked most," those in the submissive group (i.e., socially anxious) ranked last out of the four, and were tied for first with the hostile–dominant group for peers' ratings of whom they "liked least." Evidence from family studies, to be reviewed below, shows that even parents may act rejecting toward children with social phobia (Parker, 1977).

Children and adults with social anxiety disorder are typically nonthreatening, and, if anything, more likely than nonanxious individuals to try to appease others. Why then should they be the recipients of interpersonal rejection? Papsdorf and Alden (1998) hypothesize that this effect is due to perceived dissimilarity. In their study participants engaged in a conversation with a confederate, who, along with peer observers, rated the similarity of the target person to the confederate and indicated their acceptance or rejection of the target. The relationship between the target's social anxiety and interpersonal rejection from others was mediated by perception of the target's similarity (see also Heimberg, Acerra, & Holstein, 1985). Papsdorf and Alden (1998) concluded that "we reject socially anxious individuals because we perceive them as different than ourselves and that we use how uncomfortable they appear and any unwillingness on their part to reciprocate our confidence as information about exactly how different they are" (p. 365).

Interpersonal rejection plays a crucial, and perhaps etiological, role in social anxiety disorder. Spence et al. (1999) explain that children with poor social skills are likely to experience interpersonal rejection (see also Lewinsohn, 1974; Segrin, 1992). These rejection experiences lead to pessimistic expectations for social interactions, which in turn generate affective and physiological anxiety responses to social interactions. Anxious children are assumed to avoid such interactions because of these responses, and this avoidance reduces their opportunities for learning and enhancing social skills, thus returning them to the start of the cycle. Spence et al. argue that social phobia can develop if *any* stage of the model is present (i.e., poor social skills, interpersonal rejection, negative expectations, anxiety reactions, avoidance). As such, one could characterize this as a cascade model: Once any stage in the cycle is initiated in force, subsequent stages are inevitable.

GENERAL PERSONAL RELATIONSHIPS IN SOCIAL ANXIETY

The apparent consequences of problematic social skills, expectations for negative social outcomes, and interpersonal rejection are a lack of close relationships and a turbulent interpersonal environment for the socially anxious person. This pattern begins very early in life. Socially anxious children in primary school indicate that they have more negative interactions with peers (e.g., "Is there someone who teases you and makes fun of you?") than nonanxious children do (Ginsburg, La Greca, & Silverman, 1998). Similarly, adolescents who experience social anxiety report less frequent contact and intimacy with friends, compared to their less anxious peers (Vernberg, Abwender, Ewell, & Beery, 1992). A sample of socially anxious high school students who were interviewed about their friendships indicated that they received less support from their classmates, that they had fewer friends, and that their friendships were less intimate than those of nonanxious classmates (La Greca & Lopez, 1998).

The pattern of troubled personal relationships that begins in childhood continues into adulthood. Adolescents and young adults (aged 14–24 years) with social anxiety disorder exhibit impairment in social and leisure activities, in addition to problems with household and work relations (Wittchen, Stein, & Kessler, 1999). University students with social anxiety report fewer interactions with members of the opposite sex, and greater dissatisfaction with their performance in those interactions, than their nonanxious counterparts do (Dodge, Heimberg, Nyman, & O'Brian, 1987). When college students were asked to keep a diary of their social interactions, those who were classified as high in social anxiety rated the quality of these interactions (e.g., "difficult," "guarded," "many communication breakdowns," "a great deal of misunderstanding") more negatively than students who were low in social anxiety did (Vittengl & Holt, 1998). Another sample of college students with social anxiety indicated that they engaged in sexual activity less frequently than students low in anxiety, and that when they did they rated it as less enjoyable (Leary & Dobbins, 1983). Socially anxious college students evaluate themselves as generally nonassertive and socially avoidant (Alden & Phillips, 1990).

As they continue into early and middle adulthood, people with social phobia report a great deal of difficulty establishing and maintaining romantic relationships, and perhaps as a result are less likely to marry than their nonanxious counterparts (Hart, Turk, Heimberg, & Liebowitz, 1999; Turner, Beidel, Dancu, & Keys, 1986). Among those who do not marry, social dysfunction is particularly evident (Hart et al., 1999).

An unfortunate reality of social anxiety and social phobia is a lack of satisfying interpersonal relationships and interactions. The relationships that are available are often judged, at least by the socially anxious person, to be of low quality and intimacy. Like problems with social skills, these relationship problems may maintain, if not worsen, feelings of anxiety. At the same time, social anxiety itself (especially when it reaches the point of social phobia) undoubtedly has the potential to spoil opportunities for relationship development.

FAMILY-OF-ORIGIN EXPERIENCES IN SOCIAL ANXIETY

Evidence is accumulating to suggest that certain experiences in the family of origin may predispose people to develop social anxiety disorder. Hudson and Rapee (2000) have argued that the family's contribution to the development of social phobia can be organized into two distinct areas of influence: (1) child-rearing styles, and (2) parental modeling of social concerns combined with restricted exposure to social situations.

The family environment in which a child is reared can have a substantial impact on the child's concurrent and future mental health. The rates of highly rigid (low-adaptability) and enmeshed (high-cohesion) family structures in families of children with social anxiety are double those of families in the general population (Craddock, 1983). Adults with social phobia tend to recall their parents as less caring and less affectionate, but at the same time as overprotective (Bruch & Heimberg, 1994; Hudson & Rapee, 2000; Masia & Morris, 1998; Parker, 1977; but see Caster, Inderbitzen, & Hope, 1999). This noxious combination of parental behaviors is associated with a host of other psychological problems for offspring. Hudson and Rapee (2000) suggest that parental overprotection can send a message to the child that the world is a harmful and dangerous place from which the child needs protection, since the child is incapable of taking care of him- or herself.

As with other psychological disorders, an increased incidence of childhood trauma and abuse is evident among those with social anxiety disorder. Stein et al. (1996) found childhood physical abuse rates to be higher in both males and females with anxiety disorders, and childhood sexual abuse rates to be higher particularly in women with anxiety disorders. In a related study of patients with anxiety disorders (panic disorder, agoraphobia, and/or social phobia), childhood trauma was evident in 63% of the cases, as compared to 35% of controls (David, Giron, & Mellman, 1995). However, histories of sexual and/or physical abuse were found to be most specific to those patients with social phobia. Magee (1999) analyzed a representative sample drawn from the National Comorbidity Survey to explore the relationship between life experiences and various phobias. The results of this study showed that sexual assault by a relative, and exposure to verbal aggressiveness between parents, had *unique* effects on social phobia onset in women (as opposed to specific phobia or agoraphobia). The occurrence of childhood (i.e., before age 18) sexual abuse makes the development of social anxiety disorder two to four times more likely (Dinwiddie et al., 2000; Saunders, Villeponteaux, Lipovsky, Kilpatrick, & Veronen, 1992). Sexual and physical abuse, particularly when perpetrated by a relative, conveys an interpersonal message of (1) devaluation ("I am worthless") and (2) uncertainty ("I cannot trust anyone"). When people carry these psychological burdens into their future social relations, they are undoubtedly fearful of further rejection and devaluation, and suspicious of how they will be treated by others. These are key symptoms of social anxiety.

A second family-of-origin process that may contribute to social anxiety disorder involves parental modeling of social concerns. As Bandura (1999) noted, "Virtually all behavioral, cognitive, and affective learning from direct experience can be achieved vicariously by observing people's actions and the consequences for them" (p. 170). The family is a near-ideal context for modeling and social learning. Parents of children with social phobia are often excessively concerned with the opinions of others (Bruch & Heimberg, 1994). In a study of over 2,700 adolescents, Caster et al. (1999) had middle school students complete self-report instruments describing their family environments. Students who were classified as high in social anxiety described their mothers and fathers as being more concerned about the opinions of others, and more ashamed of their sons' or daughters' shyness. This study is noteworthy in that the participants were currently residing with their parents and were still in the process of being actively reared by them. Many, if not most, of the studies on family-of-origin environment and social anxiety disorder are retrospective in nature and obviously susceptible to recall bias.

Related to the modeling of parental concerns is the restricted exposure to social situations. Hudson and Rapee (2000) indicate that "if the child has limited exposure to social situations, then the child rarely has the opportunity to learn that social situations are not harmful" (p. 115). Indeed, individuals with social anxiety disorder often indicate that they were isolated by their parents when growing up, and that their mothers tended to avoid social situations that were anxiety-provoking (Bruch & Heimberg, 1994; Hudson & Rapee, 2000). The socially anxious middle school students in Caster et al.'s (1999) study also indicated that their parents were less socially active than parents of nonanxious students. Collectively, these findings reveal that people with social anxiety disorder may not have had sufficient opportunities for varied social interaction while in their families of origin. This social isolation corrupts opportunities for developing a sense of confidence and mastery in social situations.

Experiences in the family of origin can be instrumental in the development of social anxiety disorder. Specifically, emotionally distant but overinvolved and controlling parenting, physical and sexual abuse, modeling of parental social anxiety, and social isolation have all been identified at elevated rates in the histories of individuals with social anxiety disorder. Although there is some evidence to suggest an inherited genetic predisposition to anxiousness, this predisposition is not specific to social phobia (Hudson & Rapee, 2000). These authors conclude that "social phobia may in fact run in families in a relatively specific fashion. Thus if there is not a specific genetic predisposition responsible for this finding, it would seem that family environment is instrumental in this transmission" (p. 123).

COMORBIDITIES IN SOCIAL ANXIETY

Comorbidity with Loneliness

There is a notoriously strong association between social anxiety and loneliness (e.g., Moore & Schultz, 1983; Segrin, 1993b; Segrin & Kinney, 1995; Solano & Koester, 1989). Loneliness is associated with many of the same features as social anxiety—namely, a lack of optimism about interpersonal encounters, low sociability, avoidance of others, and poor social skills (Ernst & Cacioppo, 1999; Jones, Rose, & Russell, 1990). Like socially anxious or depressed individuals, lonely people devalue communication with others and view their own communication skills negatively (Spitzberg & Canary, 1985). A survey study by Riggio, Throckmorton, and DePaola (1990) showed that social anxiety was positively correlated with loneliness, and that each of these problems was negatively associated with various aspects of social skills. Another large-sample survey study showed that apprehension about public speaking and apprehension about dyadic interaction were both positively associated with loneliness (Zakahi & Duran, 1985).

Most explanations of the relationship between social anxiety and loneliness argue that loneliness is a consequence or result of social anxiety (Gambrill, 1996; Jones et al., 1990; Segrin & Allspach, 1999). Socially anxious persons tend to approach social interactions with discomfort and nervousness. As a consequence, other people tend to respond unfavorably to these awkward and reserved interactions. The disrupted and unpleasant interactions, with their attendant negative responses from others, have the obvious effect of leaving socially anxious persons longing for more satisfying and intimate personal relationships. In more extreme cases, such as full-blown social phobia, avoidance of social contact may serve as a temporarily effective means of managing and coping with the anxiety. However, this coping mechanism comes a high price. Eventually, all but the most inherently antisocial individuals, anxious or not, become painfully lonely as a result of prolonged avoidance of social contact.

Jones et al. (1990) describe four mechanisms that can cause socially anxious persons to become lonely. First, the reticent interaction style of socially anxious people may be misinterpreted as aloof or snobbish. This is thought to prompt others to avoid the anxious persons, therefore producing feelings of loneliness. Second, some people have a desire for sociability despite feeling socially anxious. Jones et al. (1990) note that sociability and shyness are distinct concepts (see also Cheek & Buss, 1981). Although it may sound paradoxical, many socially anxious people would actually like to socialize with others. The problem is that they feel such encounters will go badly, and they will in some ways be worse off than if they just avoid the encounters altogether. Therefore, among those socially anxious people with a desire for social contact, loneliness is expected to be prevalent. Third, many stressful events (e.g., moving away from home for the first time, loss of a spouse through death or divorce) present many interpersonal challenges and create feelings of uncertainty. Such events are inherently threatening and anxiety-provoking. Coping with them often requires a great deal of social skill. Of course, the people least equipped with these skills, such as socially anxious individuals, have the greatest cause for anxiety. In such cases, loneliness becomes a likely outcome. Finally, Jones et al. (1990) note that socially anxious people have a pessimistic style of social cognition that is likely to cause loneliness—namely, blaming themselves for social failures and seeing personal flaws as fairly stable, unchangeable traits. For example, if a man goes out on a date with a woman and it goes badly, if he interprets this as a result of the fact that "I'm just no good with women," it stands to reason that he should experience anxiety over such encounters in the future. The interpretation of the past failure suggests that the same outcome is inevitable in similar future encounters.

Comorbidity with Depression

There is a notoriously strong relationship between social anxiety and depression. Among those seeking clinical attention, the comorbidity between social anxiety disorder and depression is between 40% and 50%

(Ballenger et al., 1998; Faravelli et al., 2000). It is believed that social anxiety creates a predisposition to developing other psychological problems, and that it precedes the development of depression in most cases (Ballenger et al., 1998).

It is impossible to overlook the striking similarity in the interpersonal foundations of social anxiety and depression. Each is associated with poor social skills, interpersonal rejection, loneliness, and problematic experiences in the family of origin. If depression is often secondary to social anxiety, one must wonder whether the interpersonal phenomena that have been linked to social anxiety are mostly the results of comorbid depression.

Leary and Kowalski (1995a) describe three possible connections between social anxiety and depression that are worthy of consideration. First, they suggest that depression may be the result of repeated self-presentational failures. Feelings of chronic failure in social situations may produce a sense of learned helplessness that culminates in depression. This account places social anxiety (self-presentational concerns) before depression in the causal chain of events. A second possibility is that depression may predispose people to experience social anxiety. Leary and Kowalski (1995a) argue that this is due to the negative effect of depression on effectiveness in social encounters. This possibility is useful for explaining the social skills deficits that have been documented in both depression and social anxiety. Third, depression and social anxiety may each be caused by a common third variable: social exclusion. When people are excluded and isolated, they may come to simultaneously doubt their social abilities (social anxiety) and question their self-worth (depression). This proposition is a useful explanation for the interpersonal rejection that is concomitant to both depression and social anxiety.

One of the challenges for future research on interpersonal aspects of social anxiety will involve the identification of interpersonal phenomena that are caused by social anxiety, by depression, or by both problems. In most of the existing research on social anxiety, there is not often an assessment of comorbid depression, much less an attempt to control or account for its influences on interpersonal behavior. However, such a research strategy would be useful for refining our knowledge about the interpersonal aspects of both depression and social anxiety.

CONCLUSION

Social phobia or social anxiety disorder is the most prevalent of the anxiety disorders. Social anxiety exists in subclinical forms as well, and both the clinical and subclinical forms can have massive impact on the quality of people's interpersonal lives. One of the principal interpersonal theories of social anxiety predicts that it will arise when people are motivated to make a desired impression on others, but are doubtful of their ability to do so. A fundamental question then becomes this: "What causes people to doubt their ability to leave a desired impression on others?"

Research evidence shows that the roots of this self-doubt reach back as far as early childhood. Experiences in the family of origin, such as having overprotective and overcontrolling parents who are simultaneously emotionally distant, can lead to social anxiety in those raised in such families. When a child is abused by a family member, social anxiety disorder is a very likely outcome. Parents may also model excessive concern with the opinions of others and isolate their children from varied opportunities for social interaction.

Doubt about one's ability to leave a desired impression on others may also be charged by problematic social skills. Many people with social anxiety, in both clinical and subclinical forms, have problems with social skills. Although these skills deficits are to some extent overinflated in the minds of the socially anxious, evidence from observer evaluations, the use of nonverbal behaviors, and social perception skills shows that such deficits also exist in reality. If those with social anxiety are aware of (even if not mentally exaggerating) their social skills deficits, it stands to reason that they doubt their ability to impress others.

Social anxiety is marked by a pervasive tendency to expect negative outcomes from social interactions. The self-presentational model literally takes this as part of the definition of social anxiety. Sadly, these expectations are often met in social circumstances: Socially anxious individuals are often the recipients of interpersonal rejection, which can take a wide variety of forms. Problems with social skills, expectations for rejection, and actual experiences of rejection appear to culminate in low-quality, nonintimate, and generally lacking personal relationships for the person suffering from social anxiety disorder.

Finally, social anxiety often coexists with loneliness and depression. These three are something of a "holy trinity" in psychosocial problems. They share many phenomenological features, such as doubts and questions about self-worth, and have many common interpersonal correlates, such as social skills deficits and interpersonal rejection.

4

Schizophrenia

DEFINITION AND SYMPTOMS

Schizophrenia is a formal thought disorder (actually a family of disorders) characterized by symptoms such as bizarre delusions, hallucinations, disorganized speech, grossly disorganized or catatonic behavior, inability to initiate and persist in goal-directed activity, affective flattening, and impoverished and disorganized thinking evident in speech and language behavior (American Psychiatric Association, 2000). These symptoms are grouped into two classes: *positive* (an excess or distortion of normal functions) and *negative* (loss of normal functions). Such symptoms must be present for at least a month, but in some cases may persist for years. An important diagnostic criterion of schizophrenia is social/occupational dysfunction. Consequently, it is virtually true by definition that people afflicted with schizophrenia experience problems in their interpersonal relationships.

Unlike many other mental disorders considered in this book, schizophrenia is a relatively rare disorder. The lifetime prevalence of schizophrenia is estimated at approximately 1% (Kessler et al., 1994). Although it is rare, Zuckerman (1999) has recently characterized schizophrenia as probably the "most terrible" mental disorder. Relapse rates in schizophrenia are alarmingly high, and, as this chapter shows, are undoubtedly influenced by interpersonal interactions.

PREVIEW

Schizophrenia was perhaps the first psychological problem to receive intense research attention and theorizing from an interpersonal perspective. The results produced by this inquiry are a testimony to the significance of the interpersonal paradigm in mental health. Research in the domain of *family-of-origin experiences* came in two waves. In the early family-of-origin approaches, researchers identified family dynamics such as double-bind communication, mystification, and family schism. These variables are no longer considered prominent in the disorder. Contemporary family-of-origin approaches to schizophrenia have identified such abrasive phenomena as expressed emotion, communication deviance, and negative affective style in family interactions. In the area of *general personal relationships*, it is clear that people with schizophrenia experience interpersonal rejection and conflict, and have impoverished social networks. The interpersonal rejection these people encounter is linked with their difficulties in the *interpersonal communication* domain: They exhibit severe deficits in social skills, involving both the encoding and decoding of social information. (Given the magnitude of their problems in all three of the other domains, it is not surprising that patients with schizophrenia are very unlikely to form stable romantic relationships or marry; for this reason, *family-of-orientation experiences* are not considered in this chapter.) There is a high degree of comorbidity between schizophrenia and other psychosocial problems, such as depression, anxiety, and substance use disorders.

THE FOCUS ON INTERPERSONAL COMMUNICATION AND RELATIONSHIPS

The Norwegian psychologist Rolv Blakar argued almost 20 years ago that disturbed communication is at the core of schizophrenia, and he lamented the fact that such processes were not getting adequate attention in the research literature:

> Schizophrenia, like most other forms of deviant behavior and psychopathology, is manifested in interaction. The first discovery of a particular person's condition of schizophrenia is made through *interaction*. . . . Given that a common strategy in science, as well as in problem solving in general, for understanding a phenomenon or process such as schizophrenia is to take basic or core observations such as these as a point of departure, we would expect that (1) communication theory would have been the first perspective to be systematically exploited in research on schizophrenia; (2) communication theory would currently constitute a central or even predominant perspective in research on schizophrenia; and (3) communication theory would serve the function of a superordinate and integrative conceptual framework within which all pieces of relevant knowledge concerning schizophrenia . . . are put together and coherently understood. . . . The relative ignorance of the communication perspective in research on schizophrenia . . . is mainly the result

of two circumstances: First, medicine/psychiatry, which had dominated and still dominates schizophrenia research, has adopted social theories and perspectives only to a small extent, if at all. . . . Second, and even more essential, is the fact that adequate theories of communication have been lacking. (Blakar, 1982, pp. 209–210).

Blakar's observation was as accurate in 1982 as it is today: Interpersonal communication and relationships play a vital role in this most serious mental health problem. However, scientific developments in these arenas were eclipsed by parallel developments in the genetics and psychophysiology of schizophrenia, which figure prominently in the field of medicine/psychiatry. Nevertheless, schizophrenia was one of the first psychological disorders to be associated with intensive theorizing and research on its connection with interpersonal communication and relationships. The majority of such energies were originally directed toward explaining and understanding the role of family-of-origin interactions in the disorder. Although early theories probably overemphasized the role of family relationships in contributing to the disorder, family-of-origin perspectives on schizophrenia remain prominent in the literature today (e.g., Anderson, Reiss, & Hogarty, 1986; Hooley & Hiller, 1997; Miklowitz, Goldstein, & Nuechterlein, 1995). In addition to the family of origin's role, the roles of problematic social skills and impoverished personal relationships have proven to be significant in this disorder. These lines of research are beginning to converge on the type of communication theory (or theories) that Blakar alluded to and wished for.

EARLY FAMILY-OF-ORIGIN APPROACHES TO SCHIZOPHRENIA

In the 1950s and 1960s, a number of family-of-origin approaches to understanding schizophrenia appeared in the literature, sometimes with considerable prominence and acclaim. Virtually all of these approaches have since fallen into relative obscurity, now occupying no more than a footnote in most comprehensive analyses of the disorder. Why then should those seeking an understanding of the interpersonal aspects of schizophrenia take note of these early approaches? First, as noted above, schizophrenia was perhaps the first mental disorder to receive intense theorizing about its interpersonal origins and consequences. As such, the developers of these classic family approaches to schizophrenia were in some ways pioneers in the field of interpersonal relations and mental health more generally. Some of the ideas inherent in their writings and hypotheses would contribute not only to contemporary family-of-origin approaches to schizophrenia, but to the understanding of interpersonal aspects of other mental health problems.

Second, many of these classic approaches to schizophrenia would have an indelible mark on the field of interpersonal communication. The scientific study of interpersonal communication was clearly influenced by works such as *The Pragmatics of Human Communication* (Watzlawick, Bavelas, & Jackson, 1967) and "The Nature and Effects of Social Interaction in Schizophrenia" (Slotkin, 1942). Each of these outlined basic principles of symbolic interaction, language use, and nonverbal communication that are as applicable to healthy communication processes today as they are and were to disordered communication processes at the time they were written. Consider, for example, Slotkin's (1942) statement that "in a process of symbolic interaction . . . A has an idea (referent) which he wants to communicate to B; he therefore employs a culturally determined symbol which stands for the referent in question" (p. 345). Applying this basic principle of interpersonal communication to schizophrenia, Slotkin argued that "in schizophrenia, the individual develops his own symbolism" (p. 346) and "schizophrenics develop their own referents for conventional symbols" (p. 350).

Third, an analysis of the early family-of-origin approaches has additional heuristic value in highlighting the limits of clinical observation relative to large(r)-sample scientific studies. With the respect that is due to these early pioneers and with the benefit of hindsight, it can be said that many of the observations, theories, and hypotheses from the early family approaches were premature. Most were derived solely through clinical observations and employed "methods" from a field (interpersonal communication) that had not yet emerged in its own right.

Double-Bind Communication

One of the initial lines of investigation into family relationships and schizophrenia was headed by Gregory Bateson and his colleagues at the Palo Alto, California, Veterans Administration Hospital (e.g., Bateson, Jackson, Haley, & Weakland, 1956; Watzlawick et al., 1967). Out of this work emerged the well-known *double-bind* hypothesis. According to this position, communication has multiple levels of meaning; these include not only a literal content, but a metamessage at a higher level that provides information about the interpretation of the message content and/or relationship between the sender and receiver. Interactions in a family affected by a member's schizophrenia were hypothesized to contain paradoxical and contradictory communications, in which either the content of verbal messages is contradicted by the metamessages communicated nonverbally, or there is an inherent contradiction in the verbal channel (an example given by Mishler & Waxler, 1965, is "I order you to disobey me"). Such communication corrupts choice, because any potential response can be expected to produce punishing reactions from the sender, provided that the receiver cannot escape the relationship or comment on the absurdity of such messages.

Growing up in families prone to double-bind communication was thought to make logical communication impossible. Thus the illogical and severely disturbed communication of a patient with schizophrenia was presumed to be the net result of prolonged exposure to these dysfunctional family interactions. Schizophrenic communication prevents others from understanding the self, and thus avoids potentially aversive responses from senders (often parents) of double-bind communication.

This approach was originally developed deductively, and later "tested" through observations of family therapy sessions. It was based on the controversial assumption that all behavior is communication and that there is no such thing as nonbehavior (i.e., a person cannot *not* communicate). Although there were some attempts to validate the double-bind hypothesis empirically (Berger, 1965), researchers abandoned such efforts rather quickly. In a paper entitled "Double Bind Is Not A Theory of Schizophrenia," Martin Beck (1983) remarked that "no one has conclusively validated or refuted the double bind hypothesis" (p. 253). Beck also argued that it is a "widespread misconception" that the authors of the double-bind hypothesis were even proposing an etiology of schizophrenia. He concluded that the value of the concept lies in its focus on the interaction history of the family system and how it associates with the social environment.

Mystification

Another early family process concept to appear in the literature was *mystification* (Laing, 1965). Mystified communication involves ambiguities, misunderstandings, and misidentification of issues and topics. Mystification is evident in a process whereby a person responds to the other in terms of his or her own needs, but at the same time behaves as if he or she is really responding to the needs of the other. For example, an aging mother may respond to her son's nutritional needs by giving him a lot of calcium-rich foods, when in fact it is the mother who is in need of additional calcium in her diet. Such parent–child interactions were thought to have teleological significance in the development of dysfunctionally symbolic relationships that ultimately produce symptoms of the disorder.

R. D. Laing (1971) postulated that during the first years of a child's life, the members of a family develop an internalized system for interacting and relating to each other. He observed that a person who is labeled as "schizophrenic" is caught in a maze of confusion, misunderstanding, and contradictions. Laing went so far as to suggest that these mystifications reach back several generations in the family. Consequently, current family mystification may be induced by prior generations and/or a response to such family histories. It should be noted that these conclusions were based on an intensive study of few families of young patients with schizophrenia.

Laing's existential thesis was that schizophrenia is a logical reaction to an illogical family environment. He felt that our contemporary view of reality has prevented us from finding meaning and understanding in the symptoms of the disorder. He was determined to explicate this meaning in a series of influential books (e.g., Laing, 1959, 1967, 1971; Laing & Esterson, 1964). However, Laing's ideas themselves became increasingly mystified. He suggested that people with schizophrenia are on a journey back to the void, detaching themselves from reality in order to preserve their essential being, with the ultimate goal of breaking through to a higher consciousness or enlightenment. The idea of a journey back to the past became prominent in his works as he emphasized concepts such as "prebirth trauma." Laing even suggested that he had experienced prenatal intrauterine trauma, and advocated "rebirthing" therapy, complete with dance and rhythmic drumming as a treatment for such ailments (Burston, 1996). Tragically, in April 2000 in the state of Colorado, a 10-year-old girl was smothered to death during a rebirthing therapy session (Lowe, 2000). Like that of his contemporary Timothy Leary, Laing's career would ultimately languish into a condition far removed from his original innovative ideas. However, echoes of these ideas are still evident in more recent work on family communication deviance.

Family Schism and Skew

According to Lidz (1958), "the critical characteristic of schizophrenia lies in the aberrant symbolic processes—in the distortion of perception, meaning, and logic" (p. 22). He asserted that the family is the dominant force that shapes these distortions in perception and meaning. These were thought to result from blurred boundaries (i.e., parents' behaving inappropriately for both their sex and age). These family processes, Lidz argued, take the form of *schism* and *skew* (Lidz, Cornelison, Fleck, & Terry, 1957).

The schismatic pattern of family interaction entails open and hostile conflict. Schismatic parents continually attempt to undermine each other's standing in the eyes of the child. In this sense, their interactions typically could be characterized as battles for the loyalty of the child. In these families communication primarily serves the function of coercion and defiance. Family schism was believed to be most common in the families of female patients with schizophrenia (Fleck, Lidz, & Cornelison, 1963). In such a family, the daughter is caught in a bind whereby satisfying either parent is accompanied by the threat of rejection from the other. Lidz and his associates highlighted the ineffectiveness, insecurity, and paranoia between the parents as the forces driving this family process.

A skewed pattern of family interaction involves an extremely over-intrusive mother who is apparently impervious to the needs of other family members. Fathers in such families are unable to control or counterbalance the deviant parenting of the mothers. These fathers tend to be passive and often are themselves disturbed by addictions, psychosis, or other psychosocial problems. Children in such families are forced into accepting a bizarre world view that is skewed toward that of an overintrusive parent whose mental health can, itself, be questioned. In such a family, one parent supports the psychopathological distortions of the other out of dependency or masochistic needs. In contrast to schismatic families, conflict is masked in skewed families, creating an unreal atmosphere in which what is said differs dramatically from what is actually felt (Lidz et al., 1957). These families were believed to be most common among male patients with schizophrenia, and mothers were seen as often behaving in overly intrusive and at times seductive ways (Fleck et al., 1963).

Like many of the other early family-of-origin approaches, the schismatic and skewed family processes described by Lidz were based on the study of a very few hospitalized patients with schizophrenia and their families. He observed that in each family type at least one parent had significant psychopathology of his or her own. Although examples of schism and skew can be found in families of people with schizophrenia, the utility of these family processes for widespread application to and understanding of the disorder was never fully substantiated.

Pseudomutuality

Like Lidz, Wynne and his colleagues viewed the family as the crucible for the development of confused and ambiguous thought processes reflecting the overall disorganization of some family systems (Wynne, Ryckoff, Day, & Hirsch, 1958). The idea behind their approach was that children must be able to test out their identity and select roles within the family context while growing up. However, some families do not provide an adequate context for establishing healthy identities. Wynne et al. (1958) argued that "The fragmentation of experience, the identity diffusion, the disturbed modes of perception and communication, and certain other characteristics of the acute reactive schizophrenic personality structure are to a significant extent derived, by processes of internalization, from characteristics of the family social organization" (p. 215).

Where there is *mutuality*, two people recognize, appreciate, and accept (to some extent) each other's separate identities. *Nonmutuality* exists when two people minimize interaction and recognize each other only for minimal or circumscribed purposes, without ever developing any closeness. In a family affected by schizophrenia, true differences are masked by *pseudomutuality*, in which there is a preoccupation with harmony and cohesion at the expense of developing members' individual identities, and in the face of obvious differences between family members. In these families, the illusion of harmony is maintained by failing to recognize any deviations from the rigidly defined family role structure, or by reinterpreting such deviations through twisted reasoning in the service of maintaining the pseudomutuality.

The particularly noteworthy aspect of this approach is the focus on family styles of interaction that maintain the pseudomutuality and deny real differences in the family system. According to Wynne, a family affected by schizophrenia handles attention and meaning by communicating in ways that are odd, blurred, fragmented, and poorly integrated (Singer & Wynne, 1965; Wynne & Singer, 1963). In this way everyone can divert and diffuse threats to the harmonious identity of the family by being ambiguous and unclear. However, this style of interaction is presumed to come at the price of the child's healthy self-identity and psychological development. The ideas that Wynne outlined vis-à-vis this bizarre style of family interaction have stood the test of time, although they are no longer considered etiological. They are now studied under the heading of *communication deviance* and are addressed in more detail later in this chapter.

Summary of Early Family-of-Origin Approaches

Hopes for explaining the etiology of schizophrenia with these family process variables were ultimately met with disappointment. McFarlane and Beels (1988) appropriately noted that such concepts as double-bind communication, schism, skew, and pseudomutuality are no longer considered to be causal agents in the disorder. Most of these early family constructs and hypotheses were defined on the basis of small-sample clinical investigations, without matched control groups, random sampling methods, or attention to the reliability of the clinical observations (Mishler & Waxler, 1965; Shean, 1978). Presently, most of these initial interpersonal hypotheses and theories of schizophrenia are considered to be invalid accounts of the disorder's pathogenesis, and are presented here for historical context. However, some of the ideas outlined in these earlier works clearly found their way into the better-developed and tested contemporary family-of-origin variables in the study of schizophrenia.

CONTEMPORARY FAMILY-OF-ORIGIN APPROACHES TO SCHIZOPHRENIA

Contemporary investigations of family relationships and schizophrenia center more on explaining the course than the cause of the disorder. There are, however, some notable instances where researchers have employed family-of-origin variables to predict the onset of schizophrenia. Three family variables that have been, and continue to be, particularly influential in this area are *communication deviance*, *expressed emotion*, and family *affective style*.

Communication Deviance

In one of the classic family approaches to schizophrenia, Wynne and Singer (1963) noted that patients' families often have odd and unfocused styles of interacting with each other, perhaps in the service of sustaining pseudomutuality. Members of these families have difficulty establishing and maintaining a shared focus of attention through their discourse. Out of this original set of studies and hypotheses about family interaction and schizophrenia emerged a very influential line of research on *communication deviance* (CD; Miklowitz, 1994; Wynne, 1981). Wynne (1968, 1981) theorized that people learn to focus their attention and derive meaning from external stimuli through their interactions, particularly with parents, during the early years of life. Odd and deviant styles of communication among the parents were presumed to interact with biological predispositions to contribute to thought and communication disturbances in children who are unable to relate to and understand their parents.

A considerable body of evidence indicates that a family affected by a member's schizophrenia will communicate in odd, idiosyncratic, illogical, and fragmented language, even when that member is not present. Topics of conversation will often drift or abruptly change direction, with a lack of closure. Such interactions are marked by a blurred focus of attention and meaning. This characteristic style of family communication has been labeled CD (Singer, Wynne, & Toohey, 1978).

Traditionally, CD has been assessed from transcripts of parents' responses to projective tests such as the Rorschach or the Thematic Apperception Test (TAT). These responses are generally made in the absence of the child. A coding scheme originally developed by Jones (1977) classifies parents' communication behavior into such categories as *contorted peculiar language* and *misinterpretations*. More recently, Velligan and his colleagues employed an actual family interaction task based on a problem-solving discussion to assess CD (e.g., Miklowitz et al., 1991; Velligan, Funderburg, Giesecke, & Miller, 1995; Velligan et al., 1996). This measure, referred to as *interactional communication deviance* (ICD), classifies parents' discourse into categories such as *idea fragments* (e.g., "But the thing is as I said, there's got . . you can't drive in the alley"), *contradictions or retractions* (e.g., "No, that's right, she does") and *ambiguous references* (e.g., "Kid stuff that's one thing but something else is different too") (Jones, 1977). This measure has produced generally similar results, albeit with perhaps greater ecological validity, as the TAT-based coding system. Complete listings of the categories and their definitions for both the TAT and ICD procedures are provided in Tables 4.1 and 4.2.

Abundant evidence indicates that CD is higher in parents of patients with schizophrenia than it is in parents of either patients without schizophrenia or healthy controls (e.g., Miklowitz, 1994). This work shows that aspects of parental CD distinguish parents of patients with schizophrenia, although CD is evident to some extent in parents of patients with mania as well (Miklowitz et al., 1991). It is particularly intriguing that this distorted form of communication is highly reminiscent of the communication style that typifies the person who actually has schizophrenia. It is therefore unclear whether parental CD reflects a genetic effect that is evident in both parent and child, or a parental behavior that contributes to the child's problem.

An exciting development in CD research involves using the construct to predict the onset of schizophrenia. Research by Goldstein and his colleagues indicates that parental CD often precedes onset and is therefore an excellent predictor of schizophrenia among premorbid adolescents (Goldstein, 1981, 1987; Goldstein & Strachan, 1987). In one such study, parents from families with moderately disturbed teenagers each responded to TAT protocols, from which measures of CD were taken (Goldstein, 1985). Fifteen years later, the lifetime prevalence of schizophrenia in the children was assessed. High CD in the parents was strongly associated with the appearance of schizophrenia-spectrum disorders in some of the family offspring at follow-up. In a similar study, disturbed high-risk adolescents were followed over a period of 5 years (Doane, West, Goldstein, Rodnick, & Jones, 1981). By the end of the study, approximately 10% of those whose parents who were low or in-

TABLE 4.1. Thematic Apperception Test (TAT) Communication Deviance (CD) Scoring System

Factor	Definition	Examples
Contorted, peculiar language	Off-word usage, peculiar phrases; excessive verbiage	"They're trying to *make a goal of their life.*" "This man is *in the process of thinking of the process of being a doctor.*"
Misinterpretations	Gross uncertainty about percepts; attributions of intention in the cards; confusion about stimuli	"Is this a boy or a girl?" "This must be the artist's rendering of societal progression."
Flighty anxiety	Short reaction times; off-task questions and comments	"When do we finish?"
Overpersonalized closure problems	Stories left hanging; overly personalized associations	"This was me as a child."
Faulty overintellectualization	Unusual task set; complicated words used incorrectly	"He wouldn't do that *facetiously.*"
Failure to integrate closure problems	Important perceptual elements ignored; no integration of elements; "I don't know" endings	"These people have nothing to do with each other."

Note. Adapted from Miklowitz, Velligan, Goldstein, Nuechterlein, Gitlin, Ranlett, & Doane (1991). Copyright 1991 by the American Psychological Association. Adapted by permission.

termediate in CD went on to develop schizophrenia, whereas 56% of those whose parents were high in CD developed schizophrenia.

Other research on CD has examined its role in the course of schizophrenia. For example, Velligan et al. (1996) followed a group of patients with schizophrenia and their parents over the course of 1 year. Within the 12-month period of the study, slightly over 50% of the patients had experienced a relapse. Parental CD at the time of the patients' discharge was significantly higher among the parents of those who relapsed versus those who did not. However, in the assessment of parental CD at time 1, there were no differences among parents of those who did versus those who did not relapse. As it turns out, the parents of those patients who relapsed exhibited a dramatic increase in their CD over the course of the study. This investigation indicates that returning to a home with high CD will increase the likelihood of relapse.

TABLE 4.2. Interactional Communication Deviance (ICD) Scoring System

ICD code	Definition	Examples
Idea fragments	Speaker abandons ideas or abruptly ends comments without returning to them	"But the thing is as I said, *there's got . . . you can't drive in the alley.*"
Unintelligible remarks	Comments are incomprehensible in the context of conversation	"Well, that's just *probably a real closing spot.*"
Contradictions or retractions	Speaker contradicts earlier statements or presents mutually inconsistent alternatives	"No, that's right, she does."
Ambiguous references	Speaker uses sentences with no clear object of discussion	"Kid stuff that's one thing but *something else* is different too."
Extraneous remarks	Speaker makes off-task comments	"I wonder how many rooms they have like this?"
Tangential inappropriate responses	Non sequitur replies or speaker does not acknowledge others' statements	Patient: "Sometimes I work on the back yard." Mother: "Let's talk about your schoolwork."
Odd word usage or odd sentence construction	Speaker uses words in odd ways, leaves out words, puts words out of order, uses many unnecessary words	"It gonna be *up and downwards along the process all the while* to go through something like this."

Note. Adapted from Miklowitz, Velligan, Goldstein, Nuechterlein, Gitlin, Ranlett, & Doane (1991). Copyright 1991 by the American Psychological Association. Adapted by permission.

The results of an adoption study conducted in Finland illustrate the power of parental CD to influence schizophrenic outcomes in children. Children who were genetically at risk or predisposed to develop schizophrenia, by virtue of being born to mothers with schizophrenia, were especially likely to develop the disorder when reared by an *adoptive* family that was high in CD. However, among the low-risk adoptees, there was no relationship between CD in the adoptive parents and thought disorders in the children (Wahlberg et al., 1997). These findings suggest that parental CD may be a family stressor that interacts with a preexisting diathesis to influence the development of schizophrenia.

It is reasonable to wonder whether parental CD is a *response* to schizophrenia in a child. Interaction with a person afflicted with schizophrenia may possibly bring about CD. To examine such a possibility, patients with schizophrenia and their biological mothers were followed over a period of 21 to 276 days (Velligan et al., 1995). ICD was assessed from a family problem-solving discussion. Across time, the mothers' level of CD proved to be very stable, as did the patients'. Furthermore, there was no correlation between maternal CD and patient symptomatology at any point in the study. Despite the fact that patients' symptoms generally improved over the course of the study, their mothers' level of CD remained fairly stable, suggesting that parental CD is not a consequence of living in a household with someone who has schizophrenia.

In addition to distorted verbal behavior, parental CD may be accompanied by problematic use of nonverbal behavior (Goldstein, 1984; Lewis, Rodnick, & Goldstein, 1981). Parents who are high in CD also exhibit gaze aversion and rigidity in facial expression while interacting with their children (Lewis et al., 1981). These are powerfully disconfirming behaviors. At the same time, they fit well with the poor focus of attention that is the hallmark of high CD. When a high-CD parent "interacts" with a child, both verbal and nonverbal behaviors suggest that the parent's thoughts and emotions are elsewhere, and that there is some tension between the parent and child. Consequently, the child may be met with fragmented and disconfirming behavior in both the verbal and nonverbal channels when interacting with the high-CD parent.

It appears that parental CD functions as a type of stressor that affects the course and outcome of schizophrenia. When parents' communication is particularly amorphous and peculiar, children may become confused and uncertain about even basic and fundamental social realities. This confusion undoubtedly has functional significance in the course of the schizophrenia, as it is so central in the constellation of symptoms that make up the disorder. It is difficult to read the transcripts and hear the speech of a high-CD parent, and not wonder about the parent's own mental health, aside from that of the child (but see Goldstein, 1987). It is therefore understandable that when patients are discharged into the care of such parents, they offspring remain at risk for future relapse.

Expressed Emotion

Early investigations of family *expressed emotion* (EE; Brown, Monck, Carstairs, & Wing, 1962; Vaughn & Leff, 1976) identified a pattern of criticism, overinvolvement, overprotectiveness, excessive attention, and emotional reactivity that appeared to create a vulnerability to relapse and poor social adjustment among patients with schizophrenia (for reviews, see Hooley, 1985, and Hooley & Hiller, 1997, 1998). EE represents an attitude of criticism and emotional overinvolvement on the part of the parent, which is expressed during an interview with a researcher or clinician. Originally a special interview procedure, known as the Camberwell Family Interview, was employed to assess family EE. The construct is operationalized through the frequency of critical remarks, degree of hostility, and the degree of emotional overinvolvement expressed by a family member during the interview. Generally, parents who express more than six criticisms during the interview are characterized as high in EE.

Vaughn and Leff (1981) described EE as a combination of four behavioral characteristics: intrusiveness; anger and/or acute distress and anxiety; overt blame and criticism of the patient; and an intolerance of the patient's symptoms. One of their early studies (Vaughn & Leff, 1976) revealed that patients who returned to a home with high-EE relatives exhibited a 9-month relapse rate of 51%, whereas only 13% of those who returned to a low-EE family relapsed. Family therapy programs that improve communication and problem solving, thus lowering EE, have been shown to lower relapse rates significantly (e.g., Doane, Goldstein, Miklowitz, & Falloon, 1986).

Rosenfarb, Goldstein, Mintz, and Nuechterlein (1995) examined the functioning of a sample of young, recently discharged patients with schizophrenia who returned to either high-EE or low-EE families. Patients from high-EE families exhibited more odd and disruptive behavior during a family interaction approximately 6 weeks after hospital discharge than did patients from low-EE households. Relatives in the high-EE households were more critical of the patients when they verbalized unusual thoughts than low-EE family members were. Studies such as these clearly paint a picture of a vicious circle in high-EE family relations: These parents respond to a patient with a lot of criticism, because patients from these households appear to exhibit more bizarre and disruptive behavior than patients from low-EE homes. It is likely that the negative reactions they receive from their families contribute further to the potential for relapse among patients.

The EE construct has received considerable attention for its potential role in relapse among discharged patients with schizophrenia. A review of 25 studies on family EE indicated a 50% relapse rate, over a period of 9–12 months, among patients discharged to high-EE families, but only 21% among those with low-EE relatives (Bebbington & Kuipers, 1994). These findings indicate that the odds of relapse are increased by approximately 2.5:1 for patients discharged to high- versus low-EE relatives. Similar findings are evident in a recent meta-analysis of this literature, indicating an effect size of $r = .30$ for the association between family EE and relapse (Butzlaff & Hooley, 1998).

Studies on family EE show that three factors are prominent in protecting a patient with schizophrenia from relapse (Goldstein & Strachan, 1987). The first factor is low-EE in the relatives who live with the patient. For better or worse, most patients with schizophrenia are discharged back to their families of origin. When family members harbor critical and hostile attitudes toward a patient, the likelihood of relapse is high. On the other hand, low-EE, which may be indicative of greater tranquility, support, and acceptance, can greatly reduce the probability of relapse. A second protective factor is low (i.e., less than 35 hours per week) face-to-face contact with high-EE parents. Again, avoiding the agitating effect of high-EE family members appears to pay some dividends. The final protective factor identified by Goldstein and Strachan (1987) is whether a patient is maintained on medication. Obviously, those who comply with medication regimens are at reduced risk for relapse. These authors argue that of the three factors, low-EE in the family is most important in reducing relapse within a year from discharge, as it appears to have a prophylactic effect regardless of compliance with medication.

Family EE may function as a stressor that precipitates relapse among recovering patients with schizophrenia. The experience of a psychological problem as profound as schizophrenia can leave a recovering patient in a very fragile psychological and social state. Even though symptoms may be under control and in remission, the interpersonal disruption that is associated with this disorder may still be evident, leaving the patient in a precarious state of interpersonal relations. This undoubtedly increases the patient's sensitivity to criticism and hostility from others. Upon receiving these aversive interpersonal behaviors, the patient may have minimal opportunity for seeking social support and validation from other sources. The end result of this state of affairs may be relapse into an episode of schizophrenia upon being pressed by EE from family members.

There is reason to believe that parents who are particularly high in EE may have psychological problems of their own. Goldstein et al. (1992) found that lifetime rates of major psychiatric disorders were 100% in high-EE parents of patients with schizophrenia, and only 44% in parents who scored low on measures of EE. Although this 44% lifetime prevalence rate for the low-EE parents may seem high, it is comparable with rates from the National Comorbidity Study (Kessler et al., 1994) suggesting that these parents as a group are no different from those in the general population. The amazingly high rate of psychiatric disorder in the high-EE parents raises the possibility that EE may be a marker of a genetic transmission of mental illness.

Family EE is assumed to be a stressor that evokes psychiatric symptoms in a patient. Do patients find high-EE to be stressful? To explore this issue, Cutting and Docherty (2000) asked patients with schizophrenia to discuss happy and unhappy memories from their lives. Patients with high-EE parents recalled significantly fewer positive memories that involved their parents, compared to patients with low-EE parents. Overall, parents were featured in twice as many positive as negative memories. However, high-EE parents were featured in roughly equal proportions of positive and negative recollections. Cutting and Docherty's (2000) study provides at least indirect evidence that high-EE parents are experienced as stressful by patients with schizophrenia.

Research on family EE continues to flourish (e.g., Cole, Grolnick, Kane, Zastowny, & Lehman, 1993; Docherty, 1995; Mueser et al., 1993). In addition to being a useful and reliable predictor of relapse, EE may be fruitfully understood as a familial risk indicator for schizophrenia (Miklowitz, 1994). High-EE parents are especially likely to have their own history of psychopathology. Thus parental EE may signal a possible genetic transmission of psychopathology. Miklowitz (1994) also notes that high-EE parents may be especially likely to become critical of their offspring, if parents feel that their own psychological problems were overcome through internal efforts. Whether family EE is viewed as a predictor of relapse or a risk factor, one can interpret it within a diathesis–stress framework, in which this conflictual and hostile family attitude functions as a stressor on the patient (Hooley & Hiller, 1998). At the same time, however, it is important to bear in mind that EE may also reflect parents' frustration and appraisal of the burden of dealing with their son or daughter with schizophrenia (e.g., Hooley, 1998; Scazufca & Kuipers, 1998).

Combined CD and EE

Whereas EE reflects the content of communication, CD reflects the form of communication. As if to make a potentially disruptive family situation worse for patients with schizophrenia, families that are high in CD also tend to be high in EE (e.g., Miklowitz et al., 1986; Rund, Oie, Borchgrevink, & Fjell, 1995; but see Docherty, 1995). Consequently, patients may be dealt a double dose of problematic interactional exchanges with their family members. It is little wonder that patients discharged to parents high in EE, who are also likely to express unclear, odd, and fragmented ideas, are at such a high risk for relapse.

When the two variables were put side by side in the same investigation, family CD proved to be a more powerful predictor of schizophrenia outcomes (e.g., number of relapses, time hospitalized, ratings of psychosocial functioning) than family EE (Rund et al., 1995). Using a Spearman rank correlation, Rund et al. (1995) found an association between family EE and a combined index of these outcomes to be .16, whereas this same correlation for family CD was .94. However, family EE has some predictive validity above and beyond family CD. The course of the disorder is best predicted from family interaction variables when *both* CD and EE are considered (Goldstein, 1985). The combination of these two appears to have more predictive power than either on its own.

Affective Style

Affective style (AS) is a measure of the verbal behavior of family members during discussion of a conflict-laden issue with the patient present. Whereas EE is an attitude of hostility, criticism, and overinvolvement expressed by a family member during an interview in the absence of the patient, AS represents the family members' actual verbal behaviors when interacting with the patient. It may be viewed as the behavioral manifestation of the attitude indexed by the expressed emotion construct, but this relationship has been difficult to establish empirically (Miklowitz et al., 1989). Although AS and EE are closely related and perhaps overlapping constructs, a distinct body of literature exists on AS, indicating that (like EE) it is often predictive of relapse among patients with schizophrenia.

Measures of AS are typically taken from a series of brief family discussions about a current unresolved problem in the family (Doane et al., 1981). As might be expected, these conversations pull for substantial emotional expression. The conversations are then transcribed, and the family members' speech content is coded for support, criticism, guilt induction, and intrusiveness. The unit of analysis for the coding is typically six lines of uninterrupted speech by a single speaker. A complete description of the coding scheme appears in Table 4.3.

The results of the coding are used to classify families into one of three AS profiles: benign, intermediate, or poor. Benign-AS families display a lack of negative behaviors (i.e., personal criticism, guilt induction, and critical or neutral intrusiveness) during their interactions. Intermediate-AS families are those who express some negative but some positive speech behaviors (i.e., primary support) during the family discussion. Finally, poor-AS (also referred to as negative-AS) families are those in which one or both parents exhibit negative verbal behaviors, but no positive verbal behaviors.

In one of the first AS studies (Doane et al., 1981), 65 families of high-risk, disturbed, but not psychotic adolescents participated in the family conflict discussion. The adolescents were then assessed at a follow-up 5 years later. When a broad schizophrenia-spectrum diagnosis (e.g., including schizoid personality disorder) was used as the outcome

TABLE 4.3. Affective Style (AS) Codes

I.   Support
     A. *Primary support.* The parent conveys directly to the child that he or she feels genuine concern for the child him- or herself or about the child's problems or behavior. Example: "I want you to know I care about you."
     B. *Secondary support.* The parent expresses support of a less impactful nature, such as acknowledging improvements in some specific behavior.

II. Criticism
     A. *Personal criticism.* The criticism has one or more of the following qualities: unnecessary or overly harsh modifiers, reference to broad classes of behavior, or reference to the child's character or nature. Example: "You have an ugly, arrogant attitude."
     B. *Benign criticism.* The criticism is circumscribed, matter-of-fact, and directed toward specific incidents or sets of behaviors. Example: "You have a bad attitude about homework, John."

III. Guilt induction. Statements with a guilt-inducing impact have two components: They convey that the child is to blame or at fault for some negative event, and that the parent has been distressed or upset by the event. Example: "You cause our family an awful lot of trouble."

IV. Intrusiveness. Intrusive statements imply knowledge of the child's thoughts, feeling states, or motives when in fact there is no apparent basis for such knowledge.
     A. *Critical intrusiveness.* The intrusiveness contains a harsh, critical component. Example: "You enjoy being mean to others."
     B. *Neutral intrusiveness.* The intrusiveness has a neutral quality and refers to the child's emotional states, ideas, or preferences. Example: "You say you're angry [at us], but I think you're really mad at yourself."

Note. Adapted from Doane, West, Goldstein, Rodnick, & Jones (1981). Copyright 1981 by the American Medical Association. Adapted by permission.

criterion, only 8% of adolescents with a benign-AS family profile at time 1 received a schizophrenia spectrum diagnosis at time 2. Among those with an intermediate-AS family profile at time 1, 50% were diagnosed at time 2. This figure increased to 59% among those with a poor-AS family profile. Although these authors found that the best prediction of schizophrenia-spectrum disorders involved a combination of AS and CD, it is clear that family AS is a marker of risk for schizophrenia.

In a longitudinal study of even longer duration, a group of moderately disturbed teens and their families were followed over a period of 15 years (Goldstein, 1985). As in Doane et al.'s (1981) study, the families participated in the typical conflict discussion. They were then classified as either negative- or benign-AS. Results for Goldstein's study indicated that within those families classified as benign-AS, no cases of extended schizophrenia-spectrum disorders developed over the 15-year interval. However, almost all of the schizophrenia-spectrum cases observed at time 2 occurred in the context of a family where one or both parents were high in EE and AS. Like the studies on EE, the early studies on AS clearly supported the hypothesis that family expression of criticism and hostility, in the absence of any supportiveness, indicates a risk for the development of schizophrenia-spectrum disorders among high-risk adolescents. These findings are consistent with early research by Braginsky and his colleagues showing that many psychiatric patients use mental hospitals as a refuge from stressful environments, in which they seek a carefree lifestyle (Braginsky, Holzberg, Finison, & Ring, 1967; Braginsky, Holzberg, Ridley, & Braginsky, 1968).

In addition to being a risk factor in the initial development of the disorder, AS may also predict relapse. In one investigation, patients with schizophrenia whose families had benign-AS profiles at the time of their discharge from the hospital evidenced a 40% rehospitalization rate over the next 12 months, whereas those who returned to negative-AS families had over twice the rate (83%) of rehospitalization (Doane & Becker, 1993). Even more striking are the findings for AS in concert with medication compliance: Patients with negative-AS families and noncompliance with medication exhibited a 100% rehospitalization rate, compared with only 17% among those with benign-AS families and medication compliance. Of further interest is the fact that Doane and Becker (1993) tested for, and largely ruled out, the possibility that those patients from negative-AS families were sicker in the first place and therefore more likely to relapse. This finding suggests that it is unlikely that family AS is merely a reaction to the severity of a child's illness. Approximately 70% of those families characterized by excessive criticism and emotional overinvolvement at initial assessment remained that way over the course of the study, regardless of the patient's clinical status. Furthermore, about 20% of the parents became *more* critical over the course of the study, despite the fact that the patients' condition actually improved. Doane and Becker (1993) concluded that for most families AS reflects a relatively stable and enduring style of interaction, which is resistant to treatment and independent of the patients' recovery status.

The connection between family AS and rehospitalization could be the result of at least two different processes. The most straightforward hypothesis is that family AS is a stressor that pushes an already fragile individual "over the edge." Experiencing a serious psychological problem can leave a recovering patient in a delicate psychological state, as noted earlier. The criticism and intrusiveness evident in a negative-AS household have the potential to strain the already sensitive patient to such an extent that the full disorder may redevelop. An alternative but related hypothesis is that family AS is a stressor that pushes the recovering patient out of the household and back into the hospital, in an effort to seek refuge from the family. Most people would find a negative-AS household to be an aversive environment. It is understandable that almost anyone would want to get out of such an environment. For the patient with a learning history that involves being taken care of in a hospital, remission and readmission may be functional, in that it removes him or her from the stressful confines of the negative-AS family of origin.

Is negative AS specific to families of patients with schizophrenia? Several studies have been conducted to explore this issue, and these generally suggest that the problem is particularly exaggerated in such families. For example, when compared to parents of patients with bipolar disorder, the parents of patients with schizophrenia have been found to make more intrusive and critical statements toward the patients after discharge from the hospital (Miklowitz et al., 1995). When compared to families of patients with anorexia nervosa, families of patients with schizophrenia were much more likely to have negative-AS profiles (Goldstein, 1981). In this sample, only 1 of the 11 families of patients with anorexia nervosa had a negative-AS profile.

Family AS appears to have a relationship with both the onset and course of schizophrenia. At the same time, the variable has not been as widely embraced as CD or EE. Hooley and Hiller (1997) suggested that this is due to problems with reliably rating AS. Consequently, the variable appears almost exclusively in research studies of the group at or from UCLA who originally developed the construct. Nevertheless, the available research findings indicate that it is a family interaction phenomenon with potential equal to CD or EE in explaining considerable variance in the course of schizophrenia.

Summary of Contemporary Family-of-Origin Approaches

Research on family-of-origin interactions and schizophrenia is alive and well, despite a number of false starts in the 1960s and 1970s. This long-established line of research has found new life in the constructs of CD, EE, and AS. There is at least some evidence to suggest that each of these family phenomena may be an antecedent to the development of schizophrenia among at-risk adolescents, and that each may play some role in predicting relapse among recently discharged patients (e.g., Hooley & Hiller, 1997; Miklowitz, 1994). Some of these variables, such as EE, may be better suited to predicting relapse among patients in remission; others, such as CD, may be better suited to discriminating between families of people with schizophrenia and families of healthy controls (Miklowitz, 1994). Although EE, CD, and AS are not *purely* specific to families of patients with schizophrenia, each represents a potent risk factor in the course and possibly the onset of the disorder.

Unlike most of the early family approaches to schizophrenia, which often postulated a causal role for certain family variables, most of the contemporary research on CD, EE, and AS treats the variables as stressors that work in concert with a predisposition or vulnerability to produce schizophrenia. In fact, many investigators now believe that CD, EE, and AS often work in combination with each other, as well as with enduring predispositions, to affect the course of schizophrenia.

Modern conceptualizations of family interaction and schizophrenia fit well within a diathesis–stress framework. Some individuals may harbor a biological predisposition to develop schizophrenia. This predisposition is more formally known as the *diathesis*. It is unquestionably stressful to live with parents who communicate in odd and illogical ways, and who are unable to establish and maintain a shared focus of attention. It is equally stressful to live with parents who harbor as well as express attitudes of hostility, criticism, and overinvolvement. Sadly, many of these destructive and stressful family interaction patterns co-occur. The confusion and disorientation that parental CD produces, and the guilt, shame, and bewilderment about ego boundaries that parental EE and negative AS create, have the effect of combining flame and fuel among those with an existing predisposition toward schizophrenia and/or trigger relapse.

Research on CD, EE, and AS could still be characterized as being in the early stages. The precise nature of their function in the schizophrenia-spectrum disorders has yet to be determined with finality. In theory, these parental phenomena could be reactive to the condition of the patient, although there are at least some data to the contrary. Furthermore, these variables could be markers of potentially disturbed parents, thus suggesting a path of genetic transmission. As noted earlier, one could question the mental health of any parent who exhibits excessive hostility, criticism, and emotional overinvolvement toward a child, along with an inability to establish and maintain a shared focus of attention in discussions that have a bizarre tone and structure. Nevertheless, current evidence indicates that these family variables have an undeniable role in the course and in some cases onset of schizophrenia. It is not possible to fully understand and predict this disorder without at least some consideration of the family context in which a patient with schizophrenia was reared and into which he or she is discharged.

GENERAL PERSONAL RELATIONSHIPS IN SCHIZOPHRENIA

Without question, family-of-origin relations and interactions have dominated the interpersonal research on schizophrenia. However, there is reason to believe that problematic interpersonal relationships extend beyond the realm of family relations for patients with schizophrenia. For example, among patients at a residential facility, interpersonal interactions were identified as the primary cause of symptom fluctuations in approximately two-thirds of the residents with schizophrenia (Marley, 1998). The most commonly identified interpersonal interactions were with other residents, and involved arguments, irritation, and concern about having personal property stolen by these others. Residents also indicated that arguments with and criticism from staff members led to worsening of their symptoms. This kind of relational friction is very prominent in the interpersonal landscape of people with schizophrenia.

One particular area of interest for schizophrenia and interpersonal relationships more generally is social support. Patients with schizophrenia typically have smaller social networks, and report that they have fewer close friends, than healthy controls or even other psychiatric patients (Erickson, Beiser, Iaacono, Fleming, & Lin, 1989). Importantly, Erickson's research group detected a negative association between number of family members in the patients' social networks and their prognosis, whereas a greater number of friends and acquaintances in these networks was associated with better outcomes (Erickson et al., 1989; Erickson, Beiser, & Iaacono, 1998). This finding indicates that the type of "social support" that may be offered by family members actually aggravates the course of the disorder. What is obviously beneficial to the patient with schizophrenia is social support from friends. However, such support is sadly lacking in many cases. One possible reason for this lack of support may stem from the poor social skills that are often associated with schizophrenia (see below). Patients with schizophrenia and poor social skills tend to have smaller social networks (Macdonald, Jackson, Hayes, Baglioni, & Madden, 1998). The negative symptoms of schizophrenia may also inhibit the ability to secure social support from others (Macdonald et al., 1998).

The impact of social support clearly extends beyond just psychiatric symptoms for people with schizophrenia. It may literally have an impact on their long-term survival. Recently Christensen, Dornink, Ehlers, and Schultz (1999) examined the records of 133 patients with schizophrenia who were admitted to a state hospital between 1934 and 1944. Over a lengthy retrospective follow-up period, those patients with more social support available exhibited a lower expected mortality. Using survival analysis, Christensen et al. (1999) demonstrated that a 1-point increase in social support (expressed on a 5-point scale) was associated with a 25% hazard reduction over the follow-up period, which averaged 58 years. Clearly, when social support is available, it pays many dividends to people with schizophrenia—in terms of both psychiatric symptoms and longevity.

Research on social support suggests that it is difficult for people with schizophrenia to reap the benefits offered by relationships with friends. In addition to problems with friendships, schizophrenia is associated with less closeness and more conflict with siblings (Lively, Friedrich, & Buckwalter, 1995). Participants in Lively et al.'s (1995) study expressed a considerable degree of grief and stress associated with their attempts to cope with their ill siblings.

Rejection

Finally, there is evidence to indicate that, like people with depression, people with schizophrenia often elicit rejection from others. For instance, Norman and Malla (1983) asked a large sample of students to read vignettes describing a young man with paranoid schizophrenia, personality disorder, or no mental health problem. The more mentally distressed the target person was judged to be, the more respondents found him to be socially unacceptable, and the more social distance from him they desired. Similar findings are evident in a study of face-to-face interactions with patients with schizophrenia (Nisenson & Berenbaum, 1998). In this case, the more strangely patients behaved during the interaction (as rated by observers), the more negatively their conversational partners responded to them. Nisenson and Berenbaum (1998) concluded that "some patients consistently behave in ways that lead them to be responded to more or less negatively" (p. 9). This interpersonal rejection effect associated with schizophrenia may explain the difficulty such people have in building and maintaining a social support network of friends. It is also linked to the severe social skills deficits these patients have, which are described next.

INTERPERSONAL COMMUNICATION:
SOCIAL SKILLS DEFICITS ASSOCIATED WITH SCHIZOPHRENIA

In addition to being embedded in disturbed and dissatisfying interpersonal relationships, people with schizophrenia evidence serious communication problems of their own. An extensive line of research on social skills deficits associated with schizophrenia shows that the disorder is strongly associated with what are often fundamental failures in basic communication skills. Although these deficits are not ubiquitous with this family of disorders—for example, those with the paranoid subtype may be more functional—in many cases the exceptionally peculiar and disorganized style of relating to other people makes communication extremely difficult and challenging. The research on social skills deficits associated with schizophrenia has examined the expression or encoding aspects, as well as the reception or decoding aspects, of communication. Within each of these areas, distinct deficits are sometimes evident in subprocesses (speech production and use of nonverbal behavior in the case of encoding skills; and recognition of facial expressions, social information, and recognition/processing in the case of decoding skills).

Encoding Skills

Through a series of meticulously designed and controlled laboratory investigations, Bellack and his colleagues demonstrated that patients with schizophrenia have impairments in social skills that are more pronounced than those of either healthy or psychiatric controls (e.g., Bellack, Morrison, Mueser, & Wade, 1989; Bellack, Morrison, Wixted, & Mueser, 1990). In these studies, all subjects participated in a role-play assessment procedure that involved a series of interactions with a confederate, calling for skills such as conversation initiation, positive assertion, and negative assertion. The social behavior of the patients with schizophrenia in these settings tended to be less appropriate than that of either nonpsychiatric controls (Mueser, Bellack, Douglas, & Morrison, 1991) or psychiatric controls, including patients with mood disorders and schizoaffective disorder (Bellack et al., 1989, 1990; Mueser, Bellack, Morrison, & Wixted, 1990). These authors demonstrated that impairments in social skills are not just secondary to the symptoms of schizophrenia, and that they are significantly associated with more general social functioning (see also Halford & Hayes, 1995).

Further evidence of poor encoding social skills associated with schizophrenia is evident in a diverse range of studies. For example, based on clinical ratings of such social skills as acceptance of contact from others, initiation of contact with others, effective communication, engaging in activities, participating in groups, forming friendships, and asking for help, patients with schizophrenia scored significantly lower on all dimensions, compared to patients with bipolar disorder or major depression (Bartels, Mueser, & Miles, 1997). Similar findings based on clinical ratings indicate that in domains such as language development, socialization, and responsibility, patients with schizophrenia were rated more poorly than those with mental retardation, and were in about the same range as patients with organic brain impairment (Sylph, Ross, & Kendward, 1977). When using self-report instruments to assess social skills, people with schizophrenia rated themselves as less competent in their ability to initiate interactions, manage conflict, and provide emotional support to others (Semple et al., 1999). These social skills deficits were particularly associated with the negative symptoms of schizophrenia (see also Lysaker, Bell, Zito, & Bioty, 1995).

Speech Production Skills

Effective verbal communication skills are essential for conveying information, as well as for establishing and negotiating interpersonal relationships. Deficits in these skills are almost immediately evident upon interacting with an individual with schizophrenia. A frequent theme in the research on speech production and schizophrenia is the frequency of communication failures. These include such phenomena as vague or confused references, missing information in references, and structural unclarities. In conversation, people with schizophrenia will exhibit numerous communication failures (Docherty, DeRosa, & Andreasen, 1996; Docherty, Hall, & Gordinier, 1998). This makes their discourse very difficult to decode, and their train of thought almost impossible to follow. This type of speech clarity (or unclarity) is strongly related to social functioning among patients with schizophrenia (Penn, Mueser, Doonan, & Nishith, 1995). It is impossible to overlook the striking parallel between the findings on communication failures among people with schizophrenia and the findings on CD in their family members.

Another speech problem associated with schizophrenia is diminished or inhibited speech production, also known as *poverty of speech* (Davidson, Frith, Harrison-Read, & Johnstone, 1996; Glaister, Feldstein, & Pollack, 1980; Ragin, Pogue-Geile, & Oltmanns, 1989; Rutter, 1977a). This is speech that is inappropriately laconic and restricted. For example, when asked, "What was your family like when you were growing up?", a person with schizophrenia may answer, "OK, I guess." Such insufficiently elaborate responses require the conversational partner to probe continually for further information in order to get a sufficient answer. And when people with schizophrenia do speak, they tend to have poor enunciation and inflection (Todt & Howell, 1980). Such inhibited speech production is not specific to schizophrenia; it is also evident in depression (Ragin et al., 1989). However, it tends to be more chronic for people with schizophrenia, whereas it improves dramatically as symptoms remit in depression.

Nonverbal Behavior Skills

The effective use of nonverbal behavior adds considerable richness to vocal communication, conveying attitudes, emotions, and information.

People with schizophrenia regularly exhibit impairments in their use of nonverbal communication behaviors. For example, patients with schizophrenia make less eye contact with others during social interactions (Rutter, 1973), although this may be limited to certain types of interactions that are of a personal nature (Rutter, 1977b, 1978). When watching emotional films, patients with schizophrenia were found to be less facially animated than nonpatient controls (Salem & Kring, 1999). They may also be impaired in the use of paralanguage (e.g., tone of voice, speech rate, inflection) to convey emotion (Whittaker, Connell, & Deakin, 1994). In family interactions, patients with schizophrenia use fewer gestures and lean forward less toward their partners than psychiatric controls do (Simoneau, Miklowitz, Goldstein, Nuechterlein, & Richards, 1996).

Research on the encoding aspect of social skills shows that people with schizophrenia perform very poorly. Both their verbal and their nonverbal behaviors suggest disengagement, confusion, and existence in a reality that is difficult to express, much less share with others. Sadly, the extent of social skills deficits associated with schizophrenia does not stop there. An additional line of research focused more on decoding or reception skills illustrates further social deficits.

Decoding Skills

Aside from encoding or behavioral production skills, decoding skills are also vital to effective interpersonal communication. These skills are often referred to as social and emotional sensitivity (Riggio, 1986) or nonverbal sensitivity (DePaulo & Friedman, 1998). Such skills call on one's ability to perceive and read subtle cues in the discourse and nonverbal behavior of other people at a rapid pace. Obviously, these are cognitively demanding skills that are perfected over a lifetime of human interactions.

People with schizophrenia experience a multitude of decoding problems in interpersonal contexts. These interpersonal decoding skills problems are undoubtedly related to a more general problem that reveals itself equally in poor performance in decoding noninterpersonal phenomena (e.g., Weiss, Chapman, Strauss, & Gilmore, 1992). By definition, inherent in its diagnostic criteria, schizophrenia involves many serious perceptual problems that are often manifest in hallucinations and disorganized cognition and affect. They make for ineffective social perception that undoubtedly contributes to deteriorated interpersonal experiences for people with schizophrenia.

Social Information Recognition and Processing

Many people with schizophrenia appear to have social-cognitive deficits that interfere with their ability to process social cues (Corrigan, Wallace, & Green, 1992; Ikebuchi, Nakagome, & Takahashi, 1999). The inadequate recognition and processing of social cues are related to poor social skills more generally among people with schizophrenia (Corrigan & Toomey, 1995; Penn, Mueser, Spaulding, Hope, & Reed, 1995; but see Hyronemus, Penn, Corrigan, & Martin, 1998).

One common method for assessing social decoding skills is with a test known as the Profile of Nonverbal Sensitivity (PONS; Rosenthal, Hall, DiMatteo, Rogers, & Archer, 1979). This test presents a series of vignettes of nonverbal behavior through varying audio (filtered for speech content) and video clips. After each clip, subjects are presented with two alternatives and must choose the one that was conveyed in the clip. People with schizophrenia perform more poorly on the PONS than do either healthy controls (Fingeret, Monti, & Paxson, 1985; Toomey, Wallace, Corrigan, Schuldberg, & Green, 1997) or psychiatric controls (Monti & Fingeret, 1987). On related perception tests, people with schizophrenia appear to have deficits in interpersonal problem recognition and in their ability to paraphrase and summarize the feelings of an actor presented on videotape (Bedell, Lennox, Smith, & Rabinowicz, 1998).

The nature of the communication-decoding skill deficits of people with schizophrenia is such that they exhibit more false-positive responses as cues go from being more concrete to more abstract (Corrigan & Nelson, 1998). Concrete social cues are actual sights (e.g., facial expressions) and sounds (e.g., tone of voice), whereas abstract social cues are inferences about affect, rules, and goals of a social situation (e.g., "He's upset," "She's trying to get her way"). Corrigan and Nelson (1998) have suggested that this may reflect a tendency toward overinclusive thinking; that is, people with schizophrenia may falsely identify social cues and make inferences that are not consistent with the situation. An alternative hypothesis—that schizophrenia interferes with vigilance for social cues—has been effectively ruled out (Corrigan, 1997).

The ineffective processing of social information extends to schizophrenic patients' processing of their own social behavior. In a study by Carini and Nevid (1992), patients with schizophrenia rated the social appropriateness of their own behavior significantly higher than judges did. However, there were no self–other differences in the ratings of psychiatric or healthy controls. This suggests a loss of contact with social reality that may be unique to schizophrenia.

Recognition of Facial Expression

Considerable evidence suggests that people with schizophrenia experience deficits in both information processing and emotion recognition. These two deficits converge in the research on decoding facial expressions of emotion. The ability to detect and read other people's emotions is an essential social skill that contributes to effective communication and social relations. This is a specific social skill that is impaired in many patients with schizophrenia. When asked to judge emotional expressions in photographs of faces, subjects with schizophrenia perform more poorly than healthy controls, failing to detect or misreading other people's facial expressions (Dougherty, Bartlett, & Izard, 1974; Mandal & Palchoudhury, 1985; Mueser et al., 1996; Salem, Kring, & Kerr, 1996; Whittaker et al., 1994). Interestingly, this decoding skill deficit is pervasive across all facial recognition tasks, emotional or otherwise (e.g., Mueser et al., 1996; Salem et al., 1996). However, there is mixed evidence on whether patients with schizophrenia exhibit a deficit in detecting eye contact from other people (Franck et al., 1998; Rosse, Kendrick, Wyatt, Isaac, & Deutsch, 1994). There is also some evidence to suggest that such patients may be able to recognize an emotion, but that they may be unable or unwilling to use an appropriate word to describe the emotion (Mandal & Palchoudhury, 1985).

From their extensive review of the literature on facial expressions of emotion and schizophrenia, Mandal, Pandey, and Prasad (1998) conclude that two general theories explain patients' deficits in recognition of facial emotions. The first holds that these are secondary to a right-hemisphere brain abnormality. This portion of the brain has been linked with the perception of facial emotion. The second theory is based on a social-cognitive deficit that develops out of a desire to avoid social interaction and guard against exposure to arousing stimuli. In either case, it is clear that people with schizophrenia have difficulty with this basic but important social decoding skill.

Collectively, the research on social cue recognition and processing, and on perception of facial expressions in particular, clearly indicates problems with communication-decoding skills for those with schizophrenia. These poor decoding skills may make it difficult for people afflicted with schizophrenia to learn the social conventions of the culture at large (Toomey et al., 1997) and to recognize other people's emotional states accurately (Morrison & Bellack, 1987). Failure to do so may help to explain why people with schizophrenia experience such difficulties establishing and maintaining personal relationships and a social support network.

Premorbid Social Skills and Schizophrenia

Are social skills deficits just a consequence of schizophrenia? Undoubt-edly the symptoms of schizophrenia have profound effects on such pro-cesses as social cognition, communication, and message processing. However, premorbid social behavior problems and poor social compe-tence are hallmarks of risk for schizophrenia. To illustrate this phenome-non, Dworkin, Lewis, Cornblatt, and Erlenmeyer-Kimling (1994) fol-lowed groups of children who were at risk for psychosocial problems as a function of being born to a parent with a mood disorder, schizophre-nia, or no mental health problem. During childhood, there were no dif-ferences in the social competence of the three groups. However, by ado-lescence those at risk for schizophrenia had lower social competence as rated by their parents and themselves. When college students were classi-fied as being at risk for schizophrenia on the basis of scoring high on measures of perceptual aberration, magical ideation, nonconformity, and physical anhedonia, at-risk subjects performed more poorly on a role-play test of social skill and chose more odd and hostile responses on a multiple-choice test of interpersonal problem solving (Beckfield, 1985). A recent German study showed that evidence of social disability (e.g., no marriage or stable partnership) was evident during a prodromal period, as early as 2–4 years prior to formal diagnosis (Hafner, Loffler, Maurer, Hambrecht, & an der Heiden, 1999). This premorbid or prodromal social competence has proven to be a good predictor of age at first hospitalization, and of the prognosis for those who develop schizophrenia (Glick & Zigler, 1986; Glick, Zigler, & Zigler, 1985). Col-lectively, this research shows that poor social skills are already evident among those prone to schizophrenia, well before the onset of symptoms. However, since poor social skills are not specific to schizophrenia, their prodromal status must be understood as nonspecific.

Summary of Social Skills Deficits and Schizophrenia

People with schizophrenia often have serious problems with social skills. In severe cases, their social and communication behavior cannot be dis-tinguished from those with mental retardation and/or organic brain im-pairment. Among patients with certain subtypes, such as catatonic schizophrenia, social behavior may be nearly nonexistent.

The social skills deficits associated with schizophrenia involve both encoding and decoding skills. As encoders of communication, people with schizophrenia will exhibit communication failures. Their speech is difficult to understand, and their train of thought difficult to follow. Their enunciation is sometimes poor, and their use of nonverbal behavior is often inappropriate and suggestive of disengagement and a desire *not* to communicate with others. As decoders, people with schizophrenia appear to struggle to understand others. They have a difficult time recognizing basic social cues, and reading the nonverbal behaviors of others, such as facial expressions of emotion. When asked to provide information based on the behavior of others, they tend to draw unconventional conclusions that simply are not warranted by the behavior observed.

A number of prominent themes in the literature on social skills deficits and schizophrenia may explain some of these deficits. First, it is apparent that some of the problems with social behavior associated with schizophrenia are related to cognitive deficits. Communication tasks that draw heavily on cognitive processing, such as speech production and recognition of social cues, are those that people with schizophrenia have considerable difficulty with. Second, the social skills of people with schizophrenia may be impaired due to their inhibited sociability. Their social behavior is suggestive of a desire to withdraw from and avoid others, possibly because of shame and/or anxiety about interacting with other people. Rates of social anxiety and social phobia are relatively high among patients with schizophrenia (Cosoff & Hafner, 1998; Penn, Hope, Spaulding, & Kucera, 1994). Heinssen and Glass (1990) have argued that social anxiety interacts with cognitive dysfunction and skill deficiency to hamper the social performance of people with schizophrenia. Even people with reasonable social skills will experience atrophying of these skills if they do not use them with any regularity. Many people with schizophrenia may start out with poor social skills, never having fully developed them as adolescents or young adults, only to see them worsen as a result of years of social withdrawal and avoidance. Finally, psychomotor disturbances that are associated with schizophrenia, many of which have physiological/biological bases, may interfere with effective social behavior. The use of gesture, posture, facial expression, and eye contact may all be disrupted in concert with more general psychomotor disturbances that are common in schizophrenia. These may color the social behavior of patients in such a way as to impair basic social skills.

COMORBIDITY OF SCHIZOPHRENIA WITH OTHER MENTAL HEALTH PROBLEMS

It is perhaps understandable that a disorder as severe as schizophrenia is often accompanied by other psychological problems. These problems, like schizophrenia, have equally strong ties to interpersonal interaction and relationships. Results from the National Comorbidity Survey indicate that the lifetime prevalence of any mood disorder (major depression, dysthymia, and manic episode) is a staggering 73.4% among those with a primary diagnosis of schizophrenia (Kendler, Gallagher, Abelson, & Kessler, 1996). Results from this same study show a 71.4% lifetime prevalence of any anxiety disorder, and a 58.5% lifetime prevalence of any substance use disorder. For the majority of people with schizophrenia, therefore, other serious psychological problems are evident.

Why are so many people with schizophrenia depressed, anxious, or involved in alcohol or other substance misuse? Admittedly, there are cases in which these problems are evident in the prodromal stages of the disorder. However, an interpersonal perspective would explain many of these problems as features precipitated by the gross deterioration of interpersonal relationships apparent among those with schizophrenia. Presumably, as the symptomatic behaviors become more evident and bizarre, other people (including close family members) react negatively toward the person with schizophrenia. The extreme social isolation that is common among patients with schizophrenia could itself contribute to depressive symptoms. Add to that isolation delusional, and sometimes paranoid, thinking about other people, and the potential for depression is obvious. These same delusional thought patterns could also create a severe anxiety over dealing with other people. People with schizophrenia are often fearful of others, and sometimes with good reason when one considers how they may have been treated by people in the past. From this perspective, a profound social anxiety might be viewed as secondary to the amalgamation of cognitive and interpersonal problems that is an integral part of schizophrenia. Almost half of all patients with schizophrenia have some form of anxiety disorder, and approximately 17% have social phobia in particular (Cosoff & Hafner, 1998). Finally, interpersonal problems may lead people with schizophrenia to turn to drug or alcohol use, just as they do for others. People often seek consolation in drugs or alcohol as either an escape from or mechanism for regulating an abrasive interpersonal environment. From an interpersonal perspective, it is not surprising that schizophrenia is highly comorbid with problems such as depression, anxiety, and substance use disorders. These problems are clearly sensitive to troubled interpersonal relationships, and troubled interpersonal relationships are dominant in the clinical picture of schizophrenia.

CONCLUSION

Interpersonal research on schizophrenia started with a collection of family-oriented approaches. These early interpersonal perspectives emphasized various disturbances in family-of-origin interaction and relations that were thought to be etiological in the disorder. Out of this work came many provocative ideas about the association between early family experiences and later mental health. However, much of this theorizing was based on clinical observations of fairly small samples of patients and their families. Although such family process variables as double-bind communication, schism, skew, mystification, and pseudomutuality are useful for explaining the family processes of some schizophrenia patients, they are no longer considered to be prominent features in the social background of those with the disorder.

Often building on early family perspectives, the contemporary family-of-origin approaches to schizophrenia focus on the problems of CD, EE, and AS. Each of these variables rests on a sound foundation of empirical evidence linking it to the course of the disorder. Although not all of these phenomena are specific to schizophrenia, collectively they are predictive of onset and relapse, since many people with schizophrenia live with and will be discharged to their families of origin. Contemporary research on family relations in schizophrenia makes a very compelling case for attention to and consideration of interpersonal issues. A complete understanding of this most serious mental health problem is impossible without serious consideration of the family context in which a patient was reared and/or resides.

Additional lines of research on interpersonal issues in schizophrenia show that those with the disorder often have poor social support networks and few if any satisfying personal relationships. The social support that is so badly needed by people with schizophrenia appears to be something that their families cannot provide. In fact, the "social support" that their families do provide may cause more harm than good.

Perhaps related to troubles with personal relationships are the poor social skills that characterize people with schizophrenia. Of all the mental health problems in which poor social skills figure prominently, schizophrenia is tied to perhaps the most disturbed social behavior. People with schizophrenia often exhibit poor social skills in both the encoding and decoding domains of interpersonal communication.

The three interpersonal domains addressed in this chapter—poor family-of-origin relations, poor general personal relations, and poor interpersonal communication (social skills deficits)—are by no means independent of each other. If one takes as a point of departure the fact that many people with schizophrenia grow up in families marked by EE, CD, and negative AS, it is no wonder that they sometimes do not develop adequate social skills. The shame and social withdrawal evident in the interpersonal conduct of people with schizophrenia may be the direct result of such experiences in their families of origin. The difficulties in establishing and maintaining effective and satisfying personal relationships are no doubt secondary to poor social skills. Developing personal relationships requires at least some basic social skills. Without these skills, a person with schizophrenia may be doomed to a rather solitary and lonely interpersonal existence. This may leave the patient literally at the doorstep of the only interpersonal network that will accept him or her: the family of origin. In some cases, this may simply extend and protract the experience of schizophrenia.

5

Bipolar Disorder

DEFINITION AND SYMPTOMS

Bipolar disorders are a family of mental health problems whose essential feature involves oscillation between manic (or hypomanic) and depressive affective states. Originally, these problems were referred to as *manic–depressive illness* or *manic–depression*. A *manic episode* involves the experience of inflated self-esteem or grandiosity, minimal sleep, excessive and pressured speech, flight of ideas, inability to focus attention, distractibility, psychomotor agitation, and poor judgment (which often takes the form of risky behaviors such as gambling, promiscuous sexual behavior, and lavish spending) (American Psychiatric Association, 2000). A *hypomanic episode* is a milder version of a manic episode (American Psychiatric Association, 2000). On the other hand, a *depressive episode* entails the symptoms of major depression, such as depressed mood, anhedonia, insomnia or hypersomnia, psychomotor retardation, fatigue, feeling hopeless and worthless, difficulty concentrating, and suicidal ideation (American Psychiatric Association, 2000). Serious problems with school, occupational functioning, and marital and other family relationships are indicated as associated features of all bipolar disorders (American Psychiatric Association, 2000). Goodwin and Jamison (1990) wrote: "Interpersonal aspects of both mania and depression are pervasive, usually profound. Fluctuating levels of sociability, impulsivity, dependency, hostility, and sexuality are part and parcel of manic–depressive illness" (p. 315).

Based on the nature of their manic (or hypomanic) and depressive episodic experiences, patients are diagnosed with either bipolar I or bipolar II disorder. Bipolar I disorder is characterized by the experience of one or more manic episodes (often occurring immediately before or after a depressive episode), whereas bipolar II disorder involves the experience of at least one major depressive episode, accompanied by at least one hypomanic episode (American Psychiatric Association, 2000). In short, people with bipolar I disorder oscillate between full-blown mania and anything from a normal affective state to full depression, whereas people with bipolar II disorder oscillate between full-blown depressive episodes and only moderate forms of mania. Bipolar I disorder is equally common in men and women, but women are more likely than men to suffer from bipolar II disorder. Bipolar I disorder is associated with profound psychological disturbances in the form of psychotic symptoms. Completed suicide occurs in 10–15% of cases of bipolar disorders, and attempts occur in over 40% of cases (Tsai, Lee, & Chen, 1999). The 1-year prevalence of any bipolar disorder is 1.2% (Regier et al., 1993), and the lifetime risk for experiencing a manic episode has been estimated at 1.6% (Kessler et al., 1994), so these are relatively rare psychosocial problems.

Its DSM-IV-TR classification as a mood disorder and description as *manic–depressive illness* immediately invites comparison between bipolar disorder and major depression. However, bipolar disorder may be as closely related to schizophrenia as it is to depression, if not more so. Although unipolar and bipolar depressive episodes are both mood disturbances, bipolar manic episodes and schizophrenia both belong to the class of more serious psychotic disturbances. Psychotic symptoms are also far more common in bipolar depression than in unipolar depression (Goodwin & Jamison, 1990). Goodwin and Jamison (1990) also concluded that people with schizophrenia and mania do not differ in their degree of thought disorder, though there are differences in quality: Namely, mania is associated with disordered thought structure, and schizophrenia is associated with disordered thought content. On the other hand, thought disorder is rare in unipolar depression. Some of the same interpersonal variables that predict the course of schizophrenia also predict the course of bipolar disorder. In fact, patients with schizophrenia (or schizoaffective disorder) are often the ones to whom patients with bipolar disorder are compared in interpersonal studies, though some studies have compared patients with bipolar disorder to patients with unipolar depression. For this reason, it is useful for those seeking an understanding of the interpersonal mechanisms in bipolar disorder to become acquainted first with the related findings for unipolar depression and schizophrenia.

PREVIEW

In the area of *interpersonal communication*, research shows that people with bipolar disorder exhibit behavior indicative of social skills deficits.

Although no definitive early childhood experiences have been consistently linked with bipolar disorder, several *family-of-origin experiences* have been identified in the families of adults with bipolar disorder. As in schizophrenia (see Chapter 4), family members of adults with bipolar disorder exhibit relatively high rates of expressed emotion (EE), communication deviance (CD), and negative affective style (AS). Battles for control are also evident among patients and their family members. Research on *family-of-orientation experiences* indicates that people with bipolar disorder are prone to experiencing marital distress and problems in their parental role. In the *general personal relationships* domain, one finds distressed relationships and agitation by interpersonal stressors. Bipolar disorder shares many of the symptoms of, and coexists with, many other interpersonally oriented psychological problems, such as personality disorders, schizophrenia, eating disorders, and substance use disorders.

INTERPERSONAL COMMUNICATION IN BIPOLAR DISORDER: SOCIAL SKILLS AND SOCIAL STYLE

Unlike their counterparts with unipolar depression, patients with bipolar disorder exhibit social skills and styles ranging from withdrawn to obnoxiously gregarious and talkative. The features of interpersonal communication that most clearly distinguish these patients from those with unipolar depression are those associated with manic episodes. In a classic paper on mania and interpersonal relations, patients with mania were characterized as alienating, manipulative, and persuasive (Janowsky, Leff, & Epstein, 1970). Janowsky and his colleagues identified five themes evident in the behavior of people with bipolar disorder, particularly during the manic phase: manipulation of others' self-esteem, exploiting others' vulnerabilities and conflicts, projection of responsibility onto others, progressive limit testing, and alienating family members. According to Janowsky et al. (1970), each of these social-interactional styles helps to fulfill a patient's need to be taken care of. By exploiting others' vulnerabilities, projecting responsibility, and manipulating others' self-esteem, the patient with mania aims to bolster and enhance his or her own self-esteem and feelings of power and strength. Janowsky et al. (1970) explain, "As a way of maintaining self-esteem, and feelings of power and strength, the manic [patient] instigates a situation in which he is able to control and manipulate those people on whom he must rely" (p. 260). These manipulative tactics are thought to allow the patient to be taken care of by others, while still maintaining his or her self-esteem.

Unlike people with unipolar depression, patients with bipolar disorder have a communication style that is more outgoing, grandiose, and dominant. In social interactions, they show excesses of such behaviors as questions, as well as comments about their own life experiences (Grossman & Harrow, 1996). The accelerated speech rate and unrestrained commingling of ideas in their speech sometimes resemble the communication style of patients with schizophrenia. Solovay, Shenton, and Holzman (1987) interviewed patients with either mania or schizophrenia and measured their verbal behavior with the Thought Disorder Index (TDI), which codes for the presence of variables such as excessive qualification, flippant responses, vagueness, idiosyncratic symbolism, fragmentation, and incoherence. They found the TDI scores of the patients with mania to be indistinguishable from those of patients with schizophrenia, but both groups clearly scored higher than normal controls did. On some dimensions of the TDI, such as combinatory thinking (incongruous combinations of ideas, playful confabulation, flippant response, impossible/bizarre combinations), the patients with mania actually scored higher than people with schizophrenia. The authors provided the following example to illustrate the verbal response of a patient with mania, in reaction to a question about why a Rorschach image looked like a crab: "'Cause I'm Cancer the crab maybe. My sign is Cancer. My horoscope. And I'm thinking a lot about cancer, too. God forbid if anyone is dying of cancer . . . I wish it was me" (Solovay et al., 1987, p. 19). This speech style is reminiscent of the CD findings from family interactions of patients with schizophrenia.

In conversation, people with mania will talk a lot (hyperverbosity); however, they often get derailed, seemingly interrupting themselves before finishing a train of thought. This is a manifestation of their thought disorder that tends to make their discourse difficult to follow and figure out. A comparative study of speech in various groups of psychiatric patients showed that depressive speech was the most predictable and that schizophrenic speech was the least, with manic speech falling in between the two (Ragin & Oltmanns, 1983).

In some areas of social skills, patients with bipolar disorder are as functional as (and in some cases more functional than) healthy controls. Male patients with bipolar disorder were as extraverted as healthy controls, and both groups were significantly more extraverted than patients with unipolar depression (Hirschfeld, Klerman, Keller, Andreasen, & Clayton, 1986; see also Goodwin & Jamison, 1990). However, the patients in this same bipolar group were less likely than subjects in either the unipolar or control group to be married, and were equal to the patients with unipolar depression in lack of social self-confidence and assertion. On a measure of overall social adjustment, patients with bipolar disorder appeared similar to healthy controls, but reported more problems specifically in the area of family relations (Shapira et al., 1999). Patients with bipolar disorder perform even better than healthy controls at interpreting other people's nonverbal behavior (Giannini, Folts, & Fiedler, 1990). This effect may result from the hyperalertness of these patients during manic phases.

In an inpatient setting, patients with bipolar disorder were more likely than those with unipolar depression to see the staff and other patients as submissive to them (Benjamin & Wonderlich, 1994). Although the tendency to view the self as socially dominant is similar in people with bipolar disorder and healthy subjects, people with unipolar depression do not exhibit this belief. This suggests that the social style characteristic of bipolar disorder is more dominant and controlling than the submissive and inhibited style common in unipolar depression.

Summary

The research on social skills and styles of people with bipolar disorder presents an interesting mixture of function and dysfunction. If one focuses on the sheer quantity of communication behaviors, they appear quite functional: These patients are talkative, extraverted, and socially perceptive. However, sometimes these communication behaviors are taken to the point of being interpersonally intolerable. The social skills and style of patients with bipolar disorder also reflect disordered thinking: Their discourse is often laced with bizarre, idiosyncratic, and poorly formed ideas. In this regard, their interpersonal communication resembles that of patients with schizophrenia and their family members. Despite the fact that patients with bipolar disorder may possess a cunning ability to get their way with other people, they still have social adjustment problems, particularly in the areas of conflict and damage to other people's self-esteem (Wilson, Rosenthal, & Dunner, 1982). Whereas unipolar depression is associated with an avoidant, aloof, and socially withdrawn style of interaction, bipolar disorder appears to be manifested in an excessive, manipulative, and odd style of social interaction that may contribute to interpersonal conflicts.

FAMILY-OF-ORIGIN EXPERIENCES IN BIPOLAR DISORDER

Early Childhood Experiences

A series of retrospective studies tested hypotheses about early family-of-origin experiences in bipolar disorder, with mixed findings. Interviews with adult bipolar patients, corroborated by family informants, about their childhood experiences revealed some potentially pathogenic family experiences (Glassner & Haldipur, 1985). During their early childhood, the majority of patients in this study occupied special family positions, such as the first-born or youngest child, the "favorite" child, or the child assigned special responsibilities. As children these patients were also pressured for achievements, which were rewarded when accomplished. Not surprisingly, the children were also high achievers in the school setting. Glassner and Haldipur (1985) found that these children left home as perfectionists without the skills to succeed on their own. For most, symptoms emerged concurrently with their departure from their families. This pattern was more or less unique to early-onset cases, and thus may represent just one possible interpersonal path to bipolar disorder.

In some studies, patients with bipolar disorder have described their childhood experiences as similar to those of healthy controls. For example, such patients were indistinguishable from medical controls on reports of parental bonding (Joyce, 1984). They also described their family environments while growing up as similar to those of healthy controls on dimensions such as expressiveness, conflict, independence, cohesion, and control (Cooke, Young, Mohri, Blake, & Joffe, 1999). Perris, Maj, Perris, and Eisemann (1985)found no differences between patients with remitted bipolar disorder and normal controls on reports of parental rejection or overprotectiveness, although the patients reported less emotional warmth from their parents. From a sample that consisted mostly of women with bipolar disorder, Pollack (1993) found that 53% reported a history of abuse. However, a related study showed equally pronounced histories of abuse in patients with borderline personality disorder, but rates lower than 5% among a comparison sample of psychiatric controls, which included patients with bipolar disorder, antisocial personality disorder,and schizotypal personality disorder (Herman, Perry, & van der Kolk, 1989).

It is debatable whether early experiences in the family of origin are etiological in bipolar disorder. Early-onset cases may experience a particular pattern of special attention and demand for achievement, which sets up excessive needs for dependency and attention. Glassner and Haldipur (1985) explained that such experiences can lead to envy from others, competition, and ultimately loneliness. These conflicts are thought to explain the extreme mood swings in bipolar disorder: "The oscillations in mood correspond to internalization and externalization of the conflict; during the phase of depression all interest in the external environment is lost with symptoms of guilt and apathy, whereas in the manic phase the obverse is true" (Glassner & Haldipur, 1985, p. 393). This argument notwithstanding, many of the standard family environment variables that have been implicated in the origins of other mental health problems have not emerged as significant discriminators between patients with bipolar disorder and other members of the population. Consequently, the early childhood experiences of these patients are generally unremarkable.

Adult Experiences

Many adult psychiatric patients can be found still residing with their parents. Such individuals remain in the family of origin in lieu of developing a separate family of orientation, as noted in earlier chapters. Social relationships and communication in this context are powerful predictors of the course of bipolar disorder. One such predictive variable is EE, which, as described in Chapter 4, is evident in attitudes and behaviors reflective of criticism and overinvolvement. These are expressed during a standardized interview between a parent and researcher, and are implicitly assumed to be manifested in family interactions and relations.

When patients with bipolar disorder were followed over a period of 9 months after hospital discharge, those who returned to high-EE families were 5.5 times more likely to relapse than patients discharged to low-EE family environments (Miklowitz, Goldstein, Nuechterlein, Snyder, & Mintz, 1988). In a related study, families of patients with mania were as likely to be high-EE as were families of patients with schizophrenia (Miklowitz, Goldstein, Nuechterlein, Snyder, & Doane, 1987). In this study, 90% of the patients with mania who resided with high-EE relatives had poor clinical outcomes over the course of a 9-month follow-up period, in contrast to 54% of the patients who lived inlow-EE families. Another study by this team indicated a relapse rate of 92% over the course of 2 years for patients with bipolar disorder who returned to high-EE households, compared to only 39% among those who returned to low-EE households (Miklowitz, Simoneau, Sachs-Ericsson, Warner, & Suddath, 1996). The mean duration to relapse was similarly suggestive: 34 weeks for those returning to high-EE households, compared with 52 weeks for those who lived in low-EE environments. A unique aspect of this study was the inclusion of both high-EE parents and high-EE spouses. Comparisons revealed that parents scored considerably higher than spouses on the EE dimensions of overinvolvement and criticism, suggesting that EE may be especially problematic when patients reside with their families of origin as opposed to their families of orientation.

Miklowitz et al. (1987) explained that EE may reflect a parent's tendency to react negatively to disturbances presented by the psychiatric patient upon his or her return to the home. This criticism and overinvolvement are likely to be taxing for the patient, thus precipitating an exacerbation of symptoms and relapse. It is assumed that EE, as assessed in a private interview with a family member, manifests itself in the family's actual social interactions. However, this expectation has not always been borne out empirically (Goldstein, 1999; Miklowtiz et al., 1988; Tompson, Rea, Goldstein, Miklowitz, & Weisman, 2000). Family EE may also interfere with effective treatment of patients with bipolar disorder, especially in cases where family members might otherwise be able to play a role in the treatment process (Tompson et al., 2000).

Research findings on bipolar disorder and EE are remarkably similar to those on schizophrenia and EE; in both cases, EE appears to be a strong predictor of relapse. Perhaps something in the nature of these two disorders simultaneously engenders attitudes of hostility and overinvolvement in parents, and extreme sensitivity to this among patients. Regardless of the explanation for the similarity, the parallel findings on family EE and relapse for schizophrenia and bipolar disorder again illustrate how these two problems occupy neighboring positions on the continuum from extreme disturbance to complete normality.

The behavioral counterpart of EE in family interactions is AS, as also described in Chapter 4. Whereas EE is coded from an interview with a family member in the absence of the patient, AS is coded from actual family problem-solving discussions. Families are categorized as negative, mixed, or benign in their AS. Families with a negative-AS profile are prone to making harshly critical, guilt-inducing, and intrusive "mind-reading" statements during family problem-solving discussions. In the Miklowitz et al. (1987) study mentioned above, 91% of patients with bipolar disorder discharged to negative-AS families had poor clinical outcomes over a 9-month observation period, compared with 55% from benign-AS families. On the other hand, the patients who returned to benign-AS families actually showed steady improvements in their social adjustment (Miklowitz et al., 1988). As might be expected, negative AS is evident not only through relatives' verbal behaviors, but in their nonverbal behaviors as well. Negative-AS parents of patients with bipolar disorder engage in fewer affiliative nonverbal communication behaviors such as smiling, head nodding, forward leaning, and illustrator gestures during family discussions, when contrasted with benign-AS parents (Simoneau et al., 1996). These are the behaviors that people look for to feel supported and accepted by others. Collectively, these findings show that the harsh and rejecting behaviors of key relatives, as manifested in AS, are associated with a poor prognosis in bipolar disorder.

Both EE and AS may be overt signs of family stress and distress. If one adopts a systems perspective, it makes little sense to ask whether EE and AS are *responses* to a patient's illness or *causes* of it. In systems theory, all parts and their processes are related to all other parts and processes in the system. Although it has been argued that many family characteristics in cases of bipolar disorder are consequences of the patients' illness (Moltz, 1993), and indeed many may be, family dynamics such as EE and AS have been documented to predict subsequent changes in patients' symptomatology, indicating that patients' symptoms are influenced by their family interactions. Furthermore, empirical evidence indicates that patients find their parents' negative-AS behavior to be stressful (Altorfer, Goldstein, Miklowitz, & Nuechterlein, 1992; Koenig, Sachs-Ericsson, & Miklowitz, 1997). At the same time, it should be obvious that parents' social interaction behaviors are not entirely independent of and unresponsive to their children's distress and communication problems. In fact, in bipolar disorder, a *patient's* affective attitude toward a parent is predictive of the parent's AS (Goldstein, Rea, & Miklowitz, 1996). In schizophrenia, the parent's affective attitude toward the patient is thought to predict that parent's AS. Thus, in bipolar disorder, there are reciprocal interpersonal patterns that may maintain the disorder.

What makes EE and AS so stressful for recovering patients? For most people, their parents are the last line of defense against an otherwise cruel world. When there is no solace to be found in other interpersonal relationships, most expect to find at least some support from family-of-origin members. These are relationships of obligation, and during hard times, they may represent the only refuge available. When these family relationships turn hostile, overinvolved, and emotionally reactive, what was once shelter from the stresses of life becomes a stressor itself. What makes the stressor particularly caustic is the fact that it is a powerful violation of expectations and may signal the end of *any* available social support, leaving a patient with feelings of total rejection and alienation.

CD involves the use of odd, idiosyncratic, amorphous, and fragmented language during social interaction. Parents of patients with schizophrenia are prone to exhibit CD, as noted in Chapter 4; however, problems with CD may not be specific to these parents. In fact, parents of patients with mania are indistinguishable from those of patients with schizophrenia in overall levels of CD (Goldstein et al., 1996; Miklowitz et al., 1991). Certain types of CD, such as *odd word usage* (using words in odd ways, leaving words out of utterances, uttering words out of order, use of unnecessary words—e.g., "There were a number of different distinct times down the entire road when she couldn't get that act together") and *tangential responses* (failure to acknowledge others' statements—e.g., Patient: "When are we going to leave?" Parent: "That's a beautiful painting"), are actually more prevalent among parents of patients with mania. These patients, in Miklowitz et al.'s (1991) study, exhibited CD patterns similar to those of their parents.

The coding scheme used to assess CD overlaps considerably with the TDI as used, for example, in Solovay et al.'s (1987) investigation. CD is undoubtedly a manifestation of thought disorder through communication with other people. An obvious conclusion might be that parent–child similarities in CD represent genetic transmission of thought disorder. However, a social learning account would also predict a parent–child association in CD, whereby the parent models bizarre communication behavior that is then incorporated into the child's discourse. Like many other behaviors acquired through observational learning, children may just assume that if their parents engage in the behavior, it is the right thing to do. Simply interacting with a parent exhibiting CD, or observing an interaction with another family member, may lead a child to believe that "this is the appropriate way to talk to other people." In either case, parents of bipolar patients exhibit problems with CD that are of the same magnitude as the problems of parents of schizophrenia patients. In both disorders, this deviant communication pattern can also be detected in the patients themselves.

Bipolar disorder is associated with additional *family relationship problems*. The family interactions of patients with bipolar disorder are marked by a high percentage of control attempts by both patients and parents (Wuerker, 1994). This battle for control is more pronounced than in families of patients with schizophrenia. The majority of family members who care for patients with bipolar disorder report at least moderate burden, especially due to the patients' misery, irritability, and withdrawal (Perlick et al., 1999). These family relationship problems can also affect the course of the disorder. For example, 67% of patients undergoing treatment for bipolar disorder who indicated that they had good relations with their extended families had no major recurrences over a 4-year follow-up period, compared to only 20% of those patients who had poor relations with their extended families (Stefos, Bauwens, Staner, Pardoen, & Mendlewicz, 1996).

Summary

Thus far, it has been difficult to identify and replicate any particular pattern of early childhood experiences in the family of origin that is associated with later bipolar disorder. However, several interpersonal dynamics have been implicated in the families of adults with bipolar disorder. Chief among these are EE and AS, each of which negatively influences the course of the disorder. Patients and their family members also exhibit CD at levels equivalent to those of patients with schizophrenia and their families. Family members report a great deal of burden associated with caring for a patient with bipolar disorder. A generally poor-quality relationship with extended family members has been shown to increase the probability of relapse over time. In short, there are striking parallels in the family dynamics of schizophrenia and bipolar disorder. The operations of EE, AS, CD, and family burden are remarkably similar, suggesting that these are neighboring disorders both phenomenologically and interpersonally. Although questions of causality are notoriously difficult to sort out in family studies, due in part to the confounding of genes and environment, a family systems view would hold that both patients and their family members influence and are influenced by each other.

FAMILY-OF-ORIENTATION EXPERIENCES IN BIPOLAR DISORDER

Marital and Long-Term Romantic Relationships

Research on the marriages and long-term romantic relationships of people with bipolar disorder provide additional evidence of poor social adjustment. A primary finding in this area is that people with bipolar disorder are less likely than other members of the population to be married or in stable close relationships (Coryell et al., 1993; Kennedy, Thompson, Stancer, Roy, & Persad, 1983). Those patients who have ever been married are twice as likely as subjects without a history of mania to have been divorced or separated (Coryell et al., 1993). The study by Coryell et al. (1993) suggests a more pervasive problem with divorce or separation among patients with bipolar disorder (44%) than patients with unipolar depression (26%). This problem may be pursuant to the high levels of conflict and diminished mutuality characteristic of marriages in bipolar disorder (Hoover & Fitzgerald, 1981a, 1981b).

Among those patients who are currently married or in long-term close relationships, what are their relationships like? Peven and Shulman (1998) noted that "people with bipolar disorder can be effervescent, enthusiastic, attractive, and expansive at times, but sad, anergic, and anhedonic at other times. In a hypomanic state, they are charming and witty and exciting to be with. In a depressed state, they can be frustrating, unattractive, and gloomy" (pp. 18–19). This oscillation between extremes in interpersonal reactions appears to take a toll on the close relationships of those afflicted with bipolar disorder.

A survey study of patients with bipolar disorder found that they longed for more emotional contact and desired more sexual involvement from their partners (Matussek, Luks, & Seibt, 1986). In this study, these patients were more likely than those with unipolar depression to long for more togetherness with their partners; they also expressed more difficulty in standing up to their partners during conflicts. From a study of women, mostly with bipolar disorder, came results showing that 56%

experienced sexual disruption in their close relationships, and an approximately equal proportion indicated that their illness caused them to withdraw and isolate themselves from others (Pollack, 1993). Because over 50% of this sample had a history of abuse, these results might reflect the combined effect of a traumatic interpersonal history and affective illness. As in Pollack's study, themes of sexual dissatisfaction were prominent among the patients with bipolar disorder studied by Coryell et al. (1993).

Notwithstanding their feelings of dissatisfaction and lack of fulfillment, patients with bipolar disorder are not as distressed over their marriages as their well spouses are. Only 5% of such patients indicated that they would not have married had they known about the illness, compared to 53% of their spouses (Targum, Dibble, Davenport, & Gershon, 1981). Only 11% of these same patients felt that their spouses would not have married them had they known about the illness—suggesting a serious lack of awareness or denial. Although patients with bipolar disorder will express some dissatisfaction with their marriages, they tend to underestimate the burden they present to their spouses. This same lack of awareness is evident in assessments of marital conflict. Husband–wife reports of marital conflict correlated at only $r = .08$ for couples in which a spouse has bipolar disorder, whereas this same correlation was $r = .51$ for healthy control couples (Hoover & Fitzgerald, 1981a). A follow-up to Targum et al.'s (1981) study produced results that were similar in some respects but a bit optimistic in other regards. When Frank et al. (1981) asked patients with bipolar disorder and their well spouses whether they would marry the same persons if they had to live their lives over again, 81% of the patients indicated that they would, compared to only 50% of their well spouses (because of this study's small n, this difference was not significant). However, over 80% of the couples believed that their marriages were at least as good as others that they knew of. Couples in this study also described their courtships as happy and smooth, and they were indistinguishable from healthy controls in terms of the extent to which their marriages had met or failed to meet their expectations.

There is good reason to suspect that the sometimes positive and upbeat reports of marital well-being among patients with bipolar disorder are not just the result of grandiose delusions. In general, the marriages of psychiatric patients with positive behavioral symptoms, as would be expected with bipolar disorder, are more satisfying than those of patients with negative behavioral symptoms (Hooley, Richters, Weintraub, & Neale, 1987). Positive symptoms involve hallucinations, delusions, elated mood, and grandiosity, for example. These have no counterpart in normal functioning. Negative symptoms, on the other hand, involve an absence of normal functions, such as lack of emotion, depression, lethargy, and leisure-time impairment. Hooley et al. (1987) found that patients with schizophrenia and bipolar disorder were more likely to have positive symptom profiles, whereas those with unipolar depression were dominated by negative symptom profiles. They hypothesize that spouses of patients with positive symptoms do not hold their partners accountable for the symptoms, since these are seen as less controllable than negative symptoms. For this reason, spouses of patients with positive symptoms are able to maintain more positive views of their partners and marriages.

As with family relations more generally, the EE of patients' spouses has an impact on the course of bipolar disorder (Priebe, Wildgrube, & Muller-Oerlinghausen, 1989). Priebe et al. (1989) found that 79% of patients who lived with low-EE relatives (most of whom were spouses) were free of any psychotic symptoms over a 9-month period, whereas just 18% of those who lived with high-EE spouses were free of psychotic symptoms, despite an average of 12.5 years of treatment with lithium. Here again, the views of a spouse toward a patient and his or her illness proved to have a substantial effect on the course of bipolar disorder.

Suicide is a very serious problem associated with bipolar disorder, with rates far exceeding those for most other mental disorders. In an effort to understand why these patients attempt and commit suicide so frequently, Tsai et al. (1999) examined 158 patients with bipolar disorder, 68 of whom had attempted suicide. They found that the patients who had attempted suicide were 2.85 times more likely than those who had not to have experienced significant problems with a spouse or long-term romantic partner. This finding suggests that one of the key risk factors for suicide among patients with bipolar disorder may be poor relational satisfaction. Interpersonal antecedents to suicide are probably not specific to cases of suicide among these patients, however. There is no reason to believe that people with unipolar depression, for example, are less likely to weigh interpersonal issues when contemplating suicide.

Summary

Bipolar disorder significantly reduces the likelihood of getting married and staying married. The marriages of patients with bipolar disorder are characterized by a longing for intimacy and problems with handling conflict. Spouses of these patients have bleaker views of their marriages than the patients do, and the patients are unaware of this. The marriages of patients with positive symptom profiles are happier than those with negative symptom profiles, explaining why some such marriages may not be as distressed. Spousal EE can adversely affect the course of bipolar disorder, putting a patient at risk for the experience of psychotic symptoms. Troubles with marriage and similar close relationships may contribute substantially to the suicide problem among people with bipolar disorder. Collectively, these findings point to impairment of marital/ long-term romantic relations in bipolar disorder, with some heterogeneity possibly explained by the dominant symptom profile, which should covary with the bipolar I or II distinction. Whereas some of these problems are surely the result of living with a patient, spousal EE appears to be closely related to maintenance of bipolar disorder.

Parental Effects on Children

Children of parents with bipolar disorder, like children of parents with unipolar depression, are at increased risk for psychosocial problems. The lifetime prevalence of psychiatric diagnoses among children of mothers with bipolar disorder was recorded at 72%, compared to 43% in children of medically ill controls and 26% in children of healthy mothers (Hammen, Burge, Burney, & Adrian, 1990). However, 82% of the children of mothers with unipolar depression had a psychiatric diagnosis—more than any other group in this study. Children of mothers with bipolar disorder are thus at elevated risk for psychiatric problems of their own when compared to children in the general population. At the same time, they are no more likely to have such problems as children of mothers with unipolar depression, for whom this risk is exceptionally high.

In addition to psychiatric problems such as depression and anxiety, children of parents with bipolar disorder also tend to have social-behavioral problems. These involve, for example, aggression, diminished altruism and sharing with peers, less social interaction with peers, and overreactivity to stress (Zahn-Waxler, Cummings, McKnew, & Radke-Yarrow, 1984; Zahn-Waxler, McKnew, Cummings, Davenport, & Radke-Yarrow, 1984). In the Zahn-Waxler, McKnew, et al. (1984) study, in the week prior to observations of the children, the mothers with bipolar disorder were more sad, fearful, enraged, and less capable of pleasure than control mothers. These authors therefore argue that many of the problems with social behaviors driven by negative affect may be influenced by parents' own problems in these same areas.

Skeptics who feel that the emotional and social-behavioral problems found in the children in these studies are merely the results of a genetic transmission of psychosocial disorder might take note of parent–child synchrony in depressive episodes. When children of mothers with unipolar depression or bipolar disorder were followed over the course of a year, a high concordance was found for the occurrence and timing of children's and mothers' diagnoses of depressive episodes (Hammen, Burge, & Adrian, 1991). In other words, when mothers experienced a diagnosable episode of depression, their children were likely to experience one as well, in close temporal proximity. A genetic transmission model might account for parent–child concordance, but not for temporal synchrony. Hammen et al. (1991) suggest that this phenomenon may be the result of the corrosive effect of depression on parenting (which then has negative effects on the child), or of the collateral stressor effect (in which both parent and child are negatively affected by the same stressors).

Children of mothers with either bipolar disorder or unipolar depression have been shown to be particularly vulnerable to the ill effects of stress (Hammen et al., 1991). Furthermore, many of these stressors are at least partly self-generated by the children (Adrian & Hammen, 1993). Explicit comparisons of children whose mothers had unipolar depression versus bipolar disorder revealed exposure to less family conflict among children in the latter group. However, these same children experienced heightened conflict with peers, as did children of mothers with unipolar depression, when compared to both medically ill and normal controls.

Summary

The offspring of parents who have bipolar disorder are at risk for both emotional and social-behavioral problems. Rates of depression, anxiety, and aggressiveness are elevated, and altruism and sharing are diminished, among such children. These children are especially vulnerable to the ill effects of stress and may actually contribute to many of the stressors that they experience, particularly those that are interpersonal in nature. The close temporal proximity of mother–child depressive episodes among mothers with either unipolar depression or bipolar disorder suggests that these children's troubles are the result of (1) interaction with and exposure to parents with mood disorders, and/or (2) the experience of collateral stressors.

GENERAL PERSONAL RELATIONSHIPS IN BIPOLAR DISORDER: REACTIONS TO INTERPERSONAL STRESS

Bipolar disorder is activated and exacerbated, at least in part, by interpersonal stressors. When asked for their opinions of what caused their bipolar disorder, 74% of patients in one study pointed to interpersonal factors (Targum et al., 1981). There is some evidence linking vulnerability to particular interpersonal stressors with symptom severity in bipolar disorder. In particular, *sociotropy–autonomy* marks a particular predisposition predictive of negative symptomatological reactions to particular classes of stressors. People who score high on sociotropy define their self-worth and efficacy in terms of interactions and relations with other people. Conversely, people who score high on autonomy derive their self-worth and efficacy from independent and autonomous achievements. Theoretically, people who are more sociotropic would be expected to be more vulnerable to interpersonal stressors.

Hammen, Ellicott, and Gitlin (1992) followed a group of patients with bipolar disorder over a period of 18 months, after assessing their sociotropy–autonomy and their experience of stressful events. Symptoms of bipolar disorder were exacerbated as a function of experiencing interpersonally oriented stressors, and of being more sociotropic. Sociotropy appeared to place subjects at risk for heightened symptoms even if they experienced low levels of interpersonal events, whereas people who scored low on sociotropy only experienced heightened symptoms in response to high levels of stressful interpersonal events. It must be noted that in an earlier investigation, Hammen, Ellicott, Gitlin, and Jamison (1989) did not find this sociotropy–interpersonal stress–vulnerability effect, although it was evident among patients with unipolar depression. This suggests that the match between interpersonal stressful events and interpersonal vulnerabilities may be more important in unipolar than in bipolar depression. A related study also found that subjects with unipolar depression were more likely than those with bipolar depression to actually generate interpersonally oriented stressful events, such as conflicts (Hammen, 1991). In this study, the subjects with bipolar depression did not differ significantly from medically ill or healthy controls in terms of experiencing interpersonal stressful events. Although symptoms of bipolar disorder may be triggered by interpersonal stressors, particularly when a patient has a predisposition to define his or her self-worth in interpersonal terms, patients with bipolar disorder are not as likely to actually generate interpersonal stressors as are people with unipolar depression.

Social support is believed to mitigate the ill effects of stressful events. Among patients with bipolar disorder, higher levels of social support are predictive of symptom-free "survival time" (Johnson, Winett, Meyer, Greenhouse, & Miller, 1999; Stefos et al., 1996). However, social support has proven to protect against depressive episodes but not manic episodes (Johnson et al., 1999). When people are feeling depressed, social support from others may involve tangible assistance with the source of the problem, cognitive restructuring or reframing so that the problem is no longer viewed as catastrophic, and distraction to take the depressed person's mind off the problem temporarily. Each of these may be effective, at least in the short run, in alleviating some of the dysphoria felt by people who are depressed. It is interesting however, that many of these same tactics have little or no value for altering the mood of someone in a manic episode. To the extent that stressors exacerbate symptoms of bipolar disorder, social support may be helpful for minimizing some of the symptoms (depressive) but not others (manic).

COMORBIDITY OF BIPOLAR DISORDER WITH OTHER MENTAL HEALTH PROBLEMS

People with bipolar disorder have relatively high rates of the Cluster B, or "dramatic–emotional," personality disorders (i.e., antisocial, narcissistic, histrionic, and borderline) (Turley, Bates, Edwards, & Jackson, 1992). In one sample of patients with bipolar disorder, 45% had at least one personality disorder, and many had several personality disorders (Barbato & Hafner, 1998). A study of personality disorder rates in outpatients with bipolar disorder compared to controls yielded estimates of 48% and 15%, respectively (Uecok, Karaveli, Kundakci, & Yazici, 1998). Zuckerman (1999) explained the connection between bipolar disorder and borderline personality disorder by noting:

> Borderline personality disorder represents a mixture of impulsive self-damaging behavior and unstable mood with agitated depressive features, unstable and ambivalent interpersonal relationships, suicidal threats or attempts, intense inappropriate displays of anger, and transient stress-related paranoid or disorganized symptoms. In some ways it is like bipolar disorder except that the two phases are mixed and more reactive to interpersonal problems. (p. 158)

As the review in this chapter shows, however, symptoms of bipolar disorder can be triggered and exacerbated by interpersonal stressors, much like symptoms of borderline personality disorder. In both disorders, interpersonal relationships are turbulent, perhaps as both a result and a cause of the disorder's symptoms.

As noted earlier in this chapter, bipolar disorder shares some significant features with schizophrenia. It is sometimes a challenge to distinguish the two. From an interpersonal perspective, perhaps the most striking similarity is the evidence for CD and negative AS in family interactions. It is tempting to speculate that these family interaction processes may create a vulnerability to, and/or be responsive to, nonspecific psychotic symptoms such as delusions and hallucinations. In terms of social style, people with bipolar disorder, like those with schizophrenia, often communicate with other people in ways that are dramatic, odd, or grandiose. At the level of psychological and interpersonal symptoms, there is substantial overlap between schizophrenia and bipolar disorder, suggesting that the two problems occupy neighboring positions on the continuum from gross psychosocial disturbance to normal psychosocial functioning.

In addition to being highly comorbid with personality disorders, and to some extent with schizophrenia, bipolar disorder tends to co-occur with eating disorders and substance use disorders. Each of these patterns is discussed in more detail in Chapters 7 and 8. Obviously, these problems have been linked to some of the same interpersonal issues that are evident in bipolar disorder, particularly marital and family-of-origin difficulties.

CONCLUSION

The discovery of a genetic component in bipolar disorder, along with the documented efficacy of pharmacological agents for its treatment, has made biological explanations of bipolar disorder very fashionable. Attributions to biological origins are also very face-saving for patients and their families. However, as Miklowitz and Alloy (1999) point out, these biological vulnerabilities are the backdrop, in front of which interpersonal stressors and disturbances in family relations profoundly influence the course of the disorder. They conclude that "social and environmental factors may evoke or protect against biological, genetic, or cognitive vulnerabilities to bipolar disorder" (Miklowitz & Alloy, 1999, p. 555). A similar conclusion was drawn by Akiskal and his colleagues, who observed that the symptoms of bipolar disorder, which may be biologically caused, clearly lead to interpersonal impairment (e.g., divorce, rejection from others), which further exacerbates the condition's severity and chronicity (Akiskal, Khani, & Scott-Strauss, 1979; Perugi et al., 1998).

Unlike their counterparts with unipolar depression, people with bipolar disorder (at least during manic episodes) are prone to excessive talkativeness, exhibiting pressured speech, and grandiose ideas, loose associations, disorganized trains of thought, and ease of distractibility. Their excessive gregariousness may be amusing and even charming at times. However, the sheer chaos in their interpersonal communication, driven in part by thought disorder, undoubtedly interferes with competent social interaction. Other people may be annoyed, confused, and even frightened by the social behavior of these patients. There is some suggestion that patients with bipolar disorder may manipulate others, presumably in the service of fulfilling their own dependency needs.

There has not been a great deal of research on the social behavior of bipolar patients in bipolar depressive episodes. It is assumed, at least implicitly, that during such states they experience many of the same problems as patients with unipolar depression, such as social withdrawal and avoidance, interpersonal rejection, and stormy relationships.

To explore the interpersonal origins and concomitants of bipolar disorder, scientists have turned to family-of-origin studies. No clear patterns of early childhood experiences have been identified. However, a number of family-of-origin dynamics influence the course of adult patients with bipolar disorder. Some methodologically sophisticated research shows that patients discharged to families that are high in EE, and/or that have a negative AS, are more prone to relapse than those who reside in more emotionally subdued families. CD, family burden, and generally poor relations with family members are also evident among people with bipolar disorder, and may even influence its course as well. Many of these family problems may stress a patient, contributing to his or her symptoms. From a family systems perspective, these problems would be interpreted as both causes and effects of the disorder.

Like people with unipolar depression, patients with bipolar disorder have difficulty establishing and maintaining romantic and marital relationships. When they do, considerable conflict, longing for intimacy, and sexual disruption ensue. These patients appear almost oblivious to the burden they place on their spouses. Spousal EE has also proven to affect the course of the disorder. The positive symptom profile of bipolar disorder may provide a modicum of relief from marital distress, due to the external attribution that spouses make for such symptoms. In their role as parents, patients with bipolar disorder tend to raise children with psychological and behavioral problems of their own. These children are especially vulnerable to the ill effects of stress, and their symptoms appear yoked to those of their ill parents.

Finally, symptoms of bipolar disorder are responsive to interpersonal stressors. Such stressors commonly precipitate episodes of the illness. Whereas social support from others has proven to suppress depressive episodes, it does not appear effective at preventing mania.

Like two closely related mental health problems, depression and schizophrenia, bipolar disorder profoundly affects and is affected by interpersonal phenomena. Disturbed family dynamics and problems with close relationships figure prominently in the phenomenology of this severe and debilitating problem. Though biological agents have been implicated in the distal cause of this disorder, its maintenance and course are responsive to the many interpersonal problems experienced by patients with bipolar disorder.

6

Personality Disorders

DEFINITION AND SYMPTOMS

A *personality disorder* is an enduring and stable pattern of behavior and cognition that deviates from normative standards and expectations in one's culture (American Psychiatric Association, 2000). This pattern of behavior and experience has its onset during adolescence or early adulthood, and leads to tangible distress and impairment. Most people who exhibit personality disorders by definition have interpersonal problems. The official DSM-IV-TR diagnostic criteria for a personality disorder include manifestations of stable and enduring problematic behaviors and experiences in at least two of the following domains: cognition, affectivity, interpersonal functioning, and impulse control. The enduring pattern must be pervasive and inflexible across a variety of social situations, and it must lead to impairment or distress in social or occupational areas of functioning (American Psychiatric Association, 2000). The concept of *functional inflexibility* implies that the individual relates to others, expresses feelings, and resolves conflicts in a rigid fashion, with tactics that are often ill suited for the situation at hand (Millon, 1990). Symptoms of specific personality disorders are discussed in the sections that follow.

To a greater extent than views of other mental health problems such as depression and schizophrenia, scientific and clinical views of personality disorders are still under construction (see, e.g., appendices in DSM-III-R and DSM-IV-TR). Because of their relatively recent addition to the DSM and recognition by scientists, many personality disorders have not been informed by decades of principled research, as in the case of some other mental health problems. Partly for this reason, estimates of the prevalence of personality disorders in the general population are sometimes scarce. Both the Epidemiologic Catchment Area study (Regier et al., 1993) and the National Comorbidity Survey (Kessler et al., 1994) assessed the prevalence of antisocial personality disorder. The former study indicated a 1.5% 1-year prevalence rate, and the latter a 3.5% lifetime prevalence rate, for antisocial personality disorder. In conjunction with the Epidemiologic Catchment Area study, Nestadt et al. (1990) estimated the prevalence of histrionic personality disorder at 2.2% in the general population. In a college student population, the prevalence of histrionic personality disorder may be as high as 6% (Bornstein, 1999). Considering the fact that there are over a dozen personality disorders described in DSM-IV-TR (when those targeted in Appendix B for future consideration are included), it is clear that personality disorders collectively are common in the general population, with lifetime prevalence estimates on the order of 10–13% (Weissman, 1993).

Like the research on personality disorders more generally, the interpersonal research is still in the early stages of development, with a few notable exceptions. The literature on personality disorders is replete with essays based on clinical observation that advance various theories, hypotheses, and descriptions of the disorders. In contrast, large-sample, controlled scientific investigations are somewhat rare. As a result, the state of the literature on interpersonal aspects of personality disorders is similar to that of the literature on schizophrenia during the era of the 1960s and 1970s, again with a few notable exceptions.

PREVIEW

Like many other psychological problems, most personality disorders are associated with problematic interpersonal relationships, virtually by definition. Some of the most striking evidence of interpersonal disruption appears in the domain of *family-of-origin experiences*. Themes of parental abuse, insecure attachment, excessive parental attention, parental overinvolvement, and family chaos are rampant in the literature on personality disorders. Some have theorized that these early interpersonal experiences play a significant role in the pathogenesis of these disorders. Far less research has been done on *family-of-orientation experiences* than on family-of-origin experiences in the personality disorders, primarily because so few persons with these disorders do form such families; however, the existing research indicates that when these persons do marry or form stable romantic relationships, their relationships are characterized by distress and dissatisfaction. Interpersonal problems are not just confined to the various family relationships, but also extend into the domain of *general personal relationships*. Many people with personality disorders have stormy and unstable personal relationships. They often elicit interpersonal rejection, and experience conflict with others and loneliness. In the area of *interpersonal communication,* there is a tendency for people with certain types of personality disorders to use communication with others for the function of seeking attention. A powerfully complicating factor in the personality disorders is their high comorbidity with other psychosocial problems. Research studies have revealed alarmingly high rates of such problems as depression, schizophrenia, bipolar disorder, eating disorders, substance use disorders, and somatoform disorders among people with personality disorders.

INTERPERSONAL DESCRIPTION OF VARIOUS PERSONALITY DISORDERS

Currently, 10 different personality disorders (plus the residual category of *personality disorder not otherwise specified*) are formally recognized in DSM-IV-TR (American Psychiatric Association, 2000). However, over the years various diagnostic categories have been revised and added, and there is reason to suspect that this may continue in the future. One useful way to organize, describe, and map the personality disorders is with a version of Leary's (1957) interpersonal circumplex, using the dimensions of *dominant–submissive* and *hostile–nurturant* (Blackburn, 1998; Kiesler, van Denburg, Sikes-Nova, Larus, & Goldston, 1990). For example, those with dependent personality disorder are in the submissive and nurturant quadrant, while those with narcissistic, histrionic, or antisocial personality disorder are situated in the dominant and hostile quadrant. As evident from Figure 6.1, the majority of the personality disorders fall into the hostile half of the circumplex. Although all personality disorders have interpersonal implications and ramifications, Blackburn (1998) argues that the disorders projected toward the outer edge of the circumplex, such as dependent, narcissistic, and histrionic, have more evident interpersonal implications.

It should be recalled that Leary, who was a pioneer in interpersonal approaches to mental health problems, eschewed the medical disease model in favor of a more dimensional view of personality. According to such a view, personality disorders can be characterized as more extreme positions on the continuum of personality traits. Difficulty in identifying exactly where "normal" becomes "abnormal" highlights the ambiguity and imprecision that are sometimes evident in the personality disorder construct. It may be unwise to think about something like histrionic personality disorder as a disease entity, in the same way that one thinks

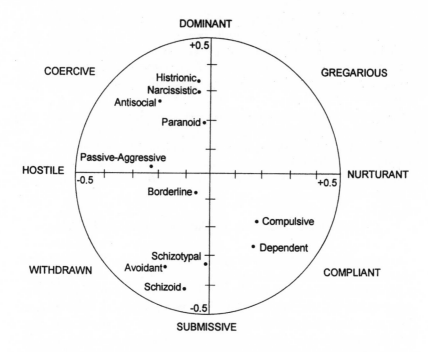

FIGURE 6.1. The interpersonal circle: Plot of correlations of Millon Clinical Multiaxial Inventory (MCMI-I) personality disorder scale with dominant–submissive and hostile–nurturant coordinates. From Blackburn (1998). Copyright 1998 by The Guilford Press. Reprinted by permission.

about Parkinson's disease or bulimia nervosa (Millon, 1990). Rather, a personality disorder may be more like high blood pressure—an exaggerated version of a normal phenomenon, with little more than an arbitrary "cutoff point" at which normal becomes viewed as pathological.

Because a thorough review of the interpersonal implications of all personality disorders is beyond the scope of this chapter, only some of these disorders are examined. The selection of disorders for presentation is guided largely by the availability of scientific research on the interpersonal implications, causes, and consequences of the various disorders. The descriptions of personality disorders presented in this chapter draw heavily on the writings of Theodore Millon, whose work has literally laid the foundation for a modern understanding of personality disorders. More comprehensive discussions and descriptions of the various disorders can be found in his principal works (e.g., Millon, 1981, 1990; Millon & Davis, 2000).

BORDERLINE PERSONALITY DISORDER

Borderline personality disorder (hereafter abbreviated as BPD) is the most frequently diagnosed of the personality disorders (Widiger & Trull, 1993). Approximately 15–25% of psychiatric inpatients and outpatients carry this diagnosis (Gunderson & Zanarini, 1987). Its principal features involve instability of interpersonal relationships, affect, and self-image (American Psychiatric Association, 2000). People with BPD exhibit intense and variable mood, ranging from irritability to euphoria to impulsive anger and even self-destructive behavior. This moodiness is combined with more generally aberrant and aloof behavior, a dissociated self-image, frantic efforts to avoid abandonment, impulsivity, suicidal behavior and threats, feelings of emptiness, problems with anger control, and occasional paranoid ideation (American Psychiatric Association, 2000). Benjamin (1996) summarized the interpersonal basis of BPD by stating, "There is a morbid fear of abandonment and a wish for protective nurturance" (p. 124). The characteristic desire of a person with BPD to fuse with another person for emotional support is a sign of ego weakness and identity disturbance (Millon & Davis, 2000). It is not surprising that BPD is highly comorbid with depression.

Commensurate with its diagnostic popularity, more research has been conducted on BPD than on any other personality disorder. Much of this research has focused specifically on interpersonal aspects of the personality disorder. Since unstable interpersonal relations and frantic efforts to avoid abandonment are part of the diagnostic criteria for BPD, it is tautological to assert that this disorder has negative interpersonal implications and consequences. As Segal (1990) noted, "Many borderline symptoms are seen as arising primarily within the context of a relationship, where the involvement of another person is the arena in which an essential component of the patient's psychopathology emerges" (p. 27). Indeed, research on BPD indicates a pervasive pattern of interpersonal problems in both adulthood and childhood that extend far beyond those outlined in the diagnostic criteria of DSM-IV-TR.

It should be obvious to even the casual observer that people with BPD have a long history of interpersonal problems both professionally and socially, and close relationships that may best be characterized as stormy (Modestin, 1987; Trull, Useda, Conforti, & Doan, 1997). Symptoms of BPD are positively associated with social conflict and feelings of loneliness (Johnson, Rabkin, Williams, Remien, & Gorman, 2000). Symptoms of the disorder are also associated with endorsing a *ludus* (game-playing) and *mania* (manic, possessive) love style (Arnold & Thompson, 1996). Accordingly, persons with BPD are less likely to find themselves in loving relationships (Benjamin, 1992).

Individuals with BPD experience a great deal of interpersonal problems and distress. Trull et al. (1997) note that these individuals have excessive interpersonal dependency needs, which make them particularly vulnerable to interpersonal losses. On the other hand, they employ manipulative tactics that often result in agitation and rejection from others. Thus persons with BPD tend to sabotage the very relationships that they so badly need. This phenomenon may be a consequence of their problems with distance regulation (Melges & Swartz, 1989). According to this hypothesis, whenever patients with BPD move close to or away from other people, they receive negative feedback. Consequently, these patients oscillate between attachment and avoidance. Sadly, people with BPD rarely learn from their interpersonal experiences and often recreate their problems as they move from one relationship to another.

A major component in the interpersonal distress produced and experienced by persons with BPD is emotion dysregulation. As noted above, anxiety about abandonment, excessive anger, and a reactive mood are all problems associated with this disorder. When compared to people with both bipolar disorder and unipolar depression, those with BPD indicated substantially more hostility in their past and present relationships—in terms of both sending and receiving hostility (Benjamin & Wonderlich, 1994; Stern, Herron, Primavera, & Kakuma, 1997). In a unique study of facial expression recognition, people with BPD performed as well as healthy controls and controls with a history of sexual abuse, with the exception of a tendency to overidentify fearful expressions (Wagner & Linehan, 1999). This suggests that BPD is associated with a hypersensitivity or readiness to identify fear in others, which could increase these individuals' own experience of fear in interpersonal contexts (Wagner & Linehan, 1999).

Like those with any of several other mental health problems, people with BPD elicit interpersonal rejection from others (Carroll, Hoenigmann-Stovall, King, Wienhold, & Whitehead, 1998). To give an idea of how potent this rejection effect is, Carroll et al. (1998) compared interpersonal reactions to BPD and narcissistic personality disorder—an intensely annoying syndrome (see below). Other people felt that the subjects with BPD were the more insecure, less powerful, more inactive, more unpredictable, and more unstable of the two groups. Carroll et al. (1998) concluded that the interpersonal consequences of BPD are even more negative than those associated with narcissistic personality disorder. Given the preponderance of interpersonal conflict, emotional lability, and oscillation between attachment and avoidance, it is little wonder that those with BPD create such negative interpersonal impressions.

Experiences in the family of origin have been a focal point in the interpersonal research on BPD (e.g., Gunderson, Kerr, & Englund, 1980;

Links, 1992). Poor maternal and paternal caring, to the point of neglect, in the family of origin are common themes among those with BPD (Gunderson et al., 1980; Nordahl & Stiles, 1997). This lack of parental caring is coupled with a greater overprotectiveness (Links, 1992), similar to that reported by other psychiatric groups. Another family-of-origin phenomenon is the perception by patients with BPD that their mothers were autonomous and hostile toward them (Benjamin & Wonderlich, 1994). This perceived hostility also spills over to perceptions of current relationships with, for example, other patients and hospital staff. A similar theme is evident in the findings of Stern et al. (1997), whose patients with BPD also rated their fathers and mothers as attacking and rejecting. However, these patients also indicated that they too were attacking and rejecting toward their parents. This illustrates how the antecedents to conflictual adult personal relationships clearly have their origins in adolescent, if not preadolescent, relationships.

Themes of separation and loss in the family of origin are common in BPD (Links, 1992; Links & Munroe-Blum, 1990). Links (1992) has argued that the predisposition to BPD is especially pronounced when this loss is due to separation or divorce rather than to death of a parent. Of course, parental conflict would also be exaggerated in such cases, and itself may contribute to the development of symptoms. In any event, such early losses predispose a child to insecure attachment, and explain the clinging attachment and fear of abandonment that are so evident in adults with BPD.

Evidence of sexual abuse in the history of many individuals with BPD indicates noxious boundary violations in the family of origin. A history of incest was evident in 19% and 35% of the cases in two samples of patients with BPD (Stone, 1990). However, the broader category of "childhood sexual abuse" is estimated to have occurred in about 70% of all patients with BPD (Paris, 1994). The relationship between childhood sexual abuse findings and treatment in the family of origin must be interpreted with several caveats. First, pooled across 21 studies, the association between childhood sexual abuse and BPD is only moderate in magnitude, with an effect size of $r = .28$ (Fossati, Madeddu, & Maffei, 1999). Furthermore, childhood sexual abuse is more strongly related to BPD when the abuse is perpetrated by a nonrelative (Fossati et al., 1999; Norden, Klein, Donaldson, Pepper, & Klein, 1995). These findings call into question whether sexual abuse in the family context is a *major* risk factor for BPD. However, the impact of such traumatic interpersonal behavior in a more general context appears to play some role in the disorder. Second, where there is sexual abuse in the family context, significant family dysfunction almost surely coexists with the behavior (Paris, 1994); this calls into question whether it is the abuse per se that contributes to the disorder or the malevolent family environment that tolerates and perhaps even encourages such conduct. Findings such as these have led to the hypothesis that those with BPD tend to internalize abandoning, neglectful, and abusive childhood relationships in such a way as to promote self-abandonment and attack in adulthood (Benjamin, 1996).

The parents of people with BPD appear to have psychosocial disturbances of their own that interfere with effective parenting (Gunderson et al., 1980). It is often the case that these problems are evident in both parents—a phenomenon characterized as "biparental failure" (Links, 1992; Shachnow et al., 1997). In a study of 30 women with BPD and their 60 parents, both parents had an Axis I or Axis II diagnosis in 73% of the families (Shachnow et al., 1997). Even 60% of their grandparents had psychiatric disorders, particularly substance use or mood disorders. A similar analysis of first-degree relatives of patients with BPD revealed that 18% of these relatives had BPD, 10% had antisocial personality disorder, 25% had a mood disorder, and about 25% had a substance use disorder (Zanarini, Gunderson, Marino, Schwartz, & Frankenburg, 1990). These staggering rates of parental psychopathology are consistent with the hypothesis that links disturbed and ineffective parenting to the development of BPD. At the same time, Zanarini et al. (1990) note that these same findings could be interpreted as support for a genetic component in the parental transmission of the disorder. The exact and relative contributions from genes and family environment remain to be established by future research. For the time being, it is apparent that mental health is far more likely to be impaired among parents of individuals with BPD than among parents in the general population. Undoubtedly, this at least has the potential to interfere with effective parenting and care.

Benjamin (1996) has described four family-of-origin processes that lead to the development of BPD. The first is *family chaos*, involving fights, affairs, intoxication, trouble with the law, and suicide attempts. This family dynamic creates a dramatic, soap-opera quality in the family of origin. Second, *traumatic abandonment* is common in these families. Children who later develop BPD are often left alone without adequate care and supervision, during which sexual abuse by others may be perpetrated. The children may interpret this abandonment as resulting from their bad behavior (Millon & Davis, 2000). Third, the families of those who develop BPD tend to *shun autonomy and promote dependency*. These children are socialized to believe that they are flawed, and that their families, miserable as they may be, are their only salvation. Finally, these families only offer *nurturance in response to misery*. These families reinforce displays of helplessness and agony by offering nurturant care in response to such displays, and at no other time. Collectively, these

family-of-origin processes are thought to promote the identity disturbance, emotional liability, fear of abandonment, and suicidal gestures
that are typical of BPD.

Summary

The interpersonal backgrounds of people with BPD are particularly remarkable. Themes of loneliness, conflict, and fear of abandonment are
prevalent. As it is for people with depression, interpersonal rejection is a
notable problem for those with BPD. This may be the result of the tendency in BPD to oscillate between clinging attachment and avoidance—a
pattern that is repulsive to even the most tolerant friend or family member. Experiences in the family of origin are commonly devoid of stability
and nurturance. Rather, one finds a lack of care, frequent abuse, rejection, and psychiatric symptoms emanating from the parents of those
who later develop BPD. It is when parental overinvolvement is combined
with neglect and abuse that symptoms of BPD are especially likely to appear (Links & Munroe-Blum, 1990). This toxic combination of parenting behaviors set the stage for the later interpersonal attachment–avoidance conflict that characterizes BPD.

NARCISSISTIC PERSONALITY DISORDER

Narcissistic personality disorder (hereafter abbreviated as NPD) has to
be one of the most interpersonally obnoxious of the personality disorders. People with NPD have an exaggerated sense of self-worth and
entitlement, coupled with a nearly insatiable thirst for attention and
acclaim. Symptoms include a grandiose sense of self-importance, preoc-
cupations with fantasies of success and power, a belief that the self is
special and should only be associated with other high-status and powerful people, a need for excessive admiration, a voracious sense of entitlement, exploiting others for personal benefit, lack of empathy, envy of
others or a belief that others envy the self, and arrogance (American Psychiatric Association, 2000). The negative effects of this behavior on
others, as well as the wrongfulness of exploiting others for personal
gain, are obscured by the arrogance of the individual. On a psychosocial
level, the person with NPD wishes for active love and protection, while
simultaneously fearing blame, being ignored, or being controlled by others (Benjamin, 1996).

The constitution of NPD dramatically interferes with the development and maintenance of intimate interpersonal relationships. Based on

clinical observations, Svrakic (1986) noted several destructive interpersonal motifs that are expressed by people with NPD. One of these is a pursuit of *metamorphosis*—that is, a fantasy that association and intimacy with powerful others will bring transformation and evolution from inferiority and insecurity. Svrakic (1986) notes that "in the core of every narcissistic personality there exists, more or less pronounced, experience of insecurity and inferiority" (p. 222). A second motif is *selective interpersonal repulsion*, or a loathing and systematic persecution of those on whom persons with NPD project their own conflicts. When such a person recognizes some unacceptable aspect of his or her own self in another individual, this individual must be cast off and put down. Finally, the *pathological intolerance of criticism* is a result of the doubly noxious nature of criticism for a person with NPD. Svrakic (1986) suggests that criticism serves to (1) threaten the person's sense of grandiosity, and (2) intensify the person's internal experience of inferiority and insecurity. Consequently, the person will respond to criticism with aggression and rage.

It scarcely bears mentioning that those with NPD rarely develop satisfying and close personal relationships. Part of this problem stems from these individuals' hostility and devaluation of others. This constitutes the so-called "narcissist's dilemma": holding others in contempt while simultaneously relying on them for positive regard and affirmation (Rhodewalt & Morf, 1995). Symptoms of NPD are negatively associated with receiving social support from others, and positively associated with loneliness and conflict with others (Johnson et al., 2000). Nevertheless, individuals with NPD may feel that there are a lot of people available who think very highly of them (Rhodewalt & Morf, 1995). Among married people, NPD is associated with domestic violence (Rothschild, Dimson, Storaasli, & Clapp, 1997) and interest in extramarital relations (Buss & Shackelford, 1997).

Among the important components of the interpersonal troubles experienced by those with NPD are the negative reactions of others to their conduct. When subjects in two studies (Carroll, Corning, Morgan, & Stevens, 1991; Carroll, Hoenigmann-Stovall, & Whitehead, 1997) viewed a person with NPD presented on videotape, they reacted with rejection and a negative mood. These findings are reminiscent of those in the literature on depression (e.g., Coyne, 1976b) indicating that depressed people irritate others and elicit rejection from them. Although people with NPD are probably rejected for different reasons, the end results are similar to those experienced by depressed persons: loneliness, a lack of social support, and conflictual interactions with others.

Rejection from others may cause great aggravation for some persons with NPD, while being of virtually no concern to others. Gabbard (1989) argued that NPD exists on a continuum ranging from an oblivious subtype to a hypervigilant subtype. Whereas a person with the oblivious subtype has no awareness at all of his or her impact on other people, the individual with the hypervigilant subtype is on the lookout for any sign of criticism or put-down from others. The interpersonal rejection that often follows in the wake of interpersonal interactions must surely contribute to substantial aggravation for the person with hypervigilant NPD.

Perhaps the most scientifically plausible account of the etiology of NPD is based on social learning theory; it places origins of the disorder in excessive and unconditional parental valuation and attention to the point of worship (e.g., Benjamin, 1996; Millon, 1981). In such an interpersonal context, the parents are viewed as devoting themselves so fully to caring for their child and making him or her feel special that they sublimate their own needs to those of the child. Consequently, the child fails to develop an awareness or appreciation for the needs of other people. Years of living in such an environment also result in an unjustified sense of self-worth that must constantly be reinforced and polished in the face of any potential failure. Benjamin (1996) has detailed this social learning phenomenon by identifying a combination of selfless, noncontingent love and adoration from the family; parental deference to the child; and an ever-present threat of a fall from grace in the pathogenesis of NPD. This account has considerable face validity for explaining the sense of grandiosity and lack of empathy that characterize this disorder.

Although a social learning account of NPD enjoys some popularity and acceptance, psychodynamic accounts of the disorder are especially prevalent, and also point to early interpersonal experiences in its etiology (e.g., Fiscalini, 1998; Svrakic, 1986). Within this literature there exists something of a controversy, based on the different assessments of Kohut and Kernberg (see Akhtar & Thomson, 1982, and Fiscalini, 1993, for more in-depth appraisals of this debate).

According to Kohut's (1968) self-psychological perspective, NPD is a manifestation of arrested development. An egocentric sense of grandiosity is seen as a normal part of early development. At this point in time, the child expects total nurturance and caring from parents, and develops *selfobjects*, which are images of other people as they relate to the self. Eventually, the infant begins to feel vulnerable upon becoming aware of the parents' inevitable shortcomings. The child then defensively idealizes the parents and returns to a sense of self-grandiosity. These are sources of strength for the child when dealing with an uncertain world. Normally, this narcissism gives way to empathy and more realistic appraisals of the self and others. However, when maternal empathy and confirmation are defective, the grandiose self perseveres as a defense against the vulnerabilities inherent in life.

In contrast, Kernberg's (1975) object relations theory holds that NPD is a compensation for early emotional deprivation and unempathic mothering. This causes the child to feel unloved, resulting in rage being projected onto his or her parents. As a defense, the child develops a *grandiose self* by combining aspects of the self that are admired by the parents, a fantasized version of the self, and an idealized version of the parents. More than Kohut (1968), Kernberg (1975) focuses on simultaneous feelings of inferiority and grandiosity in NPD. Kernberg also stresses the importance of *oral rage*, a powerful aggression originally directed at caregivers who did not provide unconditional love and approval, as a causal agent in NPD. As such, Kernberg focuses more on *pathological* psychosocial development in the etiology of NPD, whereas Kohut places more emphasis on *arrested* development (Akhtar & Thomson, 1982; Fiscalini, 1993).

Summary

NPD involves a grandiose sense of self, interpersonal arrogance and exploitation, a desire for excessive admiration, and a lack of empathy. The interactions of a person with NPD are marked by the quest for metamorphosis (rising above inferiority via association with powerful others), selective interpersonal repulsion, and pathological reactions to even the slightest criticism. Obviously these traits and qualities render intimate interpersonal relationships nearly impossible. People with NPD are trapped between a need for other people to give them attention and admiration, and contempt for others. Their interpersonal lives are marked by conflict, loneliness, and rejection from others. A social learning hypothesis holds that this personality disorder is the result of excessive parental adoration and attention. Psychodynamic accounts of NPD also stress early parent–child relations, focusing on arrested or pathological development of the self-image in relation to others.

HISTRIONIC PERSONALITY DISORDER

People with histrionic personality disorder (hereafter abbreviated as HPD) exhibit a pervasive pattern of excessive emotionality and attention seeking. Their social interactions are characterized by inappropriately seductive or provocative behavior, rapidly shifting and shallow emotions, excessively impressionistic speech that is lacking in detail, and self-dramatization (American Psychiatric Association, 1994). Persons with HPD tend to use physical appearance to draw attention to themselves, consider relationships to be more intimate than they really are, and are rather easily influenced by other people. Millon and Davis (2000) further describe these persons as resistant to being pushed into the background, and as wanting to be made to feel special, with a tendency toward anger and jealousy when not acknowledged. Using her Structural Analysis of Social Behavior, Benjamin (1996) finds that people with HPD wish for active love and protection while harboring a fear of being ignored by others. Unquestionably, the interpersonal theatrics of these people are cries for attention, and most of their symptoms are in the service of this primary goal. A distinctive quality of HPD is its inherent interpersonal quality: Interaction with others is required for expression of the disorder (Nichols, 1996).

Obviously something is seriously awry on the interpersonal terrain of persons with HPD. Although such people are often judged to be more physically attractive than their nondisordered peers, this physical attractiveness is associated with a greater reliance on immature defense mechanisms, such as projection and regression (Bornstein, 1999). These findings suggest a pattern of superficial relations based on gaining attention through physical attractiveness, in the absence of any well-developed interpersonal coping and problem-solving skills. Compared to healthy controls, persons with HPD score lower in sexual assertiveness despite their flirtations, and exhibit more phobic attitudes toward sexuality (Apt & Hurlbert, 1994). Expectedly, the subjects with HPD in this study also reported lower marital satisfaction than controls. These same respondents indicated relatively high levels of sexual preoccupation, along with sexual boredom and dysfunction. In a unique study with gay men, Johnson et al. (2000) found that symptoms of HPD were negatively correlated with receiving social support, and positively correlated with interpersonal conflict and loneliness. In their epidemiological study, Nestadt et al. (1990) found that the prevalence rate of HPD was about five times higher in divorced and separated persons than in people who were married.

Looking back at the early interpersonal experiences of people with HPD, one sees a pattern of turmoil. For example, sexual abuse is often evident in the early home environments of such individuals (Norden et al., 1995). In a similar study, people with Cluster B ("dramatic–emotional") personality disorders (i.e., antisocial personality disorder, BPD, HPD, and NPD) indicated that they experienced a pattern of parental overprotection coupled with lower parental care (Nordahl & Stiles, 1997). Although parental overprotection and sexual abuse may appear antithetical at first glance, each is indicative of poor boundary regulation. Other family-of-origin processes that are related to HPD include high achievement orientation, an intellectual/cultural orientation, and high levels of parental control (Baker, Capron, & Azorlosa, 1996).

What causes HPD? Undoubtedly this disorder, like other personality disorders, grows out of an amalgamation of temperament (which comes from genetic predisposition) and character (which is the developing aspect of one's personality that is shaped by experience) (Oldham, 1994). The character of people with HPD may be strongly tied to interpersonal interactions. Experts believe that this disorder is often preceded by rare parental punishment and unpredictable parental rewarding, resulting in the creation of behaviors that are directed toward securing rewards, developing a sense of personal competence, and seeking approval for approval's sake (Millon, 1981; Nichols, 1996).

In developing this social learning hypothesis, Millon and Davis (2000) have noted that when parents offer approval on a variable schedule, the child who will later develop HPD becomes frustrated, and learns to exaggerate his or her behaviors in the service of obtaining compliments and affection. Unless the parents recognize this conduct for what it is worth, a vicious cycle is established in which the child performs increasingly dramatic and caricatured behaviors to secure positive responses from his or her parents. Like other old habits that die hard, this pattern of conduct is carried over beyond the childhood home to adult interpersonal relations.

Psychodynamic theories of HPD originally characterized the disorder as *hysterical personality* (Breuer & Freud, 1960). It was believed that the symptoms are the results of childhood sexual abuse. Traumatic memories of the abuse were assumed to be repressed. The strong tendencies toward repression were thought to explain the vague and shallow cognitive pattern that is so characteristic of people with HPD. From the psychodynamic perspective, the sexualization of social interactions in HPD is a defense against the fear of sexual aggression and victimization. By summoning that which is feared, persons with HPD may develop a sense of mastery over this fear by replacing it with attraction. This psychodynamic perspective, notwithstanding its dubious falsifiability, clearly locates the origin and consequences of the disorder in interpersonal experiences.

Somewhere in between the social learning and psychodynamic hypotheses lies Benjamin's (1996) pathogenic hypothesis, based on her Structural Analysis of Social Behavior. Benjamin has identified three early interpersonal experiences that figure prominently in the pathogenesis of HPD. First, these people were often loved for their good looks and entertainment value as children. Second, as children, these people quickly learned that physical appearance and charm were functional for getting what they wanted from others. Finally, their early family environments were unpredictable and chaotic. However, it was this very chaos that kindled a sense of drama in their families, in which these children could play a role.

Summary

People with HPD conduct their lives in a frantic search for attention, trapped between the exploitation of sexuality and flirtation to gain this attention, and fear of its eventuality. Their interpersonal theatrics, emotional flightiness, and shallow cognitive style may have their origins in early family experiences. Proponents of both social learning and psychodynamic hypotheses converge on the belief that family dynamics such as parental boundary violation (manifested in sexual abuse and over-protectiveness) and inconsistent parental reinforcement set in motion the patterns of emotion, cognition, and social behavior that are characteristic of HPD.

ANTISOCIAL PERSONALITY DISORDER

The key feature of antisocial personality disorder (hereafter abbreviated as ASPD) is a pervasive pattern of disregard for and violation of other persons' rights (American Psychiatric Association, 1994). This pattern is manifested in failure to conform to social norms, deceitfulness, lying, impulsivity, aggressiveness, disregard for the safety of others, irresponsibility, and lack of remorse for wrongdoing to others. The pattern is evidenced by age 18 and is foreshadowed by conduct disorder before the age of 15. People with ASPD behave as if the rules and norms of society do not apply to them. Of all the personality disorders, ASPD is characterized by the greatest hostility (Kiesler, 1996).

Million and Davis (2000) note that the terms *psychopathy* and *sociopathy* have often been used to describe what DSM-IV now labels ASPD. They argue that the distinction between the two lies in the origins of the disorder: Psychopathy arises from a constitutional disposition, whereas sociopathy results from poor socialization, typically defective parenting.

Like all other personality disorders, ASPD is associated with numerous and serious interpersonal implications. In a unique comparative study, Rey, Singh, Morris-Yates, and Andrews (1997) found that adolescents who went on to develop ASPD as young adults were typified by trouble with the law, a poor work record, and early cohabitation. In contrast, those who developed other personality disorders were characterized more by social isolation and other types of problematic interpersonal relations. People with symptoms of ASPD tend to endorse a *ludus* (game-playing) love style, and score low on the *eros* (sexual) love style (Arnold & Thompson, 1996). The ludus love style appears to fit well with ASPD in that it is not an intimate means of relating to another person, and may well be seen as irritating by a large percentage of the population. This irritation and displeasure in others are obviously of little concern to a person with ASPD. On the contrary, the manipulation and "mind games" played upon others may be sources of satisfaction and amusement for such a person.

The family-of-origin backgrounds of people with ASPD are expectedly troublesome (Nichols, 1996). Poor relations with parents and a history of physical abuse have been tied to symptoms of ASPD (Norden et al., 1995). Gross neglect, to the point of abuse, is also fairly common in the family backgrounds of those with ASPD (Luntz & Widom, 1994). Parental absence is equally prevalent in these families, especially through separation, divorce, death, or incarceration (Taylor, 1993).

A provocative hypothesis that may link these dysfunctional family-of-origin experiences with adult ASPD centers around a breakdown in the normal development of empathy (Tantam, 1995). Tantam (1995) argues that during childhood, those who will later develop ASPD learn to recode vicarious fear as excitement and their victims' suffering as something akin to righteous punishment. One must entertain the possibility that this inverted emotional reaction was learned from the parents during periods of abuse and neglect. In other words, the parents of future adults with ASPD may model an emotional indifference to their children's suffering—an indifference that the children eventually internalize, and with which they then treat others.

It would be a gross oversimplification to assert that parental neglect and abuse lead to ASPD. As noted by Benjamin (1996), parental abuse may be an adequate explanation for the aggressiveness and hostility of those with ASPD, but it does not explain their resistance to control and conformity with social norms. She argues that the *combination* of parental neglect and abuse with sporadic and harsh discipline is what leads more specifically to ASPD. The parents of future adults with ASPD, who perhaps have psychosocial problems of their own, may oscillate between excessive permissiveness due to their absence, and stern discipline driven by unchecked impulse. This, according to Benjamin (1996), makes these children resent any intrusion, while placing a high premium on independence and a lack of interference from others. Like the empathy breakdown hypothesis, this formulation has considerable intuitive appeal, but has yet to be fully tested and supported empirically.

Summary

People with ASPD appear to lack a social conscience. They shamelessly exploit, manipulate, and aggress against others, with no apparent remorse. They often run afoul of the law and have difficulties in their work and personal relationships. Their orientation toward romantic relationships has more to do with playing games than establishing a mutually meaningful connection. One often finds considerable dysfunction in the family backgrounds of those with ASPD, replete with the attendant physical abuse and neglect. Sporadic and harsh parental discipline may also figure into the etiology of this personality disorder. These disordered family processes may contribute to ASPD through modeling the replacement of vicarious fear with excitement, and by creating hostility and fierce independence as a result of stern but sporadic discipline.

DEPENDENT PERSONALITY DISORDER

If ASPD can be located on the hostile–dominant quadrant of the interpersonal circumplex, dependent personality disorder (hereafter abbreviated as DPD) is almost the polar opposite, located in the nurturant–submissive quadrant. Perhaps the chief feature of DPD is a strong sense of interpersonal submission. Individuals with this disorder have a strong need to be taken care of, coupled with a strong fear of rejection. Additional symptoms include difficulty making decisions without support and reassurance from others, a need for others to assume responsibility for decisions about the self, difficulty expressing disagreement due to fear of rejection, difficulty initiating independent activities and projects, going to excessive lengths to secure nurturance from others, feeling uncomfortable when alone, urgent seeking of another relationship for support when a close relationship ends, and preoccupation with a fear of being left to take care of the self (American Psychiatric Association, 1994).

People with DPD appear ill equipped to handle mature and independent roles in life, while displaying a naive and gullible cognitive style (Millon, 1990). Because of their weak and fragile self-image, they entrust others with the responsibility for addressing major tasks and fulfilling their needs. Their delicate self-image suggests that they will not be competent or able to take on life's tasks, and therefore need others to do these for them. This excessive reliance on others appears to pay few, if any, dividends when it comes to establishing satisfactory personal relationships. People with DPD report low frequencies of positive social behaviors, reduced directness of communication with others, less positive interactions with close friends, and less helpfulness from friends than those with less dependent personalities (Overholser, 1996).

The interpersonal style of people with DPD (e.g., acting weak and submissive) is designed to pull for the complementary interpersonal response from others, particularly protection, nurturance, and control

(Millon & Davis, 2000). Millon and Davis (2000) also note that the desperate search for acceptance and approval from others is especially pronounced during times of stress. Should there even be a hint of failure to secure nurturance and care from others, persons with DPD will catastrophize, seeing themselves as totally alone and dismissed by the world.

Despite their suggestible and compliant tendencies, people with DPD report high degrees of loneliness (Johnson et al., 2000; Overholser, 1996); this calls into question the authenticity of the interpersonal connections that they may establish. Overholser (1996) has hypothesized that those with DPD may become demanding when their dependency needs are not met, and that this attention seeking may elicit interpersonal rejection from others, only further aggravating dependency needs. Consistent with this hypothesis, Johnson et al. (2000) found that symptoms of DPD were negatively correlated with receiving social support, and positively correlated with conflict.

It has been argued that parental overprotectiveness combined with authoritarianism may serve to reinforce dependent behaviors in children, while simultaneously preventing the children from developing a sense of independence and autonomy (Bornstein, 1992). By catering to children's every need, parents may inadvertently, or perhaps unconsciously, encourage dependency and inhibit the children's natural tendencies to explore the environment and develop a sense of mastery and autonomy. Although the excessive control that is pursuant to overprotectiveness may be deployed with the best intentions, it interferes with children's development of basic social competencies and a sense of security when separated from their caregivers. In fact, relative to healthy controls, those with DPD experience greater parental control in their families of origin (Baker et al., 1996). However, other examinations of physical and sexual abuse, maternal and paternal care, and maternal and paternal overprotection have found nothing unique in the family-of-origin background of those with DPD (Nordahl & Stiles, 1997; Norden et al., 1995). It must be noted that the size of the group with DPD in each of these studies was small; thus these null findings must be interpreted with caution until they can be replicated.

Summary

DPD involves a powerful need to be taken care of, resulting in clinging and submissive behaviors, as well as fear of separation. Despite their strong desire for connection with and caretaking from others, people with DPD experience less rewarding social interactions, less social support, and more loneliness than people without this disorder. A prominent interpersonal theory of DPD locates its origin in excessively over-protective parenting that fails to stimulate a sense of exploration and independence.

COMORBIDITY OF PERSONALITY DISORDERS WITH OTHER MENTAL HEALTH PROBLEMS

For most people with a personality disorder, the extent of their psychosocial problems often does not stop there. One could also say that many people with other psychosocial problems also have personality disorders. It is of interest that personality disorders are comorbid with other personality disorders (Marinangeli et al., 2000). For example, one study estimated the comorbidity of HPD and NPD at 30.4% (Watson & Sinha, 1998).

The rates of personality disorders among people with major depression are astonishingly high. As many as 20–50% of inpatients and 50–85% of outpatients with major depressive disorder have a personality disorder (Corruble, Ginestet, & Guelfi, 1996). Chief among these are BPD and HPD. Davila (2001) has explained this high rate of comorbidity by appealing to common interpersonal issues. By definition, people with personality disorders have a rigid and otherwise problematic interpersonal style. According to Davila (2001), this personality pathology can generate interpersonal stressors, leading to depression. In fact, Davila, Cobb, and Lindberg (2001) have identified interpersonal styles that play a role in stress generation in romantic contexts. These include a dependent style, which is submissive, fearful of abandonment, and reliant on others for self-esteem; and an obsessive–compulsive style, reflecting perfectionism, rigidity, and distrust in others. These personality profiles are remarkably similar to those of DPD and obsessive–compulsive personality disorder.

Personality disorders are also evident among those with schizophrenia or bipolar disorder. As many as 38% of patients with bipolar disorder meet the criteria for at least one personality disorder (Kay, Altshuler, Ventura, & Mintz, 1999). At the time of hospital admission in one study, 30–45% of patients with schizophrenia were also found to have a personality disorder (Torgalsboen, 1999). Problems as serious as schizophrenia or bipolar disorder have a profound impact on interpersonal behavior and relationships. In schizophrenia, depending upon the particular type, delusional thinking can prompt severely withdrawn and avoidant behavior, as well as conduct that reflects ambivalence about relationships with other people. Similarly, the fluctuating affective states of patients with bipolar disorder can produce interpersonal behavior that ranges from withdrawn to grandiose, dramatic, and voraciously self-entitled. One thread that connects all of these disorders is maladaptive interpersonal behavior. This behavior, which is intrinsic to personality disorders, may then perpetuate and maintain symptoms of schizophrenia or bipolar disorder because of the often negative and harmful interpersonal consequences it produces.

Alcoholism and other substance use problems are evident in as many as two-thirds of males and one-third of females with ASPD (Koenigsberg, Kaplan, Gilmore, & Cooper, 1985). This particular personality disorder generally precedes substance use disorders, since it is defined in part by a pattern of behavior that is evident before age 15 (i.e., conduct disorder), whereas evidence of full-blown substance dependence is generally not evident until later in the teens or early 20s. Problems with socialization, generally at the hands of parents, appear to be key interpersonal antecedents to both problems. Ineffective parenting, modeling of antisocial behavior, and modeling of substance use may dually predispose young children to develop both ASPD and drug or alcohol dependence.

In addition to being comorbid with depression, schizophrenia, bipolar disorder, and other personality disorders, the incidence of personality disorders is also elevated among those with eating disorders, substance use disorders, and somatoform disorders. Further discussion of these issues and their comorbidity with personality disorders can be found in Chapters 7, 8, and 9 of this book. For the time being, it should be noted that these problems, like depression and schizophrenia, share common interpersonal motifs with various personality disorders. In the case of eating disorders, substance use disorders, and somatoform disorders, there is reason to suspect that the rigid and maladaptive interpersonal behavior inherent in the personality disorders predisposes such individuals to developing these related psychosocial problems.

CONCLUSION

Personality disorders are defined, in part, by inflexible and generally maladaptive modes of relating to other people. Although the personality disorders are not as well researched and understood as many other psychological problems, interpersonal relations appear to play a prominent role in both the origins and consequences of these sometimes enigmatic disorders. A number of hypotheses, some with attendant empirical support, suggest that early experiences in the family of origin may be crucial mechanisms in the pathogenesis of some personality disorders. Family interactions involving excessive admiration and attention, physical and sexual abuse, inconsistent reinforcement, and rejection are replete in descriptions of the early childhood experiences of people with personality disorders. Perhaps as a result of these pathological interpersonal experiences, people with personality disorders develop ways of relating to other people that are extremely maladaptive and unsuitable to the needs of those in their social environment. Consequently, the persistence of interpersonal problems and distress is almost guaranteed, making personality disorders particularly intractable.

7

Eating Disorders

DEFINITION AND SYMPTOMS

The American Psychiatric Association (2000) recognizes two distinct subtypes of *eating disorders*: *anorexia nervosa* and *bulimia nervosa*. Obesity is currently considered more of a medical condition than a mental health problem. The defining features of anorexia nervosa include a refusal to maintain a normal body weight, an intense fear of gaining weight, and a disturbance in body image perception. Bulimia nervosa is defined by recurrent episodes of uncontrolled binge eating, inappropriate compensatory behaviors to control weight gain (e.g., self-induced vomiting, misuse of laxatives or diuretics), and an undue influence of body shape and weight on self-evaluations. A chief difference between the two disorders is that individuals with bulimia nervosa are able to maintain their body weight at or above normally prescribed levels, whereas those with anorexia nervosa have a body weight below 85% of what is expected. Similar to depression and alcoholism, eating disorders, especially anorexia nervosa, have a lethal component. The long-term mortality for those afflicted with anorexia nervosa is estimated to be over 10% (American Psychiatric Association, 2000). The standardized mortality ratio (observed mortality divided by expected mortality) for people with eating disorders is 3.6 for people under 20 years of age, 9.9 for those aged 20–29, and 5.7 for those over age 30 (Nielsen et al., 1998). Among females, the lifetime prevalence of anorexia nervosa has been estimated at 0.5%, and 1.3% for bulimia nervosa (American Psychiatric Association, 2000). The descriptions of these disorders in the DSM-IV-TR (American Psychiatric Association, 2000) contain references to interpersonal problems. Associated features of anorexia nervosa include social withdrawal and lessened interest in sex; episodes of binge eating associated with bulimia nervosa are often triggered by interpersonal stressors.

Research on interpersonal relationships and eating disorders has been typical of the work on interpersonal relationships and mental health more generally. The recognition of some type of relational difficulty associated with the disorder predates current investigations by at least a century (Lasègue, 1873). One of Lasègue's more notable contributions was the suggestion of "parentectomy"—hospitalization of the patients to remove them from exacerbating parental forces. Family-of-origin relationships in particular have been a focal point in this line of work (see for reviews, Kog & Vandereycken, 1985; Vandereycken, Kog, & Vanderlinden, 1989; Waller & Calam, 1994; Wonderlich, 1992). Finally, the proliferation of studies on this associated feature of eating disorders has been particularly evident within the past 25 years.

In one longitudinal investigation, patients diagnosed with anorexia nervosa were followed for a period of 5 years (Gillberg, Rastam, & Gillberg, 1994). Among the most notable features of those who did not recover over the course of the investigation (53%) were unsatisfactory family-of-origin relationships and problems with making personal contacts outside the family. Findings such as these are suggestive of the important role played by social relationships in the course of the disorder.

PREVIEW

As noted above, research emanating from the interpersonal paradigm has sought to understand eating disorders largely through a focus on *family-of-origin experiences*. Extreme levels of family adaptability and cohesion, family expressed emotion (EE), inappropriate parental pressure, low parental care, parental overinvolvement, sexual abuse, and battles for control are dominant themes in the family histories of people with eating disorders. Some models and theories suggest that these family-of-origin processes play a critical role in the development of these disorders. Some problems with *interpersonal communication* may be secondary to these pathological family processes. In particular, there is some evidence linking childhood sexual abuse to a failure to develop adequate social skills, which in turn contributes to the development of eating disorders. Recent studies on the *general personal relationships* of people with eating disorders are also suggestive of interpersonal difficulties. Interpersonal rejection and distressed personal relationships are common problems in this population. Findings on *family-of-orientation experiences* show that among those who are married, there is a strong association between eating disorders and marital distress. Like so many other psychological problems, eating disorders are situated in a network of other psychosocial problems with which they coexist, such as depression, borderline personality disorder (BPD), substance use disorders, and anxiety disorders.

FAMILY-OF-ORIENTATION EXPERIENCES IN EATING DISORDERS

Family Process Variables

Interest in the interpersonal relationships of people with eating disorders has focused largely, but not exclusively, on family-of-origin relationships. The work of Minuchin, Minuchin, Rosman, and Baker (1978) was at the forefront of this approach. These authors observed dysfunctional interaction patterns among families of patients with anorexia nervosa. The interactions in these families often minimized conflict, with a rigid, nonadaptable style. These interactions were argued to be entwined with the symptoms of the disorder. Other family systems researchers and clinicians also saw eating disorders as built into and around family relations. Root, Fallon, and Friedrich (1986) argued that "Significant others usually interact with the bulimic in ways that exaggerate relationship characteristics that were present, but in a more subtle form, before the bulimia was revealed. The bulimia becomes a symptom around which the whole family revolves. . . . While it may appear to be the individual's problem, bulimia is a signal that the environment is not meeting her needs" (pp. 4–5). In a family systems perspective, disordered eating is understood to be caused and maintained by a family's interpersonal behavior, which itself is assumed to be influenced by the disordered eating of one of its members.

Family process variables continue to receive a great deal of attention from those who seek to explain the origins and course of eating disorders (e.g., Strober & Humphrey, 1987; Wonderlich, 1992). Examples of this can be found in the investigations on family cohesion and *family adaptability*. Systems-oriented researchers have emphasized these variables as two dimensions of family relationships that are crucial to healthy family functioning, provided that neither one is too extreme (Olson, 1993). Multiple studies indicate that eating disorders are associated with perceptions of low family cohesion (Blouin, Zuro, & Blouin, 1990; Humphrey, 1986; Steiger, Puentes-Neuman, & Leung, 1991; Waller, Slade, & Calam, 1990a). Although this finding has been relatively stable across child and parent reports (e.g., Attie & Brooks-Gunn, 1989; Waller et al., 1990a), children with eating disorders give lower ratings of their families' cohesiveness than their parents do (Dare, Le Grange, Eisler, & Rutherford, 1994). Generally, daughters' ratings of family interaction have more diagnostic utility for predicting their eating disorders than mothers' and especially fathers' ratings do (Waller, Slade, & Calam, 1990b). Regardless of which family member's perception is actually "correct," the fact that a parent and a child with an eating disorder differ in their view of the family's cohesiveness is perhaps itself diagnostically significant.

Investigations of family adaptability have yielded less consistent results than those of cohesion. Some evidence indicates a negative association between family adaptability and symptoms of eating disorders (e.g., Dare et al., 1994; Waller et al., 1990a). However, a study by Humphrey (1986) found more chaos, less organization, and more poorly defined boundaries in the family, all suggestive of pathologically high levels of adaptability, among patients with eating disorders. In most studies, the families appeared to be extreme in their adaptability (either too much or too little) indicating potentially detrimental family relations.

As in schizophrenia (see Chapter 4), *family EE* is emerging as an important family process variable in eating disorders (e.g., Le Grange, Eisler, Dare, & Hodes, 1992; van Furth et al., 1996). The van Furth et al. (1996) investigation indicated that aspects of maternal EE during the interactions of patients with eating disorders and their families explained 28–34% of the variance in the patients' eventual outcome and response to therapy. The extent to which mothers made openly critical comments during family interaction assessment was a stronger predictor of patients' outcomes than a host of other impressive predictors, such as premorbid body weight, duration of illness, body mass index, and age at onset.

Inappropriate parental pressure is a phenomenon that may be particularly prominent in families of people with eating disorders. When compared to both psychiatric controls and nonpsychiatric controls, one sample of patients with eating disorders (Horesh et al., 1996) experienced excessive pressure from parents. Horesh et al. (1996) describe this phenomenon as "gender-inappropriate pressure, age-inappropriate pressure, and pressures inappropriate to the child's abilities . . . the adolescents felt that they had been forced into an exaggerated feminine style of behavior, that their parents had discussed topics (such as parental sex) before the adolescents were prepared to deal with such subjects, and that the adolescents had been made to engage in activities which reflected their parents' ambitions rather than their own" (p. 925). These authors hypothesize that this leaves an adolescent in a state of conflict between premature exposure to the world of adults and anxiety over what is involved in that world, such as sexuality and high levels of achievement. Perhaps by exerting control over their own eating, adolescents may gain some feeling of mastery or control over this conflict. Related to this, Levine's (1996) study of the families of patients with eating disorders identified four mechanisms by which family members contributed to the eating disorders, two of which are indicative of inappropriate parental pressure: high emphasis on achievement/perfection and overconcern with beauty/appearance/thinness.

In American society, it is easy to locate very young children involved in competitive activities such as gymnastics, figure skating, ballet, and beauty contests. When 3- and 4-year-olds are seriously involved in such endeavors, it is difficult to avoid wondering about whose ambition is being pursued. In cases where the motivation comes largely from the parents, and where the activity places an emphasis on physical appearance, the risk for later development of eating disorders is serious.

Excessive parental pressure may also engender a sense of *perfectionism* among children. Perfectionism involves both self-oriented aspects (expecting the self to be perfect) and socially prescribed aspects (perceiving that others expect perfection). Perfectionism has proven to be a risk factor for bulimia nervosa, particularly for women who are otherwise low in self-esteem (Joiner, Heatherton, Rudd, & Schmidt, 1997; Vohs, Bardone, Joiner, Abramson, & Heatherton, 1999). By pressuring their children to achieve, parents may inadvertently convey the attitude that anything less than "perfect" is a failure. Children who harbor such an attitude, and then perceive that they are not meeting some perfect standard of weight or body image, may engage in binge eating as an escape response to their painful self-awareness, which is then corrected with purging (Heatherton & Baumeister, 1991).

Other family process variables that have been implicated in eating disorders include *disturbed affective expression* (Garfinkel et al., 1983; Waller, Calam, & Slade, 1989), low levels of *family communication* (Neumark-Sztainer, Story, Hannan, Beuhring, & Resnick, 2000), lack of *parental care* (Webster & Palmer, 2000), excessive *parental overprotectiveness and intrusiveness* (Calam, Waller, Slade, & Newton, 1990; Rhodes & Kroger, 1992; Rorty, Yager, Rossotto, & Buckwalter, 2000), and excessive *parental control* (Ahmad, Waller, & Verduyn, 1994; Wonderlich, Ukestad, & Perzacki, 1994). This last variable has particular significance, in that the symptoms of eating disorders may be overt manifestations of a struggle for control. Particularly among women with eating disorders and a history of sexual abuse, an external locus of control (i.e., feeling little personal control over one's fate) is common (Waller, 1998). Although the struggle for control may originally be with the parents, there is reason to believe that it may extend to others with whom such women are in relationships.

The rather paradoxical nature of some of these family processes in eating disorders is nicely illustrated in a study that employed Benjamin's Structural Analysis of Social Behavior model (Humphrey, 1989). Specifically, Humphrey found that parents of patients with anorexia nervosa were simultaneously more nurturing and comforting, but also more ignoring and neglecting of their daughters, than were parents of either healthy controls or patients with bulimia nervosa. In contrast, the patients with bulimia nervosa and their parents showed signs of hostile enmeshment. Humphrey argues that these mixed messages create ambivalence about separation for daughters with anorexia nervosa.

Mother–Daughter Relationships

The ratio of females to males suffering from anorexia nervosa is approximately 10:1 (Lucas, Beard, O'Fallon, & Kurland, 1988). This may be due to the greater concerns with body image, dieting, and weight control among women compared to men (Hsu, 1989). Perhaps owing to the widely held importance of the relationship with the same-sex parent in a child's development, a great deal of attention has been granted to mother–daughter relationships in eating disorders. Girls with eating disorders have been known to describe their mothers as overprotective (e.g., Rhodes & Kroger, 1992) and less caring (Palmer, Oppenheimer, & Marshall, 1988). In light of such findings, it is not surprising to discover that mothers of daughters with eating disorders have expressed a desire for greater family cohesion than what they currently perceive (Pike & Rodin, 1991). A group of young women with eating disorders retrospectively reported maternal relations that involved more emotional coldness, indifference, and rejection, compared to a sample of controls (Rhodes & Kroger, 1992).

Some evidence suggests that dietary restraint may be passed on from mother to daughter. Hill, Weaver, and Blundell (1990) found an $r = .68$ correlation between mothers' dietary restraint and that of their adolescent daughters. In another investigation, mothers' satisfaction with their body sizes correlated $r = .77$ with that of their daughters (Evans & Le Grange, 1995). This particular sample of mothers had a history of eating disorders.

In a very carefully controlled study, Stein et al. (1999) examined rates of eating disorders in mothers of a group of probands diagnosed with bulimia nervosa, but with no history of anorexia nervosa. Their results indicated that 26% of the mothers of probands with bulimia nervosa had a lifetime diagnosis of some form of eating disorder (e.g., anorexia nervosa, bulimia nervosa, eating disorder not otherwise specified, binge-eating disorder). This rate was significantly higher than that for mothers of a control group with no history of eating disorders. Of course, family studies confound the effects of genes and environment; thus it is not entirely clear whether the association between mothers' and daughters' eating disorders is the result of maternal genetic contributions, or of the social environment to which mothers contribute.

Investigations of mothers' attitudes toward their daughters' body image paint an even more dismal picture of mother–daughter relations. Mothers of girls with eating disorders in one study thought that their daughters ought to lose significantly more weight than mothers of girls without eating disorders thought about their daughters (Pike & Rodin, 1991). Sadly, these same mothers rated their daughters as significantly less attractive than the daughters rated themselves! This is particularly amazing, given that people with eating disorders typically have low self-esteem and a negative body image (Attie & Brooks-Gunn, 1989), and hence are unlikely to inflate ratings of their own attractiveness. Data provided by mothers in an interview study indicated that mothers of daughters with bulimia nervosa were more controlling and held higher expectations for their daughters than control mothers (Sights & Richards, 1984). The effects of being in a relationship with a mother prone to such negative and excessive evaluations could be extremely caustic for an adolescent girl (see, e.g., Pierce & Wardle, 1993).

The attention granted to mothers of children with eating disorders has been criticized by feminist scholars as "mother-blaming" (Rabinor, 1994). Rabinor has argued that the tendency to see mothers as causally related to child problems is a legacy of the psychoanalytic school, which overemphasized mothers' roles and devalued the influence of fathers. At the same time, however, psychodynamically oriented theorists argue that many girls with eating disorders use food as a means of fighting a battle (both interpersonally and intrapsychically) with their overprotective but nonempathic mothers (Beattie, 1988). The data on mothers' roles in the pathogenesis of eating disorders are alluring. Whether they represent a disrespectful and misguided focus, or a theoretically and etiologically meaningful domain of inquiry, will best be resolved through future empirical investigation, particularly with comparative collateral data from fathers.

Childhood Sexual Abuse and Eating Disorders

One caustic interpersonal phenomenon that has received considerable interest in the literature on eating disorders is childhood sexual abuse. A common form of abuse reported by people with eating disorders childhood sexual abuse, represents a gross violation of boundaries, particularly when perpetrated in the family context. This abuse often causes guilt, confusion, repulsion, and distrust of others. These potentially vicious psychosocial repercussions can make intimate relations later in life very difficult.

Contrasting Findings and Possible Explanations

There is at least some evidence to suggest that histories of sexual abuse are more common among those with eating disorders, especially bulimia nervosa, than what would be expected by chance alone. However, after numerous studies on the topic, findings remain mixed. For example, some estimates indicate that rates of childhood sexual abuse run as high as 70% among patients with eating disorders (Oppenheimer, Howells, Palmer, & Chaloner, 1985). One study of such patients found that 65% had experienced physical abuse, 28% had been sexually abused, and 23% had been raped (Root & Fallon, 1988).

These statistics are shocking both for their indication of what appear to be extremely high prevalence rates of childhood sexual abuse among persons with eating disorders, and for their stark contrast to other epidemiological estimates indicating a far lower occurrence of sexual abuse in the background of such persons. For example, two reviews concluded that there was no evidence of higher rates of eating disorders among sexually abused versus nonabused women (Coovert, Kinder, & Thompson, 1989; Pope & Hudson, 1992). Furthermore, one study found that among normal-weight women with bulimia nervosa, only 7% included a history of sexual abuse involving physical contact (Lacey, 1990). Since it is estimated that the prevalence of sexual abuse in the general female population is 27% (Finkelhor, Hotaling, Lewis, & Smith, 1990), it appears as if sexual abuse was *less* prevalent in Lacey's sample than in the general population. To complicate matters further, still another review found that rates of sexual abuse were no higher among those with eating disorders than among those in the general population (Connors & Morse, 1993).

What conclusions can be drawn from the literature on childhood sexual abuse and eating disorders? First, some of the variance in these prevalence estimates can be explained by wildly discrepant operationalizations of "sexual abuse." Second, the samples on which these estimates are based are also nonequivalent. For example, it is reasonable to expect a greater history of childhood sexual abuse in clinical samples than in samples with eating disorders drawn from the general population. Third, there is some consensus that childhood sexual abuse is neither necessary nor sufficient for the development of eating disorders in later life (Kinzl, Traweger, Guenther, & Biebl, 1994). This may explain the high rates of sexual abuse in some samples, and the lower rates in others.

Interpersonal Communication (Social Skills) Deficits as a Mediating Factor?

Many investigators now view childhood sexual abuse as a risk or vulnerability factor in the development of eating disorders (e.g., Connors & Morse, 1993; Vanderlinden & Vandereycken, 1996). One particularly well-developed yet parsimonious model of this process has been proposed by Mallinckrodt, McCreary, and Robertson (1995) (see Figure

7.1). According to this model, childhood sexual abuse, particularly in-cest, is expected to contribute to (and result from) dysfunctional family environments and parent–child attachments. The combination of these poor family environment variables with the sexual abuse is thought to inhibit the development of social competencies in a child. Mallinckrodt et al. (1995) define *social competencies* as a sense of self-efficacy, an ability to communicate emotional needs, an ability to experience inti-macy, and the capacity to use relationships with other people to regulate negative affect. The failure to develop these basic social competencies is thought to be the causal link between sexual abuse and eating disorders. An eating disorder becomes the means by which a child develops a sense of self-efficacy and affective regulation, albeit through dysfunctional, noninterpersonal means. The results of Mallinckrodt et al.'s (1995) in-vestigation provide compelling evidence for the validity of their model. For example, they observed eating disorders at a rate of 39% among in-cest survivors, but only 17% among those with no childhood abuse. As an aside, the rate of eating disorders was 47% in their clinical sample of incest survivors, and 24% in the student sample with a history of incest, again suggesting higher rates of abuse in the background of clinical sam-ples. Those incest survivors in this study who reported little emotional warmth and expressiveness from their mothers were most likely to have developed an eating disorder. Furthermore, people with a history of in-cest scored lower on a number of social competency indicators than did those with no history of childhood sexual abuse.

Perhaps the cornerstone hypothesis of Mallinckrodt et al.'s (1995) model is that incestuous family environments do not provide an ade-quate context for the development of social competencies and skills. They offer two lines of reasoning for this hypothesis. First, incest inter-

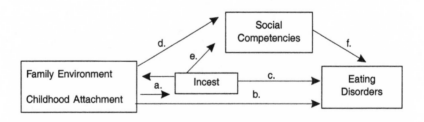

FIGURE 7.1. Conceptual model of relations among family environment, attachment, incest, social competencies, and eating disorders. From Mallinckrodt, McCreary, & Robertson (1995). Copyright 1995 by the American Psychological Association. Re-printed by permission.

feres with developmental processes by destroying the emotional comfort and "felt security" that allow for healthy attachment bonds. Thus children with a history of incestuous abuse have a difficult time forming attachment relationships with others. Second, Mallinckrodt et al. (1995) argue that sexual abuse may also "interfere with introceptive awareness, which is the ability to perceive and label internal emotional states and hunger" (p. 179). Those who are unaware of their own emotional reactions may have difficulty appropriately regulating their own social behavior, and thus may have problems with developing social skills. Similar hypotheses involving social skills deficits are prevalent in the psychopathology literature more generally. However, Mallinckrodt et al.'s (1995) model is unique in postulating an origin of those social skills deficits—namely, a dysfunctional family environment that includes sexual abuse.

Although the literature on problematic social skills is not as extensive for eating disorders as it is for other mental health problems, there is some suggestive evidence of social skills problems in this population. For example, one theme that has been identified on multiple occasions is difficulty with assertion (e.g., Williams, Chamove, & Millar, 1990). This research group noted a strong negative correlation between eating disorder symptomatology and assertiveness. Similar findings show that women with anorexia nervosa tend to inhibit the expression of their thoughts and feelings when they are in conflict with those of other people (Geller, Cockell, Hewitt, Goldner, & Flett, 2000). Clinical observations indicate that "eating-disordered clients typically have poor communication skills" (Riebel, 1989, p. 69). Riebel (1989) describes the typical client as having "porous ego boundaries. She admits too much from others (in the form of opinions and requests), resulting in harsh introjects and a tendency to caretake because she cannot tell where others' needs leave off and hers begin" (p. 70). In a dissertation study, Espelage (1998) observed deficits in social competence among women with eating disorders across such domains as relationships, family concerns, and academic concerns. This study is especially unusual in that the social competence assessments were based on behavioral observation. Another study has found evidence for social skills deficits of a different sort: Adolescent girls with eating disturbances and/or dietary restriction are three to four times more likely to be involved in aggressive behaviors such as robbery with a weapon or aggravated robbery (Thompson, Wonderlich, Crosby, & Mitchell, 1999). This type of aggression against others is to be expected among those with a history of abuse. Though there would be great value in additional research on the social skills of people with eating disorders, there is at least tentative evidence at this time that they experience deficits in some social skills, and that these problems may be the developmental consequences of childhood sexual abuse.

Precisely how childhood sexual abuse factors into the development of eating disorders may never be fully understood (but see the discussion of *desexualization* theory, below). This is because such abuse is hopelessly confounded with dysfunctional family environments (Connors & Morse, 1993; Kinzl et al., 1994; Schmidt, Humfress, & Treasure, 1997). There is an almost tautological relationship between the two phenomena. A family that either perpetrates or tolerates the sexual abuse of its children surely has other drastic problems. These other problems may be sufficient on their own to contribute to the development of eating disorders in such a family's affected children. A vital study on this issue showed that even after family psychosocial factors (e.g., family communication, parental monitoring, parental caring) were controlled for, youths who reported sexual abuse were still at increased risk for disordered eating (Neumark-Sztainer et al., 2000). At this time, childhood sexual abuse appears to be a risk factor for the later development of eating disorders. This relationship may be mediated by the poor social skills that result from a history of such abuse.

Summary

Scientific research findings on family environments, mother–daughter relationships, and childhood sexual abuse point very clearly to the family of origin in the etiology of anorexia nervosa and bulimia nervosa. The architecture of these families' relationships and interaction patterns suggest considerable dysfunction. Extreme and abnormal levels of adaptability, cohesion, and EE are common in families of children with eating disorders. Excessive and inappropriate pressures for achievement are also evident in many of these families. There is reason to believe that the parents of children with eating disorders may actively and aggressively project their ambitions onto their children. A history of psychiatric problems is evident in as many as 48% of the families of patients diagnosed with either anorexia nervosa or bulimia nervosa (Pantano et al., 1997). Findings on mother–daughter relations show that girls with eating disorders often have mothers with elevated body image concerns, excessive dieting, and eating disorders of their own. Finally, childhood sexual abuse is evident in the backgrounds of some people with eating disorders. Although not necessary or sufficient for the development of eating disorders, this abuse is believed to impair the development of social competencies, leading to inappropriate eating as a mechanism for regaining control and regulating affect.

GENERAL PERSONAL RELATIONSHIPS
AND FAMILY-OF-ORIENTATION EXPERIENCES IN EATING DISORDERS

Dating/Romantic and Other Personal Relationships

As noted earlier, not all research on the interpersonal relationships of people with eating disorders has focused on the family-of-origin context. The other personal relationships of these people also appear to be problematic (e.g., Herzog, Pepose, Norman, & Rigotti, 1985; Schmidt, Tiller, & Morgan, 1995). Symptoms of eating disorders are associated with lower satisfaction and closeness in dating/romantic relationships (Evans & Wertheim, 1998). O'Mahony and Hollwey (1995) conducted an intriguing study comparing the interpersonal problems of patients with anorexia nervosa to those of women who had an occupation or hobby that stressed physical conditioning and appearance (e.g., dance, athletics, professional models), as well as to women from the general public. The group with anorexia nervosa scored significantly higher on a measure of loneliness than either of the comparison groups. In addition, the correlation between loneliness and eating problems was higher in the group with anorexia nervosa ($r = .65$) than in either the weight-concerned group ($r = .47$) or the group from the general public ($r = .28$).

A study of women with bulimia nervosa indicates that such individuals perceive less social support from friends as well as family members (Grissett & Norvell, 1992). These women felt less socially competent than a group of controls in a variety of social situations, particularly those that involved seeking out social encounters and forming close relationships with others.

Some of these interpersonal problems may stem from distorted views of personal relationships by people with eating disorders. For example, characteristics of eating disorders are positively associated with a possessive, dependent love style, and negatively associated with a relatively more healthy passionate and friendship-based love style (Raciti & Hendrick, 1992). In a related study, women with high scores on the Dieting and Bulimia–Food Preoccupation subscales of the Eating Attitudes Test tended to endorse *ludus* (game-playing) and *mania* (dependent, possessive) love styles (Worobey, 1999). Women with symptoms of eating disorders also view sexual expression as exploitative (Evans & Wertheim, 1998), and see relationships with men, but not with women, as difficult and dissatisfying (Thelen, Farmer, Mann, & Pruitt, 1990). Studies such as these suggest that people with eating disorders, or at least a propensity toward eating disorders, have characterological attitudes toward love and romantic relationships that are unlikely to lead them into stable and soothing relationships. It is tempting to speculate that the development of these dysfunctional attitudes toward close relationships may have been shaped by earlier family-of-origin interactions that produced distorted models of such relationships.

As with depression, eating disorders may be associated with negative interpersonal responses from other people (Sobal & Bursztyn, 1998). This may partially explain some of the loneliness and lack of relational involvement among certain people with eating disorders. In Sobal and Bursztyn's (1998) study, over 700 university students were asked an open-ended question about what they thought it would be like to date someone with either anorexia nervosa or bulimia nervosa. The responses revealed mostly negative expectations. Themes that were prevalent in the answers included difficulty, stress, frustration, and disliking. Students were also asked for their views toward involvement with someone who has anorexia nervosa or bulimia nervosa, starting with just studying with the person, to dating the person, all the way up to getting engaged. There was a very clear and strong linear relationship between reported discomfort and level of involvement: The more deeply involved the relationship was, the more respondents reported discomfort with the idea of involvement. Sobal and Bursztyn's (1998) study has added an important component to the understanding of eating disorders and personal relationships: People tend to harbor negative attitudes toward getting involved, especially in intimate relationships, with others who have an eating disorder.

Like people with depression, those with eating disorders elicit interpersonal rejection. Also like their depressed counterparts, people with eating disorders actually appear to seek and elicit such negative interpersonal responses. Testing hypotheses derived from self-verification theory, which argues that people prefer information consistent with their self-concept, Joiner (1999) found symptoms of bulimia nervosa and body dissatisfaction to be positively associated with interest in negative feedback from others in such domains as intellect, social skills, and even physical appearance. Joiner noted that the drive for self-verification among women with bulimia nervosa causes them to seek the very interpersonal responses that serve to maintain or exacerbate their condition.

Marital Relationships

People often associate eating disorders with adolescence. However, cases of anorexia nervosa and bulimia nervosa are easily found among those in their 20s and 30s. Somewhat surprisingly, many of these people are able to maintain at least the semblance of normal adult relations through marriage and child rearing. However, the marriages of people with eating disorders are sadly distressed. Physical intimacy is a problematic theme in the literature on marriage and eating disorders (Heavey, Parker,

Bhat, Crisp, & Gowers, 1989; Morgan, Wiederman, & Pryor, 1995). For example, an examination of case records from a large sample of patients with anorexia nervosa (Heavey et al., 1985) showed that among those who were married, only 10% indicated some interest in sexual matters, and 72% indicated active avoidance of sexual activity. These authors also found a high degree of sexual conflict and conflict avoidance in these patients' families of origin. Here again, there is reason to suspect that problems bred in earlier family-of-origin interactions were transported into the marital relationships of these women with anorexia nervosa. It is unfortunate that these problems with physical intimacy in the marital relationship persist several years after remission of an eating disorder: Morgan et al. (1995) found that approximately 40% of the women in their sample had clinically significant sexual discord with their mates, despite being asymptomatic for 2 years on average. They also noted that diminished involvement in marital (or any romantic/sexual) relationships was more common among people who had anorexia nervosa than among those with bulimia nervosa or control subjects without eating disorders.

Marital problems have also been documented in the marriages of people with bulimia nervosa, however. Compared to healthy controls, people with bulimia nervosa report greater marital distress (Van Buren & Williamson, 1988). In fact, the degree of distress in these marriages did not differ significantly from those of people seeking marital therapy. Assessments from the spouses in Van Buren and Williamson's (1988) investigation were also suggestive of marital distress. The women with bulimia nervosa in their study exhibited poor problem-solving skills and conflict avoidance, which may partially explain the state of their marriages.

Summary

Taken as a whole, currently available evidence indicates that the other personal relationships of people with eating disorders are as disturbed as their family-of-origin relationships. They tend to hold dysfunctional attitudes toward love and romance, and, in the case of anorexia nervosa, avoidance of physical intimacy and involvement. The quest for self-verification may cause people with eating disorders to seek the very interpersonal responses that will worsen their condition. Among those who do get married, relational distress is still evident. It is impossible to overlook the potential connections between the distressed relationships in the families of origin and the adult romantic or marital relations of people with eating disorders. In many instances, people with anorexia nervosa or bulimia nervosa appear to be set up for interpersonal trouble by their experiences in their families of origin. As noted earlier, these family interactions are often marked by poor handling of conflict, excessive cohesion, and what are sometimes gross boundary violations. Not surprisingly, children from such households go on to develop possessive and dependent attitudes toward love, poor conflict resolution skills, and a fearful avoidance of physical intimacy. The implications for satisfaction with personal relationships are obvious. And if their own personal problems were not enough of a barrier to healthy relationships, other people appear reluctant and uncomfortable getting involved in a close relationship with those who have eating disorders.

THEORETICAL ACCOUNTS OF INTERPERSONAL
MECHANISMS IN EATING DISORDERS

The process of *modeling* has been identified as a potential causal mechanism in eating disorders. Maternal modeling in particular has been implicated in the etiology of eating disorders by a number of writers (e.g., Silverstein & Perlick, 1995). Social learning theory (Bandura, 1977) indicates that people can learn behaviors through imitation of a model. This process of learning is enhanced when, among other features, the model is perceived to hold high status and is similar to the target. Each of these conditions is intact in the typical mother–daughter relationship. Findings reviewed earlier indicate that daughters' concerns with dieting and body image are strongly associated with those of their mothers (see also Paxton et al., 1991). Mothers of daughters with eating disorders often themselves have symptoms of eating disorders. According to social learning theory, girls may observe their mothers' restrictive eating behaviors and imitate them, perhaps because they perceive that their mothers were rewarded for such dieting. No student of communication could ever rightfully overlook the possibility that the mass media also play a powerful role in this process of social learning: Unusually thin and attractive models are commonly depicted as the recipients of social rewards (e.g., Harrison, 1997; Harrison & Cantor, 1997).

Psychodynamically oriented theories (including object relations and attachment theories) continue to occupy a conspicuous presence in the literature on eating disorders and family-of-origin relations (e.g., Beattie, 1988; Dolan, Lieberman, Evans, & Lacey, 1990; Rhodes & Kroger, 1992). These accounts emphasize the symbolic significance of food in the adolescent girl's struggle for control in her relationship with her mother. Abuse of food is seen as a means of covertly expressing dissatisfaction with the mother–daughter relationship. Refusing to eat food may represent a rejection of the mother's overprotectiveness and overinvolvement in the child's life. Rhodes and Kroger (1992) contributed further to this approach by suggesting that the adolescent girl with an eating disorder may be struggling with a second separation–individuation process, similar to that which infants are hypothesized to experience in their relationships with their mothers. They present some supportive data indicating that women with eating disorders had higher levels of separation anxiety and lower healthy separation scores, while simultaneously experiencing greater maternal overprotectiveness, than their counterparts with eating disorders. Bulimic behaviors and a pursuit of thinness can also be predicted by dependency conflicts and a diminished sense of individuality (Friedlander & Siegel, 1990), further highlighting the importance of separation–individuation.

Observations of what appear to be elevated rates of childhood sexual abuse among those with eating disorders, in both research and clinical contexts, have led to what could be characterized as a *desexualization* theory of eating disorders. Several writers have noted that some individuals develop eating disorders, especially anorexia nervosa, as a means of avoiding sexual contacts and repelling would-be perpetrators (e.g., Hall, Tice, Beresford, Wooley, & Hall, 1989; Rorty & Yager, 1996). According to this perspective, anorexia nervosa becomes a means to make the self sexually unappealing to others. In this sense, it may be understood as serving some greater interpersonal function (i.e., protection from sexual abuse), despite its personal destructiveness. Some intriguing support for this position can be found in a study of so-called "sexual barrier weight" (Weiner & Stephens, 1996). These authors found that patients with eating disorders tended to avoid weights that they associated with certain traumatic events. For instance, if a woman had been sexually abused at a time that she weighed 110 pounds, that weight would trigger memories of past traumatic events. This appeared to motivate compulsive or restrictive eating to avoid the weight. Weiner and Stephens (1996) present some compelling data indicative of radical changes in weight coincidental to sexually traumatic events. On its face, the desexualization approach is a more adequate account of anorexia nervosa than of bulimia nervosa, as those with the latter disorder generally maintain a normal body weight. With that stated, Rorty and Yager (1996) argue that bulimia nervosa can be activated by anger, presumably against a perpetrator and against those who fail to provide protection, and may also be tied to a desire to make the self look unappealing. They note that difficulty handling emotions such as anger and depression is common among people with bulimia nervosa. This, they suggest, leads to disturbed eating behavior as a mechanism for coping with posttraumatic distress.

A second version of the desexualization approach suggests that it is pursuant to a fear or denial of sexual maturation and upcoming sexuality (Crisp, 1988), rather than a reaction to sexual trauma. Accordingly, eating disorders are thought to be triggered by anxiety associated with the meaning of and uncertainty about physical changes that occur during adolescence. Functionally, anorexia nervosa in particular becomes a way to preserve the preadolescent form and avoid having to address the self as a sexual being. As such, it is viewed as a psychobiological regression from sexual maturity (White, 1992). Like the "reactive" version of the desexualization hypothesis, this approach assumes a powerful concern over sexual relationships with other people—to the extent that concerned individuals physically damage their own bodies through disordered eating to cope with these concerns.

Among current approaches to understanding the role of the family in eating disorders, perhaps the most widely accepted is a variant of the *diathesis–stress* model. This position draws heavily on the literature that documents disturbances in personality traits and temperaments associated with bulimia nervosa and/or anorexia nervosa (e.g., Brookings & Wilson, 1994; Steiger, Stotland, Trottier, & Ghadirian, 1996; Vitousek & Manke, 1994). These pathological traits may be passed on from parent to child (Steiger et al., 1996) and create a predisposition or vulnerability to an eating disorder. The ultimate manifestation of the eating disorder is thought to be triggered by, among other things, disturbed family-of-origin relations (e.g., Strober & Humphrey, 1987). Thus the interaction of predisposing traits and temperaments with problematic family and social relationships is thought to be what ultimately brings about the eating disorder.

Although the diathesis–stress model predicts the development of an eating disorder as the result of stress brought about by family interaction, the nature of the predisposition, or diathesis, to develop an eating disorder when stressed is not well understood. After all, one can find problematic family-of-origin interactions in the backgrounds of people with many other forms of psychological problems, and even among some people who have no psychological problems. Some might argue that the predisposition to develop an eating disorder is part of one's genetically determined temperament. However, there may be some unique qualities of the stressor (e.g., dysfunctional family relations) that pull more for eating disorders than for other psychosocial problems. When parents are overly involved and overcontrolling with a child, this creates an obvious battle for control. When the parents are emphatic about achievement and perfectionism, this often motivates the child to engage in extraordinary behaviors. When these conditions are put on a developing adolescent, in the context of a society where thinness is still glamorized and portrayed as something of an ideal, the development of an eating disorder in particular—as opposed to other problems, such as depression, social anxiety, or alcoholism—becomes more understandable. Food intake is one thing the child can control. Maintaining a thin body form can create a sense of "achievement" in the restrictive eater. In this sense, restrictive eating may be a "functional" response to the particular nature of the family stress.

COMORBIDITY OF EATING DISORDERS WITH OTHER MENTAL HEALTH PROBLEMS

Given the often disturbed parent–child relationships associated with anorexia nervosa and bulimia nervosa, it is not surprising that a number of other mental health problems tend to covary with these disorders. Chief among these are depression (Blouin et al., 1990; Wonderlich & Swift, 1990a), BPD (Waller, 1994; Wonderlich & Swift, 1990b; Wonderlich et al., 1994) substance use disorders (Watts & Ellis, 1992), and anxiety disorders (Bulik, 1995). It is important to note that these related mental health problems may in some cases be (1) secondary to the eating disorder, and (2) more strongly associated with poor family relationships than with the eating disorder per se (see, e.g., Head & Williamson, 1990). The elevated incidence of BPD among patients with eating disorders (running as high as 40%) is also notable, in that symptoms of this disorder include difficulties with personal relationships, poor anger control, impulsivity, and affective instability. Also notable is the fact that childhood sexual abuse has been implicated in both BPD and bulimia nervosa (e.g., Claridge, Davis, Bellhouse, & Kaptein, 1998).

There is some evidence to suggest that the eating disorder–personality disorder comorbidity is different for different types of eating disorders. In particular, bulimia nervosa is associated with a high rate of BPD, whereas anorexia nervosa is associated with a relatively high rate of avoidant personality disorder (Skodol et al., 1993). These differing rates of personality disorders may reflect different interpersonal mechanisms in bulimia nervosa (e.g., approach–avoidance conflicts) versus anorexia nervosa (e.g., concern with social evaluation).

Rates of anxiety disorders also run very high among those with eating disorders (Bulik, 1995). Among probands diagnosed with bulimia nervosa in one large-scale study, the comorbidity with anxiety disorders was 42% for phobias, 11% for generalized anxiety disorder, and 9% for panic disorder (Kendler et al., 1991). Bulik (1995) has argued that in most cases the anxiety comes first and is followed by the eating disorder. Her analysis further concludes that a particular type of self-conscious social anxiety—one that causes people to be ultraconcerned with appearance and thinness—may strongly contribute to the development of an eating disorder. In this case, again, a concern with interpersonal or social relations appears to be the common link between the anxiety and the eating disorder. The comorbidity of eating disorders with other interpersonally oriented mental health problems suggests that eating disorders reside in a nomological network that also holds problematic interpersonal relationships and functioning in close proximity.

CONCLUSION

There is an undeniable association between eating disorders and past (i.e., childhood) as well as concurrent interpersonal relationship problems. Distressed and dysfunctional family-of-origin interactions are common antecedents to both anorexia nervosa and bulimia nervosa. Families of people with these problems have difficulty setting and respecting appropriate boundaries, adapting to change, and containing their criticism of each other. In extreme cases, boundary violations in these families may take the form of childhood sexual abuse, particularly in the case of those who go on to develop bulimia nervosa. Parents in these families also sometimes exert inappropriate and excessive pressure to achieve on their children.

Sadly, interpersonal problems do not always end when offspring with eating disorders leave their families of origin. These young adults depart from their families with dysfunctional attitudes and beliefs about close relationships with other people. They may eschew physical intimacy with others, partly out of their dissatisfaction with their own bodies, and partly out of anxiety about sexuality. Unfortunately, other people do not appear particularly eager to develop romantic or other relationships with those who have an eating disorder.

When people with anorexia nervosa or bulimia nervosa do get married, they are likely to find themselves in dissatisfying marriages. Still evident at this advanced stage of interpersonal development and experience are avoidance of physical intimacy and poor conflict-handling skills. Not surprisingly, the spouses of people with eating disorders are also unhappy with the state of their marriages.

The pervasiveness and seriousness of interpersonal problems associated with eating disorders may explain why family and interpersonal therapies are so effective for their treatment (e.g., Fairburn et al., 1995; Russell, Szmukler, Dare, & Eisler, 1987). Therapies that focus on understanding and improving the interpersonal landscape of patients with eating disorders, even though they do not focus on the disorders per se, tend to be more effective for treating such disorders than traditional cognitive or behavioral therapies are. If some sense of order can be brought to these patients' interpersonal and family relations, symptoms of eating disorders may dissipate without any specific attention being paid to them.

A number of very useful interpersonal theories have been developed to explain and describe eating disorders. These include the modeling of inappropriate dieting and eating behaviors by a parent; the psychodynamic explanation of food's symbolic significance in the battle for separation–individuation between the mother and daughter; attempts to "desexualize" the self, either in reaction to sexual abuse or as a means of avoiding upcoming sexual maturity; and a diathesis–stress model, which indicates that certain preexisting temperamental patterns may combine with the experience of stressors (perhaps from the family of origin) to promote eating disorders.

Both anorexia nervosa and bulimia nervosa tend to coexist with several other psychosocial problems, including depression, BPD, and anxiety disorders. Even a brief perusal of the literature associated with these disorders will reveal a number of common interpersonal antecedents and concomitants. Among these are rejection from others, childhood abuse and trauma, and uncaring family relations.

Finally, it is important to note that not all people with eating disorders have grossly disturbed interpersonal and family relations. Like any mental health problem, eating disorders may be caused by a variety of factors, only some of which are interpersonal. However, a full appreciation of the experience of anorexia nervosa or bulimia nervosa demands a careful consideration of the social/interpersonal context in which these problems are deeply embedded.

8

Alcoholism and Other Substance Use Problems

DEFINITION AND SYMPTOMS

Substance use disorders in DSM-IV-TR are divided into two groups: *substance dependence* and *substance abuse* (American Psychiatric Association, 2000). Substance dependence involves a maladaptive pattern of substance use, associated with symptoms such as tolerance (the need for increased amounts to achieve the desired effect); withdrawal (physical and psychological distress associated with cessation); taking more of the substance, or taking the substance for longer periods of time, than intended; a persistent desire to ingest the substance; spending a great deal of time securing the substance for use; disruption of social, occupational, or recreational activities as a result of the substance use; and continuation despite awareness of problems associated with the substance use (American Psychiatric Association, 2000). As evident from these diagnostic criteria, interpersonal impairment (in the form of reduced or abandoned social, occupational, and recreational activities) is a fundamental symptom of substance dependence, although it is not necessary for a diagnosis.

The primary feature of substance abuse is a maladaptive pattern of substance use that is associated with adverse effects. These adverse effects include, for example, failure to fulfill important occupational, social, or domestic roles; using the substance in such a way as to create physical hazards (such as driving a car while intoxicated); legal problems associated with the substance use; and continued use of the substance despite interpersonal problems that are caused or exacerbated by its use

(American Psychiatric Association, 2000). Here again, interpersonal problems figure in the symptoms of substance abuse.

Alcoholism is a specific class of the more general diagnosis of substance use disorders. The term *alcoholism* is generally used to refer to alcohol dependence and/or alcohol abuse. The defining features of alcohol dependence are the same as those of substance dependence more generally (American Psychiatric Association, 2000; see above). What distinguishes alcohol dependence from alcohol abuse is the presence of tolerance, withdrawal, and alcohol-related compulsive behavior in the person who is dependent on alcohol. In both cases, however, the substance is used in ways that culminate in physical, occupational, and interpersonal impairment. In many cases, these impairments may be evident before the onset of symptoms, leading to the observation that some people may use alcohol and/or other drugs to cope with the very problems that their heavy use exacerbates.

Results from the Epidemiologic Catchment Area study indicate that among people over 18 years of age in any given year, 7.4% will experience some form of alcohol use disorder, and 9.5% will experience some form of substance use disorder, alcoholism included (Regier et al., 1993). Lifetime prevalence estimates from the National Comorbidity Survey are 14.1% for alcohol dependence and 9.4% for alcohol abuse (Kessler et al., 1994). The lifetime prevalence for any substance abuse or dependence is nearly 27%. Among 17-year-olds, the point prevalence of substance abuse or dependence is just over 10% (Kilpatrick et al., 2000), and surveys of American high school students show that drug use has been on the rise since the early 1990s (O'Malley, Johnson, & Bachman, 1999). Substance use disorders are about twice as common in men as in women. For men, the lifetime prevalence for any substance abuse or dependence is a staggering 35.4%.

There is an interesting relationship among gender, depression, and alcohol abuse/dependence (see Swendsen & Merikangas, 2000, for a discussion of the comorbidity between depression and substance use disorders). When men become depressed, they often seek solace in alcohol. Consequently, when their distress brings them to the attention of government authorities or health care professionals, they are prone to be diagnosed as having alcoholism rather than depression. This may, in part, account for the 2:1 ratio of female to male diagnoses of major depression. In a unique study of mood disorders among the Amish, an American subculture in which alcohol use is prohibited, the rates of such disorders were found to be one-half of what they were in the general population, and virtually identical in males and females (Egeland & Hostetter, 1983). An obvious conclusion is that in the general population, alcoholism may mask depression in males.

PREVIEW

Interpersonal difficulties tend to be prolific in the lives of people with substance use problems. Research on *interpersonal communication* indicates that many such individuals have difficulties with social skills. This may make them unable to resist peer pressure to initiate substance use, and/or may cause them to seek consolation in substance use when they have trouble resolving issues with other people. A distinct literature has emerged on alcoholism and *family-of-orientation experiences*. Problems such as poor distance regulation, parenting problems, interpersonal conflict, and marital distress are clearly evident in families affected by an adult member's alcoholism (sometimes referred to as "alcoholic families"). Paradoxically, for some such families, alcohol consumption may actually bring temporary stability to their interactions. The interpersonal conflict that is evident in family interactions also spills over into *general personal relationships,* such as those with peers and coworkers. Another distinct literature exists on adolescent substance use. This literature is dominated by a focus on *family-of-origin experiences* (although factors in the other three domains may play roles as well). Many young people who use and misuse drugs come from families with low cohesion and excessive adaptability; histories of maltreatment and parental modeling of the substance use behavior are also evident in their family backgrounds. Interpersonal problems associated with substance use disorders may be complicated by comorbidity with other psychological problems that are disruptive to interpersonal communication and relationships, such as depression, anxiety, bipolar disorders, and personality disorders.

THE SOCIAL CONSTRUCTION OF USE AND MISUSE

Most of the research reviewed in this chapter focuses on substance or alcohol *dependence* or *abuse*. Substance *use* studies are only considered for adolescent populations, as these are thought to identify the mechanisms that lead to abuse and/or dependence. The distinction between substance use and misuse is a social construction, and one that our society is still struggling with. American society permits (and in some cases sanctions) the use of certain drugs, such as caffeine, nicotine, and alcohol. However, some people believe that when children or adolescents are involved, the use of any drug is problematic and takes on the quality of a drug "problem." Regardless of the veracity of this assumption, this is part of the reason why there has been considerable research attention paid to substance *use* in adolescents. Similarly, some feel that the use of any illegal drug by adults or children is problematic, again blurring the use and abuse distinction. Also, the diagnostic criteria for substance abuse (e.g., failure to fulfill important occupational, social, or domestic roles as a result of substance use) may not be valid when applied to adolescents.

A distinct body of literature exists on interpersonal concomitants of alcoholism, and this research is examined separately from that on other substance use problems. As noted above, alcohol is for the most part a socially accepted substance, so long as its use falls within certain parameters. There is reason to suspect a priori that the interpersonal consequences of alcohol abuse/dependence may differ from those of other substance abuse/dependence, due to the greater social stigma and lesser social tolerance of such substances as cocaine, heroin, and amphetamine. However, it is again important to remember that the different interpersonal reactions to people who are dependent on alcohol versus other drugs are not due to inherent differences in the nature of the substance, but rather are the results of social convention.

INTERPERSONAL FEATURES OF ALCOHOLISM

Interpersonal Communication in Alcoholism: Social Skills Deficits

Like other mental health problems, alcoholism has been associated with poor social skills in some studies. However, unlike the literature on other mental health problems, social skills deficits in this population have received only limited scientific attention, and the associated findings are more equivocal.

Contact with inpatients in an alcohol treatment program led Foy, Massey, Duer, Ross, and Wooten (1979) to note that many of these inpatients reported having interpersonal problems. In particular, they appeared to have deficiencies in social skills in the context of interactions with coworkers and bosses (e.g., being underassertive, engaging in "explosive" verbal behavior). For many patients, work-related problems led to problem drinking. Another study of inpatients with alcoholism found that they performed poorly on a facial expression decoding task (Philippot et al., 1999). This unique investigation of social decoding skills found that these inpatients exhibited a general bias to overestimate the intensity of emotion conveyed by various facial expressions, and to interpret happy facial expressions as indicative of negative mood. Finally, Buhr and Pryor (1988) found those with alcoholism are more likely than those without to experience anxiety over communication with other people.

In a rare study of adolescents with problem drinking, Hover and Gaffney (1991) discovered a fairly linear association between 13- to 16-

year-olds' social skills and their drinking behavior. A group of teens who did not drink had the highest social skills scores, followed by those who drank to some extent, and then those with problem drinking. In this study, 11% of those who drank and 50% of those with problem drinking were in the "incompetent" range on the social skills measure.

Although some people with alcoholism may exhibit social skills deficits, it is also evident that some are quite functional socially. For example, Twentyman et al. (1982) conducted an extensive assessment of social skills in inpatients with alcoholism through a series of role plays that called for such responses as alcohol refusal, assertion, and expressing positive sentiments. Compared to a group of firefighters who served as a control group, the inpatients were rated as being less skillful in the alcohol refusal situations, but not in other social contexts. Furthermore, the inpatients actually performed better than the control group on an index of speech dysfluencies during their role plays. In a similar study, subjects with alcoholism performed better than psychiatric controls on role-play tests of social skills (Monti, Corriveau, & Zwick, 1981). When alcoholic subjects were asked to give their "typical" response in role-play social skills tests, they performed worse than controls, but when admonished to "give the very best response," they were indistinguishable from controls (Patterson, Parsons, Schaeffer, & Errico, 1988).

Research on social skills and alcoholism shows that poor social skills may be a problem in some cases of alcoholism. However, there is good reason to suspect that these skills deficits are not global or pervasive. Rather, they may be limited to social contexts such as negative assertion and refusal of alcohol when offered. In addition, when those with alcoholism do have problems with social skills, the problems may be due more to poor execution of the skills than to a lack of capacity for such skills. It is also possible that in such cases, prolonged problem drinking may deteriorate people's motivation and energy for producing interpersonally skilled behavior.

Family-of-Orientation Experiences in Alcoholism

General Family Interactions

Perhaps nowhere in the mental health literature has family systems theory had more of an impact than in the area of alcoholism (Steinglass, 1985). Family systems theory is a conceptual model, rather than a true theory, that locates causes and consequences of problematic behavior in the larger family system in which it is embedded. Family behavior is thought to be responsive to regulatory mechanisms that maintain the status quo, as well as a tendency to grow and change in response to dynamic qualities within and outside of the family. Viewing a family as a system suggests that a disturbance in one part of the system will have an impact on other parts of the system. Applying family systems concepts to alcoholism, Steinglass (1985) noted that some families organize their lives around the alcoholism of an adult member, just as other families might organize their lives around children or work.

In an early investigation of adults with alcoholism and their family members (Steinglass, Weiner, & Mendelson, 1971), the expression of previously inhibited positive affect between family members became extremely pronounced during drinking periods. This and later studies revealed that interactions in such families were actually more patterned, organized, and predictable while the adults with alcoholism were intoxicated (Steinglass, 1979, 1981b; Steinglass & Robertson, 1983; Steinglass et al., 1971). Thus alcohol ingestion serves an adaptive function in family relationships through a stabilizing phenomenon. This prompted Steinglass et al. (1971) to suggest that there is an "alcoholic system" in some families, in which drinking is an integral part of the family system that actually maintains and stabilizes the family. Similar positive effects on the family were evident in a study where family members viewed and rated a videotape of their own interaction, in the absence of actual drinking (Schweitzer, Wilks, & Callan, 1992). Both mothers and adolescent children in families with paternal alcoholism rated family members as less anxious and their interactions as more friendly than those of families without alcoholism. Unfortunately, drinking and intoxication may provide only a temporary "solution" to a family's problems, at the cost of what may be more serious long-term ill effects.

Although drinking can temporarily inject positivity into some family relationships, several laboratory investigations have also documented negative effects associated with drinking. For example, Jacob, Ritchey, Cvitkovic, and Blane (1981) had families with an alcoholic father discuss items from various questionnaire inventories while the fathers were drinking or not drinking. During their discussions, the families expressed more negative affect during the drinking versus the no-drinking condition (see also Billings, Kessler, Gomberg, & Weiner, 1979). The nature of interactions in families without paternal alcoholism was not affected by the drinking conditions.

The ill effects of parental alcoholism on family interaction and child rearing may begin to have an impact on family members as early as 1 year of age (Eiden, Chavez, & Leonard, 1999). In this study, families with alcoholism in at least one parent were observed interacting with their 12-month-old infants for 5 minutes in a room filled with toys. Observations of the parents' behavior indicated that the parents with alcoholism were less sensitive to their infants during the free play; such fathers in particular made fewer verbalizations, expressed more negative affect, and were less responsive to their infants. Self-report measures further indicate that the parents with alcoholism were more aggressive toward their spouses than those without alcogolism were. The family observation study by Eiden et al. (1999) was unique in showing that parents with alcoholism were far more depressed than those without, and that this depression mediated the relationship between parental alcoholism and sensitivity to the infants during interaction. So for many adults with alcoholism, effective parenting may be disrupted directly by the alcoholism, or by comorbid problems such as depression that in and of themselves have a negative impact on parenting behavior (see Chapter 2).

Different subtypes of alcoholism have been identified to explain the variable effects of alcohol consumption and alcoholism on family interactions and relations. In one such instance, Jacob, Krahn, and Leonard (1991) characterized subtypes of alcoholism as *episodic* or *steady* drinking. During family interactions, adults with episodic drinking exhibited more negativity than those with steady drinking. In addition, Jacob et al. (1991) found evidence of more positive behaviors from children, and greater problem solving by both children and mothers, in the families affected by steady versus episodic drinking.

Another useful distinction in alcoholism is that between *high-antisociality and low-antisociality* subtypes (Jacob, Haber, Leonard, & Rushe, 2000). These subtypes are defined on the basis of a measure that taps into negative social consequences of drinking, feelings of alienation, interpersonal disruption, and negative attitudes toward authority (higher scores = higher antisociality). Home observations of family dinner conversations revealed that wives, husbands, and children in families with high-antisociality alcoholism were all less positive, and less inclined to communicate disagreement, than were control family members. Although family interactions in the high-antisociality condition were characterized by diminished positivity, they appeared to have a "cautious" appearance as well, in that family members were careful to avoid open disagreement with each other.

This pattern of interaction could have interesting implications for the genesis of alcoholism. For the person who develops alcoholism, the tendency to avoid communicating disagreement may lead to the internalization of problems with other family members. Instead of airing complaints, the individual is left to ruminate over them on his or her own— perhaps without seeing any change in the offensive behavior by other family members, since they may be unaware of the problem. For this individual's family members, the tendency to be cautious and avoid disagreement may inadvertently cause his or her problem drinking behavior to go unchecked. In some cases, families have some ability to regulate problem drinking through punishing responses in reaction to the behavior. However, in a family system affected by high-antisociality alcoholism, this regulatory function may be inoperative.

Recognizing considerable diversity in alcoholism's effects on family interactions, Steinglass (1981a) proposed a *family alcohol phase* model. According to this perspective, a family moves through various phases that correspond to the drinking behavior of the member with alcoholism. The *stable–wet* phase is marked by consistent drinking, whereas the *stable–dry* phase is marked by general abstinence. The family is in a *transitional* phase either when a period of abstinence begins, or when a period of abstinence ends with episodes of drinking. Steinglass (1981a) found that *content variability* (the range of affect and decision-making behavior in verbal interaction) in family interactions, as well as *distance regulation* (use of space and rate of movement in the home), varied as a function of phase. In the stable–wet phase, families maintained the greatest distance, interacting only for purposeful reasons, while exhibiting midrange variability in their interactions. Families in the stable–dry phase exhibited a great deal of content variability in their interactions, with midrange distance regulation. Finally, those families in the transitional phase showed a decrease in distance regulation, manifesting physical closeness, with a slight decrease in the content variability of their interactions. A 2-year longitudinal study suggested that families in the stable–wet phase were the most likely of the three to dissolve their marriages (Steinglass, Tislenko, & Reiss, 1985). In particular, those families in the stable–wet phase that exhibited the least intrafamily engagement during home observations of family interaction were most likely to break up over the course of the study.

Summary. It has been noted that "in families of alcoholics relationships change when parental drinking occurs" (Seilhamer, Jacob, & Dunn, 1993, p. 194). However, sometimes these changes are positive and sometime they are negative. Where there are positive or adaptive outcomes, these may be somewhat short-lived. Researchers have been working to identify different subtypes of alcoholism that are associated with more negative family consequences. The poorest family processes and outcomes appear to be associated with the episodic (vs. steady), high-antisociality (vs. low-antisociality), and stable–wet (vs. stable–dry or transitional) alcoholism.

Marital Interactions

Alcoholism has a powerful and unavoidable impact on marital communication and relationships. In a pioneering study of marital relations and alcoholism, Gorad (1971) placed married couples in a game simulation in which they could win money individually through competitive moves or collectively through cooperative moves. Gorad also included a possibility in which partners could "secretly" compete with each other without making their competitive moves known. The men with alcoholism in this study made more secretly competitive moves than either their wives or any of the men without alcoholism did. This finding is thought to be characteristic of attempts by people with alcoholism to avoid taking responsibility for their behavior in close relationships, where alcohol provides an external, uncontrollable attribution.

Like the literature on alcoholism and family interaction more generally, examination of the marital interactions of those with different subtypes of alcoholism has been profitable. For instance, men with episodic alcoholism engage in less problem solving, and their wives exhibit more negativity, than men with steady alcoholism and their wives do (Jacob & Leonard, 1988). It is interesting to note that these group differences were only evident on occasions during which the men were drinking. Also of interest is the fact that steady drinking was associated with more problem-solving communication on drinking nights, indicating that alcohol may actually activate conflict resolution skills in those with this drinking subtype. This, of course, could reinforce the alcohol consumption. An interesting possibility is that the drinking brings about more problem-solving behavior because it motivates spouses to present complaints to their partners with alcoholism. In other words, the drinking could be a reminder of, or could prime the spouses for presenting, complaints about drinking-related problems. So long as the partners respond to these complaints, one would see elevated problem solving coincidental to drinking occasions.

Another useful distinction in the alcoholism literature concerns typical drinking locations, characterized as *in-home* and *out-of-home*. Marital relations appear most strained in couples where husbands engage in out-of-home drinking. In such couples, the husbands' alcohol consumption is negatively associated with wives' marital satisfaction (Dunn, Jacob, Hummon, & Seilhamer, 1987). Dunn et al. (1987) also found that the alcohol consumption pattern during out-of-home drinking was more variable and chaotic, whereas consumption during in-home drinking was reinforced and associated with more positive outcomes. One might speculate that those who drink outside the home may be seeking an escape from what they perceive to be bad marriages. On the other hand, spouses of those who drink at home may find the drinking behavior to be more predictable, less stressful, and associated with less suspicion about the behavior.

Negative marital interactions are especially prevalent when a husband with alcoholism is physically aggressive (Murphy & O'Farrell,

1997). When couples affected by husbands' alcoholism were discussing a marital problem, those with aggressive husbands showed a higher base rate of negative communication behaviors (e.g., blaming, criticizing, put-downs) and more negative reciprocity in their communication than did the couples with nonaggressive husbands. This suggests that some of the negativity in marital interactions when a husband has alcoholism may be the result of aggressiveness, which covaries to some extent with alcoholism, as opposed to the alcoholism per se. Negativity in marital interactions is also pronounced when a wife has alcoholism. In a rare comparison of couples affected by female versus male alcoholism, the female-alcoholism couples were found to be more negative in their conversations than either the male-alcoholism or no-alcoholism couples when *no* drinking took place (Haber & Jacob, 1997). When drinking occurred, differences from male-alcoholism couples disappeared. For concordant couples (in which both husbands and wives had alcoholism), negativity in communication behaviors escalated when the spouses were allowed to drink. This latter finding suggests that at least one spouse without alcoholism may be a prerequisite for adaptive outcomes associated with drinking. However, marital differences in female- versus male-alcoholism couples remain mixed; some studies show that wives with alcoholism express more positive communication with their husbands, and that husbands with alcoholism express more negative communication with their wives, relative to controls (Noel, McCrady, Stout, & Fisher-Nelson, 1991). Because wives with alcoholism are very likely to have been divorced or deserted by their husbands (Corrigan, 1980), such couples who find their way into research studies with their marriages still intact may represent particularly well-functioning marriages.

The spouses of those with alcoholism tend to suffer ill effects from the social and physical consequences of their partners' drinking. Steinglass (1981b) found a strong relationship between psychiatric symptomatology in a spouse without alcoholism and the social and physical consequences of the other spouse's drinking. Jacob, Dunn, Leonard, and Davis (1985) partially replicated this finding, but with weaker associations. Spouses of those with alcoholism have also been shown to be low in extraversion and high in neuroticism (Suman & Nagalakshmi, 1993). These same spouses were significantly more inhibited and withdrawn in interpersonal relationships than were spouses of those without alcoholism. An obvious inference is that the phenomenon of alcoholism and its associated features (e.g., trouble with the law, moodiness, missed work, deterioration of physical health) causes psychosocial distress for the spouses of the affected individuals. However, the cross-sectional nature of the data on which this conclusion is based cannot rule out an alternative interpretation: Perhaps individuals with alcoholism increase their drinking, with the attendant consequences, in response to their spouses' increased distress. Considering that this is a population prone to maladaptive use of alcohol for coping purposes, this hypothesis deserves at least some exploration and consideration.

Research findings on the spouses of those with alcoholism warrant consideration of at least one additional hypothesis. In the depression literature, there is some evidence to favor an assortative mating effect (see Chapter 2): Some depressed people appear to seek relationships with others who have depressive tendencies. Similarly, people who engage in problem drinking, or are prone to alcoholism, may be attracted to other people who are introverted and at least mildly distressed themselves. Perhaps this allows the alcoholism-prone individuals to engage in downward social comparison and not feel so bad about themselves. Perhaps the potential assortative mating effect in alcoholism is driven by something as simple as the "misery loves company" effect.

Another phenomenon indicative of interpersonal friction is the failure of those with alcoholism and their spouses to come to mutual agreement about personal and family issues. In one investigation, subjects with alcoholism described themselves as *more* loving, affectionate, and understanding than subjects without alcoholism described themselves (Neeliyara, Nagalakshmi, & Ray, 1989). However, the spouses of the subjects with alcoholism sharply disagreed with their partners' self-perceptions, perceiving them as less loving and more aggressive. In the areas of affective involvement (e.g., "We are too self-centered") and behavior control (e.g., "Anything goes in our family"), persons with alcoholism and their spouses showed very low agreement, although they did exhibit higher agreement on descriptions of family problem solving and general functioning (McKay, Maisto, Beattie, Longabaugh, & Noel, 1993). These differing perceptions among intimates are a potent recipe for distress.

Summary. The literature on alcoholism and marital and family relations (see Jacob & Seilhamer, 1987, and Jacobs & Wolin, 1989, for reviews) clearly indicates that for at least some families, alcohol brings stability and temporary positivity. These outcomes contribute to a family maintenance of the alcoholism. At the same time, other research evidence indicates that increased negativity in family relations is also quite possible as a result of drinking (e.g., Billings et al., 1979; Jacob et al., 1981), although it is not always reciprocated between spouses (Jacob & Leonard, 1992). Certain subtypes of alcoholism, such as the out-of-home drinking pattern, physically aggressive alcoholism in males, and concordant alcoholism in marriages, are particularly associated with negative communicative exchanges. Those with alcoholism appear to hold beliefs about themselves and their families that their spouses sharply disagree with. These spouses also appear to exhibit psychosocial problems and distress of their own. An intriguing issue in need of further clarification is the extent to which distressed family relations contribute to problem drinking, as well as the extent to which problem drinking can cause deterioration in family relationships. Currently, there appear to be no data that directly disconfirm either of these causal routes.

Children of Parents with Alcoholism

Children of parents with alcoholism—or "children of alcoholics (COAs)," as they are commonly known—have received a great deal of research attention as an at-risk population (e.g., Sher, 1991; Windle & Searles, 1990). Concern with this population stems from the belief that parental alcoholism leads to disrupted and dysfunctional family environments that have ill effects on children. These ill effects may be driven by parental modeling of dysfunctional and destructive behaviors, corruption and deterioration of parenting behaviors, or an amalgamation of both processes (Curran & Chassin, 1996; Jacob & Johnson, 1997). Indeed, results of a large-sample cross-sectional study with rigorous sampling techniques indicated that COAs exhibited significant differences from non-COAs: greater involvement in alcohol use; more drug dependence; more depression, agoraphobia, social phobia, and generalized anxiety; less behavioral control; lower self-esteem; lower scores on tests of verbal ability; and lower academic achievement (Sher, Walitzer, Wood, & Brent, 1991). Differences between COAs and non-COAs in this investigation were small to moderate in magnitude. Other findings indicate that COAs are more depressed, less satisfied with their own marriages, and more likely to drink for coping purposes (Domenico & Windle, 1993); that they are more susceptible to the ill effects of conflict with their parents (Barrera & Stice, 1998); and that they experience less intimacy in their close relationships than non-COAs do (Martin, 1995). Taken in isolation, findings such as these suggest rather pervasive deficits among COAs.

Perhaps the problem most strongly linked with being a COA is a risk for alcoholism (Chassin, Pitts, DeLucia, & Todd, 1999; Jacob, Windle, Seilhamer, & Bost, 1999; Pollock, Schneider, Garielli, & Goodwin, 1987). COAs are far more likely to have alcohol problems themselves than are members of the general population. Consideration must certainly be given to the influence of genetic mechanisms in the familial transmission of alcoholism. At the same time, however, it is plausible to assume that social learning processes also contribute to the increased risk. Children who observe parents using alcohol as a means of relaxation, coping with stress, celebration, and so forth would naturally be expected to imitate this behavior that their parents regularly modeled during their formative years.

Notwithstanding some of the significant problems that appear to be associated with being a COA, a substantial body of literature is emerging that questions the distinctness and at-risk status of the COA population. For example, studies have found no differences between COAs and non-COAs in alcohol-related problems, suicidal ideation, personal control, and perceived social support (Wright & Heppner, 1991); anxiety (Clair & Genest, 1992; Velleman & Orford, 1993); social skills (Jacob & Leonard, 1986; Segrin & Menees, 1996); social maladjustment (Dinning & Berk, 1989); use of nonverbal communication behaviors (Senchak, Greene, Carroll, & Leonard, 1996); personality traits such as expressiveness, alienation, defensiveness, independence, impulsiveness, sociability, and extraversion (Baker & Stephenson, 1995; Berkowitz & Perkins, 1988; Havey & Dodd, 1993; Lyon & Seefeldt, 1995; Velleman & Orford, 1993); object relations deficits and compulsive behavior (Hadley, Holloway, & Mallinckrodt, 1993); self-esteem (Menees, 1997), fear of intimacy (Giunta & Compas, 1994); or depression (Reich, Earls, Frankel, & Shayka, 1993). The list of such studies is too long, and the breadth of dependent variables too extensive, to dismiss these findings to sampling error or other artifacts. Such results are interpretable as good news for the COAs. Although parents who have alcoholism may raise children with psychosocial problems of their own, this is not a deterministic relationship. Dysfunction may be more evident in those COAs seeking attention through self-help groups and professional contacts (Chafetz, Blane, & Hill, 1971; Hinson, Becker, Handal, & Katz, 1993; Sheridan & Green, 1993). In general, researchers are converging on the conclusion that COAs are a complex and heterogeneous population who are not always distinguishable from those in the general population (Harrington & Metzler, 1997; Harter, 2000; Jacob & Johnson, 1997; West & Prinz, 1987).

It is notable that although many COAs are as functional as their non-COA counterparts, most still describe their early family environments as distressed and dysfunctional. For example, compared to non-COAs, COAs describe their families of origin as more conflict-laden (Garbarino & Strange, 1993; Giunta & Compas, 1994), less harmonious (Velleman & Orford, 1993), more troubled and stressed (Jones & Houts, 1992), and less cohesive (Dinning & Berk, 1989; Havey & Dodd, 1993; Sheridan & Green, 1993). To a large extent, parents with alcoholism and their spouses describe similar dynamics in the family environment (Moos & Moos, 1984). This pattern of findings speaks favorably to the validity of family environment assessments from people with alcoholism, their spouses, and their children: All see troubles in the family context. Even though COAs often describe a negative atmosphere in their families of origin, many are still indistinguishable from non-COAs on a variety of psychosocial outcomes. Wright and Heppner (1993) found that the family environments in which COAs are raised are as varied and diverse as those in which there is no parental alcoholism. Since parents with alcoholism are themselves a diverse and heterogeneous group, it stands to reason that the family environments that they help to create are reflective of that heterogeneity. Taken one step further, it may be understandable why their children are an equally heterogeneous group.

The new frontier in research on COAs entails the search for mediators and moderators of the effects of parental alcoholism on the children's psychosocial adjustment (Sher, 1991). The advice to researchers has been clearly stated: "We must move beyond COA–non-COA contrasts to systematic analyses of within-group variance in order to better understand the conditions under which family history of alcoholism results in adverse outcomes" (Jacob & Johnson, 1999, p. 170). Recognizing this, researchers are attempting to discover the family factors that enhance risk or resiliency in the face of parental alcoholism. For example, some models of the influence of parental alcoholism on children's adjustment suggest that variables such as *marital strain*, *social isolation*, *role reversals*, and *medical problems* may moderate this relationship (Seilhamer & Jacob, 1990). COAs are more likely to have experienced *physical or sexual abuse* while growing up (Bensley, Spieker, & McMahon, 1994). However, when abuse history is controlled for, the effects of parental alcoholism on offspring's social maladjustment become nonsignificant (Harter & Taylor, 2000). When parents with alcoholism create dysfunctional family environments, *attachment to the parents* mediates the relationship between family and interpersonal distress in young adult children (Mothersead, Kivlighan, & Wynkoop, 1998). Specifically, family dysfunction tends to reduce parental attachment, which in turn is associated with increased levels of interpersonal distress in COAs. Also, COAs who have a *predisposition toward social deviance* (e.g., problems with authority, unresponsiveness to discipline, social alienation) are especially prone to developing alcohol problems themselves (Finn, Sharkansky, Brandt, & Turcotte, 2000).

In their review of the literature on COAs, West and Prinz (1987) noted: "Parental alcoholism does not occur in a vacuum. Other adverse familial and environmental factors can influence child outcomes to varying degrees" (p. 206). A brief review of the diagnostic criteria for alcohol abuse or dependence reveals that problems with the law, physical health, and occupational performance are, by definition, part of each disorder.

Each of these could precipitate a host of stressors that could have a malevolent impact on family members. COAs are between two and four times more likely than non-COAs to be exposed to *parental divorce, separation, unemployment,* or *death,* in addition to their parents' alcoholism (Menees & Segrin, 2000). Each of these stressors could independently have deleterious effects on the psychosocial adjustment of children. The Menees and Segrin (2000) study was one of the few studies in the literature on COAs to control extensively for comorbid stressors; the findings indicate that once these are taken into account, family environments of COAs are not described differently from those of children of nonstressed control families. Therefore, where COAs appear to be psychologically or socially disadvantaged, family stressors that covary with parental alcoholism may be as responsible for the disadvantages as parental alcoholism per se, if not more so (see also Heller, Sher, & Benson, 1982; Velleman, 1992).

Some family and interpersonal factors that protect COAs from distress have recently been identified. Jennison and Johnson (1997) found that for adult COAs, *dyadic cohesion* and *agreement in marital communication* (e.g., household management, self-disclosure, consensus, etc.) greatly diminished the association between parental alcoholism and their own problem drinking. Similarly, families that are able to maintain *family rituals* (e.g., birthday celebrations, evening meals) are less likely to raise offspring with alcohol problems, despite parental alcoholism (Wolin, Bennett, Noonan, & Teitelbaum, 1980). Also, *social support from friends,* but not from family members, is associated with a lower risk of alcohol and drug misuse among COAs (Ohannessian & Hesselbrock, 1999).

Summary. Recognition of the interpersonal consequences of alcoholism has brought considerable attention to COAs. Although they were originally considered to be an at-risk population, research findings show that COAs are a heterogeneous population, not particularly distinct from non-COAs. In cases where COAs experience problematic psychosocial outcomes, a generally distressed family environment, rather than parental alcoholism per se, may be the causal agent.

INTERPERSONAL FEATURES OF OTHER SUBSTANCE USE PROBLEMS

The emphasis in this part of the chapter is on the development and maintenance of drug use problems among adolescents. As noted earlier, the bulk of the research on this topic has focused on *family-of-origin experiences.* Parental modeling, family-of-origin discord, and physical and sexual abuse within the family may all play roles in the development of adolescent substance misuse. However, factors in the other three major domains considered in this book may also be important: *general personal relationships* (peer modeling and maltreatment perpetrated by nonrelatives as paths to substance use), *interpersonal communication* (social skills deficits in adolescents themselves as either causes or effects of substance misuse), and eventual *family-of-orientation experiences* (inconsistent nurturing by significant others as a factor maintaining substance misuse).

Social Paths to Substance Use

Modeling by Peers and the Family of Origin

Few people stumble into drug use by accident. Considering the elaborate and varied steps involved in the procurement, preparation, and ingestion of different drugs, the likelihood that people acquire these behaviors on their own is extremely low. Rather, most people learn about drugs, and learn how to take drugs, by observing other people. In fact, most adolescents who begin to use drugs and alcohol do so after first observing this behavior in their peers (Beisecker, 1991; Kandel, 1978). Substance misuse may thus be a unique mental health problem, in that it can literally be learned from others. Consistent with this idea, research findings show that drug and alcohol use by peers and parents is one of the most powerful predictors of adolescent drug and alcohol involvement (Johnson & Pandina, 1991; Kandel, 1978; Kandel & Andrews, 1987). For this reason, the most compelling account of drug use initiation can be found in social learning theory (Bandura, 1977, 1986).

As noted in connection with eating disorders in Chapter 7, social learning theory posits that one mechanism by which people acquire behaviors is observational learning, or *modeling*. Modeling works because it gives people a template or guide for their own behavior. Bandura (1986) refers to this as "making the unobservable observable" (p. 66). He notes that people cannot observe their own behavior; however, the observation of others' behavior gives people a mental picture of how a behavior can and should be performed. When people see others rewarded for performing a behavior, they are more likely to enact that behavior. Bandura explains that people learn if–then relationships by observing others. For example, an adolescent may learn that "if I smoke marijuana, then I will look cool and feel great." This could be learned by observing peers who use the drug with the support and camaraderie of other friends, and who extol its positive effects.

Social learning theory is currently one of the major theories of adolescent substance use initiation (Howard, 1992; Simons, Conger, & Whitebeck, 1988; Strickland & Pittman, 1984). As predicted by the theory, association with peers and/or parents who use substances has a powerful impact on adolescents' own substance use behavior (Hawkins, Catalano, & Miller, 1992; Kandel, 1978). For example, a study of high school students revealed a correlation of approximately $r = .50$ between students' substance use and that of their parents (Malkus, 1994). In another study of prisoners enrolled in substance misuse treatment programs, 54% indicated a family history of parental alcohol or other drug problems (Sheridan, 1995). A national household probability sample of over 4,000 adolescents showed that a history of family drug use increased the odds of adolescents' abuse or dependence on alcohol, marijuana, or "hard" drugs by factors of 1.89, 4.14, and 7.89, respectively (Kilpatrick et al., 2000). In other words, adolescents whose family members use drugs are anywhere from two to eight times more likely to be abusing and/or dependent on drugs themselves than are adolescents in families without a history of drug use.

In addition to the family, association with peers who use drugs may also provide a source of further observational learning of substance use. Spending time with such peers, and developing friendships with them, are associated with a greater likelihood of drug use (e.g., Bahr, Hawks, & Wang, 1993; Kandel, 1973; Kandel & Andrews, 1987). However, this finding is complicated by the fact that adolescents who use drugs tend to select peers who use drugs as friends (Bauman & Ennett, 1994). Similarity is a major determinant of interpersonal attraction, so it stands to reason that such friendships will develop.

The varied findings on associations with peers who use drugs have provoked equivocal conclusions about their impact on the development of adolescent substance use. For instance, some investigators state that "peer use of substances has consistently been found to be among the strongest predictors of substance use among youth" (Hawkins et al., 1992, p. 85), while others assert that "peer influence appears to be less significant than previously thought in predicting either drug use . . . or drug abuse" (Weinberg, Rahdert, Colliver, & Glantz, 1998, p. 255). Longitudinal studies reviewed by Kandel (1978) indicate that perceived drug use in peers and perceived favorable attitudes toward drug use among peers are both precursors to adolescent substance use. These phenomena may normalize substance use in an adolescent's mind. If a young person feels that his or her friends are taking drugs, and that his or her friends think it is cool to take drugs, it follows that drug use will be viewed as normative conduct. This cognitive and attitudinal socialization into drug use makes it difficult to rule out the peer influence hypothesis. Ultimately, Kandel (1978) points out that both of these processes (the influence of peers who use drugs, and the selection of such peers) may be simultaneously operative.

Family-of-Origin Discord

Aside from the effects of parental modeling, certain negative family dynamics and atmospheres may predispose adolescents toward substance use. The families of teens who use substances tend to be less cohesive, to be less adaptable, and to exhibit less togetherness than families of teens who do not use (Malkus, 1994). Negativity and conflict in the family are also positively correlated with adolescent drug use (Shek, 1998). These results notwithstanding, some of these family dynamics may actually be related to parental drug use. Bahr et al. (1993), for example, found that after they controlled for parental monitoring and family drug use, the association between family cohesion and adolescent drug use was not significant.

The family may also influence adolescent substance use through problematic or ineffective parenting (Hawkins et al., 1992). For example, inconsistent parental discipline and skewed parenting, in which one parent is overinvolved and the other is overly permissive, are risk factors for initial drug use in adolescents (Kandel & Andrews, 1987; Ziegler-Driscoll, 1979). A combination of low parental support and high parental control has proven to be a particularly noxious combination of parenting behaviors that is also predictive of adolescent substance use (Barnes, Farrell, & Cairns, 1986). In addition, excessive maternal expressed emotion (criticism) is associated with a threefold increase in the risk for at least one of the following childhood problems: depression, substance abuse, or conduct disorder (Schwartz, Dorer, Beardslee, Lavor, & Keller, 1990). The effects of paternal hostility on adolescent alcohol use are equally powerful (Johnson & Pandina, 1991).

Some noteworthy longitudinal studies indicate that defective parenting behavior may precede offspring's substance misuse by many years. A landmark study by Shedler and Block (1990) found that mothers of children who were frequent users of marijuana at age 18 were underresponsive to their children and gave them little encouragement during an observation at age 5. Similarly, parents who exhibited less directive control and assertiveness while interacting with their 4-year-old children were more likely to have adolescents who used marijuana heavily some years later (Baumrind, 1991).

These parenting behaviors and family environments may push an adolescent away from the family—causing him or her to reject traditional family beliefs and values such as religion, work, and education, and to move toward socialization with deviant peers (Blackson, Tarter,

Loeber, Ammerman, & Windle, 1996; Harbach & Jones, 1995). Note-worthy in the Harbach and Jones (1995) study is the finding that parents of at-risk adolescents held beliefs and values similar to those of other parents, but that their children did not share these values. This suggests a breakdown in the process of parenting and/or and overwhelming influence of deviant peers.

Interpersonal Maltreatment

As with so many other mental health problems, a history of interpersonal maltreatment (including physical and sexual abuse) is predictive of later substance misuse. Although this phenomenon may be an extension of the aversive family-of-origin environments described above, such maltreatment need not be perpetrated by family members in order to increase risk for substance use. In addition, the assessment of childhood maltreatment in this literature does not always identify the relationship between the perpetrator and the child. Therefore, this set of social stressors is discussed separately from family-of-origin environment issues, although it is acknowledged that there may be a considerable interrelation between family-of-origin environment and these stressors. (It is also acknowledged that other social stressors, such as rejection by peers, may play a role in adolescent substance use/misuse; however, the present discussion focuses on physical and sexual abuse.)

In Sheridan's (1995) study of prisoners in treatment for substance misuse, 67% had a history of physical abuse, and 37% had a history of sexual abuse. A large national probability sample of adolescents revealed that a history of sexual assault increased adolescents' odds of alcohol, marijuana, and hard drug abuse/dependence by factors of 3.93, 3.80, and 8.59, respectively (Kilpatrick et al., 2000). In this study, adolescents with a history of sexual assault were over *eight times* more likely to have a drug use problem than were those without a history of sexual assault. Moreover, among the adolescents with substance use in this study, those who were sexually abused started using at a younger age than those who were not. A large national survey of adult women also indicated that a history of childhood sexual abuse increased the odds of using illicit drugs by a factor of 2.52 (Wilsnack, Vogeltanz, Klassen, & Harris, 1997).

The research findings on childhood physical and sexual abuse cast the parental modeling hypothesis and findings in a different light. In addition to modeling drug use and misuse, parents who use drugs are also more likely to abuse their children physically and sexually than are parents with no history of substance use (Kilpatrick et al., 2000; Sheridan, 1995). Thus parental substance use may affect adolescent substance use/

misuse both directly, through modeling, and indirectly through the effects of maltreatment.

A number of hypotheses have been developed to explain the relationship between childhood maltreatment and adolescent substance use (e.g., Jarvis, Copeland, & Walton, 1998; Kilpatrick et al., 2000). The *self-medication hypothesis* holds that survivors of physical or sexual abuse engage in substance use to cope with the emotional trauma of the abuse. This may take the form of sedating or dulling the senses with depressants, or maintaining a state of hypervigilance and watchfulness with stimulants. The *self-esteem hypothesis* suggests that people turn to substance use to combat the effects of the damaged self-esteem resulting from maltreatment. For some people, drug use may bring a temporary feeling of acceptance from peers, and a ready means of socializing without developing any real intimacy. An additional and related explanation for the association between physical or sexual abuse and substance misuse could be characterized as a hypothesis of *perceived non-risk*. People with a history of such abuse sometimes feel damaged and worthless. To such individuals there may be fewer deterrents to drug initiation, since they feel that they have less to lose. Unfortunately, as Jarvis et al. (1998) note, adolescent substance use in response to prior maltreatment may create a vicious cycle. Substance use or misuse can itself increase the risk of subsequent maltreatment, due to impaired judgment, socializing with deviant peers, and inhabitation of dangerous environments. Therefore, many young people may find themselves in a cycle of maltreatment, substance use, more maltreatment, further substance use, and so on.

Sheridan's (1995) intergenerational model of substance misuse and family abuse/neglect provides a useful connection between findings indicating that parents who misuse substances are more likely to maltreat their children, and that survivors of childhood maltreatment are more likely to get involved with substance use. According to this model, substance misuse may be passed on intergenerationally, in part, through child maltreatment. As illustrated in Figure 8.1, *parental substance misuse (substance abuse in the figure)* has negative effects on overall *family competence* (e.g., cohesion, parenting quality, respect for boundaries) and positive effects on the likelihood of *child abuse/neglect*. The poor family competence and abuse/neglect are expected to predispose the offspring to *adult abuse/neglect*, due to their learned "victim" roles and developing excessive dependency needs. The continuation of this abuse and neglect into late adolescence or adulthood then leads to *offspring substance misuse*, perhaps for reasons such as self-medication and coping. As adults, these offspring then become parents themselves, and the whole cycle starts anew. Sheridan (1995) presents some provocative data in support of this model (see also Henderson, Albright, Kalichman, &

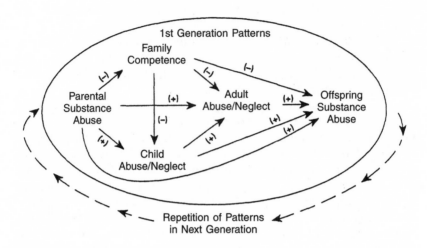

FIGURE 8.1. Proposed model of intergenerational substance abuse, family functioning, and abuse/neglect. From Sheridan (1995). Copyright 1995 by Elsevier Science.
Reprinted by permission.

Dugoni, 1994), which provides an intriguing theoretical account of the
interpersonal transmission of substance abuse in a family context.

Summary

The origins of substance use appear to be largely interpersonal. Modeling, family-of-origin discord, and the social stressors constituting childhood maltreatment, are all interpersonal processes and mechanisms
associated with substance use in adolescents. It is apparent that drug *use*
(and its initiation, in particular) is associated with family and peer influences, but that drug *misuse* may be related more to biological and psychological processes (Kendler, Karkowski, Neale, & Prescott, 2000;
Weinberg et al., 1998). Nevertheless, it would be naive to overlook family-of-origin environments and other chronic social stressors as contributory factors in drug misuse. Unlike problems such as depression or
schizophrenia, which are in some cases characterized as "endogenous,"
substance misuse is a phenomenon that almost always originates in interactions with other people. These people demonstrate the problematic
behavior. A predisposition to engage in the behavior, and its maintenance, may be activated by a tumultuous family-of-origin environment
and interpersonal maltreatment.

Adolescent Substance Use and Interpersonal Communication (Social Skills) Deficits

There is a tendency to think of young people who are involved in drug and alcohol use as poorly socialized, interpersonally disconnected, and behaviorally lethargic. Is this an accurate characterization? The answer is not entirely straightforward.

The multiple interpersonal factors that lead to and maintain substance use/misuse per se may also affect the social/interpersonal development of the individual. Among adolescents, substance use is associated with aggressiveness (Braucht, Brakarsh, Follingstad, & Berry, 1973; Kellam, Brown, Rubin, & Ensminger, 1983), low assertiveness (Rhodes & Jason, 1990), and poor social skills (Webb & Baer, 1995). Deficits in social skills create a sense of low self-efficacy, which in turn promotes involvement in substance use (Webb & Baer, 1995). When the social skills for coping with stress are not available, substance use is more likely to occur as a means of reducing stress. In addition, people with poor social skills do not have a strong sense of self-efficacy for the ability to control or resist drug and alcohol use. Therefore, social skills deficits may be said to have an indirect effect on adolescent substance use, through diminished self-efficacy.

Although adolescents who use drugs may present some interpersonal problems, the extent to which these are causal agents deserves careful attention and consideration. Substance use can cause a deterioration of social skills and competence over time (Pentz, 1985). At least some of the interpersonal problems that may be evident among adolescents experienced in drug use may be the *results* of drug use. At the same time, social maladjustment generally predates drug use in young people. In Shedler and Block's (1990) 15-year longitudinal study, index cases of heavy drug use at age 18 could be traced back to a profile of alienation, emotional distress, failure to develop close relationships, and an inability to get along with friends as early as age 7. Consequently, these authors concluded that "problem drug use is a symptom, not a cause, of personal and social maladjustment" (p. 612).

The relationship between interpersonal deficiencies and drug use is complex: Such deficiencies predispose young people to get involved with drugs, but at the same time, heavy drug use has deleterious effects on interpersonal competencies. As if to complicate matters further, the relationship between social maladjustment and drug use is not linear. In their longitudinal study, Shedler and Block (1990) compared three groups they referred to as "abstainers," "experimenters," and "frequent users." In terms of the quality of their interpersonal relations, "experimenters" scored highest, followed by "abstainers" and then "frequent users." Visually, the pattern of association between drug use and quality of interpersonal relations in this sample as a whole took the form of an inverted U. Looking back to their childhood, eventual "abstainers" appeared unresponsive to humor, shy, reserved, obedient and compliant, nontalkative, and dependent on adults for direction. Many of these interpersonal qualities persevered through their late teens. This study shows that while the frequent use of drugs in adolescence is associated with poor social competence, so too is complete abstinence from drugs, although to a lesser extent.

Why do those who abstain from drugs have lower-quality interpersonal relations than those who experiment with them? First, those in the former group may be globally overcautious. The same anxious cognitions and emotions that may keep an adolescent from ever trying drugs may also prevent him or her from approaching classmates who are relative strangers and attempting to develop interpersonal relationships with them, or from asking people out on dates. These interpersonal processes require a certain degree of adventurousness and risk taking; the adolescent who abstains from drugs may not have these traits. Second, experimentation with drugs is ordinarily a social phenomenon; adolescents will often engage in the behavior at the urging of, or with the aid of demonstrations by, peers. People with interpersonal skill deficits may simply be less likely to find themselves in such contexts, and therefore may be less likely to experiment with drugs, since the social facilitation is generally lacking in their lives.

Social Paths to the Maintenance of Substance Use and Misuse: A Family-of-Orientation Hypothesis

Interpersonal problems are widely recognized as risk factors for the initiation of adolescent substance use. It is equally well accepted that once a pattern of drug use/misuse is underway, the biological and psychological characteristics of addiction may be largely responsible for its maintenance. For this reason there has been very little research attention paid to interpersonal mechanisms that might perpetuate substance misuse, despite the fact that systems oriented therapists who treat alcohol and drug dependence routinely address the interpersonal milieu surrounding the problem behavior.

Recently, Le Poire and her colleagues (Le Poire, 1992, 1994; Le Poire, Hallett, & Erlandson, 2000) developed and tested a theory of substance misuse maintenance, based on the notion of inconsistent nurturing. In short, their *inconsistent-nurturing-as-control* theory predicts that the significant others of those who misuse substances may actually play a role in maintaining the substance abusing behavior. Significant others tend to oscillate between punishing their partners for drug-related behavior (e.g., conflict, fights, withdrawal) and rewarding them for it (e.g., cleaning up after them, taking care of them) (Le Poire, Erlandson, & Hallett, 1998). The rewarding behavior allows a significant other to feel needed and included in such a relationship. However, this same behavior is what perpetuates the substance misuse of the partner. According to this theory, the competing goals of nurturing the partner and controlling the drug-misusing behavior result in a schedule of intermittent reward and punishment, which has the paradoxical effect of strengthening the drug abusing behavior.

Empirical tests of inconsistent-nurturing-as-control theory have yielded generally supportive results (Le Poire et al., 1998, 2000), indicating that the course of substance misuse may be influenced by the nature of interactions with significant others. Individuals who misuse substances, and who find themselves in relationships with partners who have the codependent tendency to nurture and control them, may inadvertently and paradoxically be reinforced for their drug-misusing behavior. This theory is a departure from traditional models of substance misuse maintenance, which are sharply focused on biological and psychological factors.

COMORBIDITY OF ALCOHOLISM AND OTHER SUBSTANCE USE PROBLEMS WITH OTHER MENTAL HEALTH PROBLEMS

The *signal hypothesis* holds that excessive alcohol or substance use is a sign of distress. The comorbidity of other psychological problems with drug and alcohol misuse is testimony to the validity of this hypothesis. Before these are discussed, it should be noted that drug use problems are highly comorbid with alcohol use problems: About half of all those who misuse hard drugs also suffer from alcohol dependence (Brooner, King, Kidorf, Schmidt, & Bigelow, 1997; Manley, 1992).

Rates of alcoholism and other substance use disorders are very high among those with mood disorders (e.g., Kandel et al., 1999; Swendsen & Merikangas, 2000). As noted earlier in this chapter, a study by Egeland and Hostetter (1983) showed that rates of mood disorders are equal for men and women in the American Amish community, where the use of alcohol is prohibited. This suggests that alcoholism may mask depression in men in the general population, since men are thought to have about half the rate of depression than women do. In fact, there are very few people who have *just* drinking problems. Such individuals often have a number of related problems, such as depression and anxiety. In some cases, the drinking may be a misguided attempt to "cope" with these disorders, and in other cases, these other psychosocial problems may be consequences of problem drinking.

Chapter 5 has noted that many patients with bipolar disorder also have substance use problems. About a quarter to half of all such patients have some substance use disorder (Pini et al., 1999; Sonne & Brady, 1999). Substance use disorders are also highly comorbid with personality disorders, as noted in Chapter 6. Almost 60% of all people with substance use disorders have a comorbid personality disorder (Skodol, Oldham, & Gallaher, 1999).

The pattern of comorbidity with alcoholism and other substance use disorders reveals close associations with other disorders that have strong links to interpersonal relationship problems. One plausible account of this comorbidity may be that the substance use is secondary to the primary psychological problem, initiated in an effort to regulate and cope with a deteriorating interpersonal environment. Problems such as depression, anxiety, and personality disorders can rapidly decay interpersonal relationships. The feelings of loneliness, damaged self-esteem, and lack of direction that often accompany and follow the deterioration of interpersonal relationships may prompt some people to turn to substance use. In such instances, the substance use may be an attempt to regulate interpersonal interactions (e.g., taking cocaine in effort to go out in public and have a good time) or to cope with feelings of emptiness and rejection (e.g., drinking alcohol to "escape" dysphoric feelings).

In other cases, substance use disorders may precede other psychological problems that stem from destroyed interpersonal relationships. Once substance use is initiated, some people continue and escalate it because of chemical addiction. However, it is virtually a foregone conclusion that as the substance use becomes more pervasive, interpersonal relationships are damaged and ultimately destroyed. This effect happens partly because excessive drug and alcohol use interferes with competent interpersonal behavior; it focuses individuals almost exclusively on substance ingestion, at the expense of maintaining mutually rewarding relationships with other people. When this focus is taken to extremes, a person may steal from others to get money to buy drugs, lie, and become excessively abrasive. These behaviors reliably damage interpersonal relationships, and problems such as depression and anxiety may follow— not necessarily because of the substance use disorder per se, but because of the interpersonal consequences of the substance use. Consequently, much of the comorbidity between substance use disorders and other psychosocial problems may be explained by aversive interpersonal experiences. These are the experiences with the power and impact to link the problems.

CONCLUSION

At least a quarter of the population will experience significant problems with substance abuse or dependence in their lifetimes. This class of problems generally has its origins in adolescence, and substance use is currently on the rise in this cohort. Within the substance use disorders, alcoholism has received a great deal of interpersonally oriented research attention.

People who are dependent on alcohol exhibit problems with some social skills, such as negative assertion and refusal of alcohol from others. However, these interpersonal skills deficits are not broad-based, and may be due more to low motivation to use the skills than to not possessing them. Alcoholism has complex associations with family interactions. In some cases, alcoholism can bring positivity and stability to family relations. In other cases, alcoholism is associated with increased family troubles. Scientists are learning that alcoholism is a heterogeneous phenomenon, and that persons with certain subtypes of it are more inclined than others to have more severe family problems. In particular, those with episodic (vs. steady), high-antisociality (vs. low-antisociality), and stable–wet (vs. stable–dry or transitional) alcoholism tend to have the most disrupted family environments and interactions.

As in the family more generally, the marital relationship can influence and is influenced by spousal alcoholism. Alcoholics may harbor feelings of hostility and competitiveness toward their spouse. At the same time, drinking can in some cases activate positivity and problem solving in marital interaction. The marriages of those who drink at home tend to see more positive consequences of drinking than the marriages of those who drink outside the home.

A great deal of attention has been paid to COAs in both the scientific and lay press. Problems for COAs are thought to represent the interpersonally destructive consequences of parental alcoholism. Although they are clearly at risk for developing problem drinking themselves, COAs are not easily distinguished from non-COAs. When they are, a more general negative family environment mechanism may explain their troubles better than the specific effects of parental alcoholism do.

The architecture for adult substance abuse or dependence is often intact by the end of adolescence, and is largely established through interpersonal interactions. Young people learn to use drugs and alcohol by observing their friends and family members perform the behaviors; this process is known as *modeling*. High levels of family-of-origin discord and interpersonal maltreatment may predispose young people to get involved with and continue to use drugs and alcohol. Undoubtedly, many such youths are self-medicating and seeking an escape from interpersonally inflicted trauma. Although adolescents who are involved in substance use and misuse have some interpersonal problems of their own, these problems are in some cases the consequences of substance use. Some evidence also suggests that codependent interpersonal relationships can even maintain substance misuse.

All those with habitual substance use, abuse, or dependence seek to alter their consciousness, and often to escape a negative mood state. No one is born with the knowledge or behavioral ability to use drugs and alcohol for these or other purposes. Rather, this knowledge and behavior comes from interpersonal interaction. Drug and alcohol use is socially learned. The path from substance use to substance abuse and/or dependence is often strewn with the wreckage of destructive interpersonal interactions and relationships, such as conflict and hostility in families of origin and orientation, rejection by peers, sexual abuse, and marital discord. Alcohol and other substance abuse and dependence are both causes and consequences of interpersonal distress.

9

Somatoform Disorders and
Psychogenic Sexual Dysfunctions

The two groups of psychosocial problems discussed in this chapter—somatoform disorders and psychogeic sexual dysfunctions—are distinct types of disorders that, in the abstract, have similar manifestations. Each somatoform disorder or sexual dysfunction represents a constellation of "physical" symptoms in the absence of any identifiable physiological or medical condition to which the symptoms could be attributed. Both classes of problems are associated with patterns of friction in interpersonal relationships: Somatoform disorders are prominently linked with troublesome interactions in the family of origin, and psychogenic sexual dysfunctions are strongly tied to disturbances in family-of-orientation (i.e., marital) relationships.

SOMATOFORM DISORDERS

Definition and Symptoms

Somatoform disorders entail the expression of some symptom or symptoms that suggest a medical problem, but are not fully explainable by a medical condition (American Psychiatric Association, 2000). These symptoms, such as severe back pain or chronic digestive problems, tend to cause significant distress or impairment for the individual expressing them. The experience of these physical symptoms is very real for the afflicted individual, and they are not intentional, as in the case of malingering or factitious disorder. Three of the more common types of somatoform disorders are *pain disorder* (the experience of pain that is severe enough to warrant clinical attention and interfere with social and occupational functioning, in the absence of any obvious medical cause), *hypochondriasis* (a preoccupation with fears of having a serious disease based on misinterpretation of one or more bodily signs or symptoms), and *somatization disorder* (a chronic pattern of pain, sexual, gastrointestinal, and pseudoneurological symptoms) (see Ford, 1995, for a description of these and other somatoform disorders). Somatization disorder includes what has in the past been referred to as *hysteria* and *Briquet's syndrome.*

Results from the Epidemiologic Catchment Area study suggest that somatization disorder is somewhat rare, with an annual prevalence of only 0.2% (Regier et al., 1993). A more recent study of over 3,000 adolescents and young adults indicated that the risk of any specific somatoform disorder was 2.7% in that population, the most prevalent being pain disorder and conversion disorder (Lieb, Pfister, Mastaler, & Wittchen, 2000). However, these authors found that the use of a new and thorough diagnostic technique yielded an overall lifetime prevalence rate of 12.6% for any somatoform disorder. These disorders are more common in women than in men, and typically have their origin in adolescence; they are also highly comorbid, with 50–75% of patients also afflicted with such problems as depression, eating disorders, and substance dependence (Lieb et al., 2000).

Preview

Somatoform disorders may serve a variety of functions in the *family of origin*, the *family of orientation*, and even *general personal relationships*. For many people, a somatoform disorder brings a "solution" to a systemic problem within the family or marriage by shifting attention away from conflicts. It may also serve as a means of securing various types of support and attention. In research on somatoform disorders, antecedent *family-of-origin experiences* have received much attention. These often include low parental care (coupled with parental overinvolvement), family conflict, physical and sexual abuse, and other adverse experiences; disrupted attachment; and parental modeling of somatization. Somatoform disorders may also be understood as distorted forms of *interpersonal communication*: Many people express their physical symptoms as a means of indirectly communicating their distress to others. Somatoform disorders tend to be highly comorbid with personality disorders, further complicating the clinical and interpersonal picture of these disorders.

Functions of Somatization in Families of Origin/Orientation and in General Personal Relationships

Why would an individual experience and express "physical" symptoms in the absence of any precipitating medical or biological cause? Many have argued that there are social functions and perhaps even social causes underlying this phenomenon. In a comprehensive review of the relationship between social-psychological factors and somatic symptoms, Davidson and Pennebaker (1996) argued that "perceptions and reports of physical health may function as non-verbal indices of social health" (p. 114). Numerous possible etiological explanations for somatization have been suggested (Barsky & Klerman, 1983; Ford, 1986; Stuart & Noyes, 1999). Many if not most of these explanations entail some significant issue(s) in the area of interpersonal relationships, such as primary or secondary gains; a solution to a systems problem in a family; or a means of communicating when other, more direct forms of expression are blocked (signal function). Ford (1986) argues than many people with somatization disorder turn to health care professionals for social support that is otherwise lacking in their lives.

The concept of *secondary gain* has figured prominently in the literature on somatization. When one is "sick," he or she is freed from normal and typical obligations and is generally absolved from any responsibility for being in the sick condition (Barsky & Klerman, 1983; Ford, 1986). The expression of physical symptoms also brings attention, sympathy, and support from others, not to mention more instrumental types of assistance, such as disability payments. For the individual who is unable or unwilling to solicit or secure social support from others through more standard means of social interaction, assuming the sick role may be a covert mechanism for effectively achieving this interpersonal goal.

In the traditional psychodynamic approach, somatization is thought to have primarily intrapsychic functions, with secondary interpersonal consequences. However, the interpersonal perspective would interpret the "secondary" interpersonal effects as primary. That is, the person exhibits, and indeed experiences, the physical symptoms primarily as a mechanism for attaining particular interpersonal outcomes.

Somatoform disorders may also bring a temporary *solution to a system-wide problem*. For example, a child's physical symptoms may temporarily divert attention from an otherwise contentious family conflict. As parents shift their attention toward the welfare of the child, they may actually behave in a more cooperative fashion and reduce their conflict. Just as intoxication can bring temporary stability to a household affected by alcoholism, somatoform disorders may temporarily stabilize a family setting and subdue conflict.

According to the *signal function* hypothesis, somatic symptoms may be the nonverbal expression of an emotional and/or interpersonal problem. As Brodsky (1984) pointed out, "Somatization is communication, consciously or unconsciously coded in the language of the body" (p. 673). For a variety of reasons, some people may not be comfortable expressing their interpersonal or emotional distress to others; for them, expression of physical symptoms may be a more socially acceptable means of expressing their feelings to other people and soliciting social support from them. From this perspective, a somatoform disorder can be interpreted as a sign of psychic distress in the afflicted individual. This point is discussed in greater detail later.

Family-of-Origin Antecedents to Somatoform Disorders

As for any mental health problem, there are multiple, and often interacting, experiences in the family of origin that can give rise to somatoform disorders. Although the etiologies of these problems are not as widely understood as those of anxiety or depression, for example, there is good reason to suspect at least three sets of causal mechanisms: a range of adverse childhood experiences, parental modeling, and disrupted attachment (Barsky & Klerman, 1983; Brodsky, 1984; Stuart & Noyes, 1999).

Adverse Childhood Experiences

Exposure to adverse childhood experiences may begin with uncaring parents. Patients with somatoform disorders and somatic symptoms often have a history of insufficient parental care (Craig, Boardman, Mills, Daly-Jones, & Drake, 1993; Russek, Schwartz, Bell, & Baldwin, 1998). Relationships with parents are often lacking in intimacy and in boundary regulation (de Gruy et al., 1989). Excessive and dysfunctional conflict in the family of origin is also evident among those with somatoform disorders (Hurrelmann, Engel, Holler, & Nordlohne, 1988). An interview study conducted in Switzerland showed that respondents with psychogenic pain problems were more likely to indicate that their parents were physically or verbally abusive toward each other, and that they tried to deflect the aggression of one parent away from the other and onto themselves (Adler, Zlot, Hurny, & Minder, 1989). These subjects also had more concurrent problems with interpersonal relationships than did patients with organically identifiable pain or disease (Adler et al., 1989). The findings on deflection of aggression illustrate the system-wide problem hypothesis: As a child the patient was unable or unwilling to confront an aggressive parent, or intervene in the conflict, so he or she exhibited somatic symptoms that at least temporarily preoccupied the conflictual parents and calmed the family household.

Studies of patients with myofascial disorders (muscular aching and tenderness in localized sites, in the absence of organic pathology) identified family-of-origin relationships that were overly involved and overly focused on success and achievement (e.g., Malow & Olson, 1984) as factors discriminating such patients from medical controls. Findings such as these illustrate some of the ingredients in the secondary gain hypothesis: When the family places an excessive emphasis on success and achievement, the somatic symptoms relieve the patient from living up to these strict standards, with minimal loss of face. In such a context, the symptoms might be viewed as a form of self-handicapping.

Reports of childhood physical and sexual abuse are rampant in the literature on somatization (Adler et al., 1989; Barsky, Wool, Barnett, & Cleary, 1994; Morrison, 1989). Morrison (1989) found that 55% of patients with somatization disorder had a history of childhood sexual abuse, compared to 16% of a group with mood disorders. There appears to be a fairly linear association between the degree of childhood sexual abuse and somatization (Kinzl, Traweger, & Biebl, 1995). As noted earlier, childhood abuse is the tip of the iceberg in dysfunctional families. Although people with somatic symptoms often present a history of sexual abuse, they also indicate that their families were less cohesive, expressive, and sociable, and more enmeshed and conflictual (Nash, Hulsey, Sexton, Harralson, & Lambert, 1993). When these authors statistically controlled for these pathogenic family environment variables, the relationship between sexual abuse and psychiatric symptoms became nonsignificant, leading them to conclude that "impairment may be an effect not only of abuse but of the context in which it is embedded" (Nash et al., 1993, p. 282).

Parental Modeling

Children may learn that the expression of somatic symptoms brings support and attention from others. People with somatoform disorders are particularly likely to have witnessed a history of parental illness, in addition to their own history of increased illness (Bass & Murphy, 1997; Craig et al., 1993). These disorders may be learned from parents who teach their children to interpret minor physical ailments as signs of more serious physical illnesses (Barsky & Klerman, 1983; Brodsky, 1984). When children frequently witness their parents expressing physical symptoms, they may pick up on the style and language of these presentations, and incorporate them into descriptions of their own well-being.

Should children witness positive responses to parental illness (in the form of caregiving, time off work, etc.), they are then more likely to enact these somatizing behaviors themselves. To a child who has been otherwise neglected or poorly cared for, parental expression of somatic symptoms, and its attendant response from the social environment, might suggest the ultimate tool for securing much-wanted attention and social support.

Disrupted Attachment

Two intriguing theoretical accounts of somatization attribute the phenomenon to poorly formed socioemotional connections with other people. Invoking the traditional concepts of attachment theory, Stuart and Noyes (1999) have argued that aversive childhood experiences such as family conflict, neglect, and abuse interfere with the formation of secure attachments. Throughout adulthood, such people are hypothesized to engage in excessive care-seeking behavior during times of stress, in an effort to achieve some level of comfort and security. Of course, this may often take the form of somatization, particularly when it has been previously associated with caregiving responses. Unfortunately, these care-seeking behaviors often culminate in ambivalence, frustration, and rejection from both significant others and health care professionals, due to the persistence of the complaints and lack of connection to any obvious medical problem. According to the attachment-based theory of Stuart and Noyes (1999), people prone to somatization find themselves in a downward interpersonal spiral of care-seeking behavior; this is eventually met with interpersonal frustration and rejection, which only serve to pull for more care-seeking behavior.

A related interpersonal account of somatization, which is even more explicitly rooted in the psychodynamic tradition, also argues that somatization has its origins in a problematic relational history (Blaustein & Tuber, 1998). These authors suggest that somatization results from inadequate parenting, and from patients' inability to effectively manage and express the affective aspect of their relational challenges. To Blaustein and Tuber (1998), somatization signifies a disrupted relational history and impaired adult object relations. They assert that "for some people, somatization may be specifically and temporally linked with their inability to fully tolerate either their longings for empathic connection to others, or the disappointments when those desires are not satisfied. In other words, the affective trigger for a psychosomatic eruption may have an intrinsically relational dimension" (Blaustein & Tuber, 1998, 355).

According to Blaustein and Tuber (1998), somatization functions in several ways to help people cope with their inability to be close to others. In some cases, somatic eruptions are disguised messages of emotion that the patient is unable or unwilling to put into words. Thus somatization allows for the communication of distress without coming right out and stating it plainly to a partner (see below). In cases where the partner might be the source of the distress, somatization may be a way of conveying distress without risking harm to the relationship by directly confronting the partner with complaints. These authors have also argued that somatization may function to bring some relatedness to other people into the patients' lives through contact with physicians and health care providers. When a person experiences difficulty in relating to others in his or her life, somatization may serve to bring attention from people and create at least some feeling of being cared for.

Both Stuart and Noyes's (1999) attachment approach, and Blaustein and Tuber's (1998) object relations account of somatization, conceptualize the problem as rooted in poorly formed early caregiving relationships that cause people to express their anxious and negative affect about subsequent relationships through the expression of somatic symptoms. At the core of each of these theories is a difficulty in establishing and maintaining substantial and effective interpersonal relationships. Though formal longitudinal tests of these theoretical accounts have yet to be conducted, each is consistent with existing data on early parent–child relationships and adult interpersonal dysfunction of people with somatoform disorders.

Interpersonal Communication in Somatoform Disorders

Maladaptive Attempts at Communicating Distress

Somatoform disorders are often a means of expressing psychological and/or interpersonal distress to others. The audience for these displays may well be the same individuals who were instrumental in creating the distress. Evidence for this cause of somatoform disorders can be found in research showing that (1) people with these disorders have obvious interpersonal distress, and (2) the expression of these symptoms has implicit communicative value.

Studies of General Personal Relationship Distress. Studies in the somatoform literature show that people with hypochondriasis often exhibit symptoms of social phobia and fear of criticism from others (Schwenzer, 1996), as well as elevated loneliness (Brink & Niemeyer, 1993). Patients with somatic symptoms not attributable to organic causes report greater interpersonal and social problems than those with organically caused pain (e.g., Adler et al., 1997; Kisely, Goldberg, & Simon, 1997). The Kisely et al. (1997) study was a multinational investigation with an *n* of over 5,000, in which the association between psychological distress and symptoms without a medical explanation was generally consistent across different cultural groups.

Studies of specific types of somatic symptoms present an equally compelling case for distressed interpersonal relationships at their core. Faucett and Levine (1991) compared people with myofascial disorders to those with medically documented arthritis. The patients with arthritis indicated that they had more available family and network support than those with myofascial disorders, who also appeared to experience significantly more conflict with members of their social networks. The extent to which patients' personal relationships were supportive rather than conflictual was significantly, and negatively, correlated with their reports of pain. A similar pattern of findings is evident in a study of elderly people (Hays et al., 1998), whose rated satisfaction with social interaction protected against the experience of somatic symptoms that are commonly associated with depression (e.g., trouble falling asleep, diminished appetite).

Studies of Family-of-Orientation Distress. One can find vigorous somatization in distressed marital and other family-of-orientation relationships. Early family studies of patients diagnosed with hysteria (somatization disorder) showed a high prevalence of separation, divorce, and sexual dysfunctions (Briscoe, Smith, Robins, Marten, & Gaskin, 1973; Woerner & Guze, 1968). The elevated incidence of sexual problems and impairment in social roles among married patients with pain disorder led Hughes, Medley, Turner, and Bond (1987) to conclude that "the chronic illness or pain becomes a 'scapegoat' towards which the couple can direct their energies rather than to the underlying marital dysfunction, so affording the marriage a degree of stability" (p. 169). In the family context, individuals with somatization are also more likely to be married to spouses with alcoholism, to abuse or neglect their children, and to have serious marital problems (Zoccolillo & Cloninger, 1986). Patients who perceive high levels of criticism in their families have been known to report poorer physical health and to make more office visits to physicians than those reporting less family criticism (Fiscella, Franks, & Shields, 1997).

A unique experimental study with married couples shows that the experience of physical pain can be exacerbated by interpersonal stress. Schwartz, Slater, and Birchler (1994) randomly assigned patients with chronic back pain and their spouses to discuss an issue that was stressful or to simply describe some line drawings to each other. After this manipulation, subjects were instructed to ride an exercise bicycle at a steady pace, aided by feedback from their spouses, for 20 minutes or until they felt too much pain to continue. Over twice as many subjects in the stressful-interaction condition as in the nonstressful-interaction condition terminated the bicycle ride prior to the 20-minute time limit. This rare experimental investigation shows that interpersonal stress can precipitate the experience of pain and the avoidance of physically demanding activities.

The expression of somatic symptoms and complaints tends to be synchronous with feelings of negative affect (Craig et al., 1993). In this longitudinal study, depression and anxiety improved and worsened in conjunction with physical symptoms. Since these symptoms often had no physiological basis, these findings suggest that the symptom expression may have been a proxy for more direct expression of psychological distress. A key assumption is that such symptoms are not mere artifacts of inner distress, but that they are interpersonally functional indicators of that distress.

A report by Walker, Garber, and Greene (1994) also suggests that somatic symptoms may be an alternative to direct communication of distress. Among children with low levels of social competence at time 1, there was a positive relationship between the experience of negative life events and somatic complaints at time 2. However, there was no such relationship for children with higher levels of social competence. Socially competent children have good communication skills and satisfactory relationships at their disposal. Presumably such individuals can cope with the experience of stress through expressing their reactions and concerns to others and through soliciting social support. However, these mechanisms are unavailable to the child lacking in social competence; hence the expression of somatic symptoms.

Alexithymia

People with somatization disorder often suffer from *alexithymia* (Lesser, Ford, & Friedman, 1979; Nemiah, 1977). Alexithymia is a difficulty in describing emotions and feelings verbally. People with this problem tend to focus on external events rather than on inner emotions and wishes. In this context, physical symptoms may be a means of communicating some emotional distress when the person is unable to express it verbally. For example, anxiety and fear are often accompanied by a number of bodily sensations that may include stomach pain and muscle tension. Rather than convey feelings of fear to other people, an individual with alexithymia will focus on his or her physical symptoms, complaining of muscle aches and stomach pain, instead of talking about the feeling of anxiety and what is causing that feeling.

The alexithymia hypothesis has received some empirical support. Oxman, Rosenberg, Schnurr, and Tucker (1985) obtained 5-minute speech samples from patients at a family practice center. Those with somatization disorder used many words in the "not" category (e.g., "not," "cannot," "never"), suggesting a preoccupation with negativism, and very few words from emotion categories (e.g., "angry," "happy"), compared to patient controls. A further analysis of this data set revealed that the patients with somatization were 4.5 times more likely to make statements that involved "I am," such as "I am going off deep," "I am tired," and "I am going to fall," than a group of patients with paranoia (Oxman, Rosenberg, Schnurr, & Tucker, 1988). These examples illustrate the equation of self with negativity in the discourse of patients with somatization disorder.

Cultural Idioms of Distress

The role of culture in the somatoform disorders cannot be overlooked. Somatic symptoms have been described as cultural idioms of distress (e.g., Kirmayer, Dao, & Smith, 1998; Kirmayer & Young, 1998; Nichter, 1998). Cultures vary in their acceptance of individuals who express and experience largely "emotional" problems. In some cultures, it is more appropriate to have physical symptoms than psychological problems. Accordingly, the somatic symptoms of people in these cultures and subcultures are considered to be idioms of distress—their own unique and culturally accepted, if not prescribed, mechanisms for expressing their emotional distress. Asian cultures are often held up as examples of contexts in which depression and other psychological disorders are not tolerated to the same extent as physical problems. Consequently, a high prevalence of somatization is expected in such cultures, although this notion has been challenged (Lee, 1997). Kisely et al. (1997) have also questioned the role of culture in promoting somatization, given the ubiquity of the relationship between psychological distress and somatic symptoms across the range of cultures that they studied (see also Kirmayer & Young, 1998). Although this is obviously a hypothesis that is in need of more attention and evaluation, somatization may be a socially and culturally constructed mechanism for communicating psychological distress to others.

Comorbidity of Somatoform Disorders with Other Mental Health Problems

Somatoform disorders are often accompanied by other psychological problems. A study of over 1,000 adolescents indicated that almost half of those with a somatoform disorder also had at least one other documentable psychological disorder (Essau, Conradt, & Petermann, 1999). Among adults with somatization disorder, 23% had one personality disorder, and 37% had two or more (Rost, Akins, Brown, & Smith, 1992). The most frequently occurring personality disorders among the patients with somatization disorder in this study were avoidant, paranoid, self-defeating, obsessive–compulsive, histrionic, and antisocial. Some have estimated the rate of personality disorders to be as high as 60–70% among people with somatoform disorders (Bass & Murphy, 1995).

From an interpersonal perspective, the coincidence of somatoform disorders and personality disorders is understandable. Bass and Murphy (1995) explained: "In most patients with somatoform disorders, illness behaviour is a lifestyle in which the sick role is a mode of relating to self and others. . . . in relation to others the role provides strategies for eliciting care and exercising control" (p. 424). Recall that, by definition, personality disorders involve inflexible and maladaptive patterns of behavior, with problems in the interpersonal domain (see Chapter 6). People with personality disorders often related to other people in ways that are ill suited for the situation. The same reasons for this maladaptive relating to others undoubtedly also cause the somatization. In fact, somatization could be understood as an interpersonal manifestation of a personality disorder. Instead of communicating with others directly and openly, the person with a somatoform disorder develops symptoms in an effort to convey a message (neediness, desire for attention, etc.) to other people. It is easy to envision how somatization could be a "functional" form of communication for persons with avoidant personality disorder, who shun direct communication with others; those with histrionic personality disorder, who have a taste for drama; or those with dependent personality disorder, who want to be taken care of.

Conclusion

Somatoform disorders involve the experience and expression of distressing physical symptoms in the absence of any medical cause. The expression of distress through physical symptoms serves a number of social functions, such as secondary gain, signaling intrapersonal and interpersonal distress, and providing a temporary solution to a systemwide problem.

Scientists have documented several interpersonal processes that predict the development of somatoform disorders, the majority of which are rooted in childhood experiences. Many people with somatoform disorders have a history of adverse childhood experiences, ranging from growing up in a family characterized by conflict, poor boundary regulation, little intimacy, excessive control, and exaggerated demands for success, to outright physical and sexual abuse. As in the case of substance use problems and eating disorders, modeling may play a role in the pathogenesis of somatoform disorders. Many such patients witnessed serious illness in their parents, and have a history of illness themselves. Two psychodynamically oriented theories of somatoform disorders postulate that insecure attachments prompt excessive care seeking in the form of physical symptom expression.

Many investigators see somatoform disorders as maladaptive attempts to communicate psychological and interpersonal distress. Research findings reveal a number of interpersonal problems that tend to covary with somatoform disorders, although some of these problems may be due to psychological distress more generally, rather than to somatoform disorders in particular (Chadda, Bhatia, Shome, & Thakur, 1993; Hiller, Rief, & Fichter, 1997). Alexithymia is a communicative phenomenon that is common among people with somatoform disorders; it entails an inability to express emotions and feelings to other people. This condition may contribute to the expression of distress through physical symptoms. At a sociological level, somatoform disorders may represent cultural idioms of distress. In many cultures, it may be more socially acceptable to have a "physical" illness than to express psychological distress. In such cultures, the expression of physical symptoms may be a proxy for conveying emotional distress to others.

Finally, somatoform disorders tend to be comorbid with personality disorders. In many cases, the somatization may be a manifestation of the maladaptive interpersonal styles that are inherent in personality disorders.

PSYCHOGENIC SEXUAL DYSFUNCTIONS

Definition and Symptoms

Psychogenic *sexual dysfunctions* are a subgroup of sexual disorders whose origins appear to be psychological in nature, and are not adequately accounted for by medical or organic causes. These dysfunctions involve a disturbance in sexual desire or in the psychophysiological changes associated with the human sexual response (American Psychiatric Association, 2000). This disturbance causes both personal and interpersonal distress. Included in this class of problems are hypoactive sexual desire disorder, male erectile disorder, and the sexual pain disorders, for example. (Another subgroup of sexual disorders consists the *paraphilias*. These involve recurrent and intense sexual urges, fantasies, or behaviors that include unusual objects, situations, and activities; these symptoms cause personal and interpersonal stress, occupational impairment, and sometimes legal troubles. This section of the chapter is focused on sexual dysfunctions, however.) Psychogenic sexual dysfunctions are clearly caused by, and cause, profound problems in interpersonal relationships.

The incidence and prevalence of psychogenic sexual dysfunctions are not well known. These disorders are often overlooked in major epidemiological studies of mental health problems. Given the preponderance of individuals seeking treatment for them, it is likely that sexual dysfunctions are among the more common classes of psychosocial problems (e.g., Watson & Davies, 1997). A recent U.S. national survey of adult women supports a lifetime prevalence estimate of approximately 11% (Wilsnack et al., 1997).

Kaufman and Krupka (1973) were at the forefront in suggesting that many sexual problems are produced by interpersonal processes gone awry. Specifically, they suggested that early deprivation, guilt over seeking sexual gratification, sexual relationships transformed into power struggles, unexpressed anger, and unrealistic expectations of the self and others can each lead to the experience of sexual difficulties. Interpersonal problems such as these continue to occupy a dominant presence in the literature on psychogenic sexual dysfunctions (e.g., Horowitz, 1978; Metz & Dwyer, 1993; Zimmer, 1983). Such themes are clearly evident in the writings of those such as Zimmer (1983), who argued that "both clinicians and researchers have considered relationship factors to be of major importance in the development and maintenance of sexual distress" (p. 251); Purine and Carey (1997), who stated that "most theoretical models of human sexuality emphasize the importance of interpersonal communication in maintaining sexual adjustment" (p. 1017); and Clulow (1984), who concluded that "sexual dysfunction is therefore not viewed as an isolated complaint but as evidence of emotional disturbance in the relationship as a whole" (p. 371).

Preview

A dominant theme in the research findings on psychogenic sexual dysfunctions is that of problematic *family-of-orientation experiences* (i.e., the relationship with the spouse). (Although sexual dysfunctions can of course arise in the context of some *general personal relationships*—that is, in dating/romantic relationships—the vast majority of research on such dysfunctions has been done with marital or quasi-marital couples; therefore, general personal relationships are not discussed in detail here.) Within marital relationships, sexual dysfunctions are linked with breakdowns in *interpersonal communication*. As such, they may serve two functions that resemble functions of somatoform disorders: They may provide a temporary solution to a system-wide problem, and they may serve as a method of communicating unhappiness indirectly. Sexual dysfunctions are also linked with many forms of marital conflict. The conflict may be both a cause and a result of the dysfunction; in any case, it is patently obvious that psychogenic sexual dysfunctions and marital distress go hand in hand. Research on *family-of-origin experiences* has identified a number of early interpersonal experiences that may be etiological in this class of disorders. For example, many people with psychogenic sexual dysfunctions have a history of childhood sexual abuse, and/or exposure to parental modeling of dysfunctional attitudes and behaviors surrounding sexuality.

Family-of-Orientation Experiences in Sexual Dysfunctions

Interpersonal Communication Breakdown in Couples

Significant problems with basic communication processes are abundantly evident in sexually distressed couples. In most cases, a psychogenic sexual dysfunction is part of a larger relational problem with establishing and maintaining intimacy (McCabe, 1997). To illustrate, Zimmer (1983) compared sexually distressed and nondistressed couples on a number of specific communication skills that are important in close relationships. Partners in sexually distressed couples exhibited a greater proportion of disapproval to approval, less empathic reaction to each other, and more indirect as well as hostile expression of anger, in comparison to control couples. Analysis of a 10-minute marital interaction indicated that couples with sexual dysfunctions were less behaviorally engaged and assertive than control couples. A study with similar subject groups found that couples with sexual dysfunctions were more likely to have experienced instability and a general lack of communication in their relationships than those in more functional relationships (McCabe, 1994). These findings are consistent with those that more generally indicate a powerful relationship between interspousal sexual communication and marital adjustment (Banmen & Vogel, 1985; Cupach & Comstock, 1990; Ferroni & Taffe, 1997).

Roffe and Britt (1981) developed a unique typology of marital interactions among couples with sexual dysfunctions; their work is reminiscent of the pioneering work of Olson and Fitzpatrick on different marital and family types (e.g., Fitzpatrick, 1988; Olson, Sprenkle, & Russell, 1979). Their analyses yielded four couple groups: the *conflict-centered relationship*, which harbors a hostile and dominant spouse (this group is actually split into two subgroups, one in which the husband is dominant and one in which the wife is dominant); the *passive–constrained relationship*, composed of introverted spouses who are withdrawn and emotionally inhibited; and the *congenial–affectionate relationship*, characterized by some anxiety and discouragement, but with similar attitudes toward spontaneity, compassion, and emotional self-absorption. The conflict-centered and passive–constrained relationships, which collectively accounted for approximately 50% of the sexually dysfunctional couples in Roffe and Brit's (1981) sample, had obvious marital communication problems. The congenial–affectionate group is perhaps the most functional, and the couple type for which the prognosis is best.

A sense of mutuality is an important component of any healthy personal relationship. Accordingly, agreement and a sense of understanding between partners play an important role in sexual adjustment (Purine & Carey, 1997). Purine and Carey's (1997) survey study of cohabiting couples indicated that agreement between partners' sexual preferences was a key predictor of their sexual adjustment, as was men's (but not women's) understandings of their partners' preferences. The role that communication plays in creating this understanding cannot be overstated or overlooked.

Functions of Sexual Problems in Couples

Sexual dysfunctions may actually serve two purposes for couples that are similar to functions of somatoform disorders: (1) They may temporarily deflect attention away from serious or chronic problems in a marriage, particularly when attention to these problems becomes a threat (Clulow, 1984); and (2) they may serve a signal function, enabling spouses to communicate distress indirectly. Admittedly, a sexual dysfunction itself can become a serious problem for a marriage. However, despite its seriousness, it may allow members of a couple to draw their attention away from a long-standing conflict that they are otherwise frustrated with and/or exhausted by, and express unhappiness without doing so openly. Consider, for example, a husband and wife who cannot agree on whether or not they would like to have more children. If they both feel strongly, and are truly at odds and unable to come to a resolution of this issue, a sexual dysfunction (1) takes attention away from the more abstract and philosophical disagreement, and gives the couple a more immediate focus of attention; (2) can covertly sustain the position of the partner who does not want more children; and (3) can be a means of expressing distress and dissatisfaction with each other without having to rehash the actual conflict about family size.

Sexual problems have proven to be a reliable barometer of more general marital satisfaction or distress (Rust, Golombok, & Collier, 1988). In one study of couples seeking treatment for sexual problems, researchers found that the incidence of sexual dysfunctions was actually fairly low, but that couples generally had more general interpersonal problems (Snyder & Berg, 1983). Apparently for some couples, seeking treatment for a "sexual" problem substitutes for addressing more general relational problems, when it may be these problems that are causing the dysfunction. Viewed this way, they are seeking help for the symptom, not the cause, of the condition.

Conflict in Couples

One interpersonal problem to emerge frequently in the literature on sexual dysfunction is marital conflict. Sexual relationships sometimes get transformed into power struggles, and may be depreciated by unexpressed anger between the partners (Horowitz, 1978). Research shows that subjects who experience sexual dysfunction are more likely to experience increased conflict in their marriages or close relationships, compared to their more functional counterparts (Hartman, 1980; McCabe, 1994). In a unique comparison of couples with sexual dysfunctions and couples in which one partner had been convicted of a sexual offense (referred to by the authors as "sex offender couples,") Metz and Dwyer (1993) had couples complete a measure of relationship quality and the Styles of Conflict Inventory, which measures respondents' appraisals of and styles for handling marital conflicts. In terms of both relationship quality and effective conflict management, satisfied couples scored the highest, followed by those with sexual dysfunctions, and then the "sex offender couples." In terms of the intensity of conflict experienced, "the sex offender couples" and dysfunctional couples did not differ from each other, and both were higher than satisfied controls. The couples with sexual dysfunctions were also less likely to attribute blame for the conflict to the self, showed more problems with assertion and aggression, and perceived more verbal aggression in their partners than satisfied controls.

Members of the general population, as well as those seeking treatment for sexual dysfunctions exhibit similar patterns of association between relational conflict and sexual dysfunctions (McCabe, 1994). This study was noteworthy in that McCabe assessed conflict about sexual and nonsexual matters separately. Each type of conflict was positively and significantly correlated with sexual dysfunctions. This indicates that the heightened relational conflict in a couple with a sexual dysfunction is not merely conflict about the dysfunction itself; it is obviously more broad-based.

The effects of unresolved, poorly resolved, or poorly handled conflict corrode the sense of intimacy that should be inherent in a close relationship. One way in which this is manifested is in disrupted sexuality, often to the point of bona fide dysfunction. Of course, a sexual dysfunction itself may propagate conflict in many cases. However, there is reason to believe that the conflict prevalent among couples with such dysfunctions is not isolated to matters of sexuality.

Family-of-Origin Antecedents to Adult Sexual Dysfunctions

Modeling of Parental Beliefs and Attitudes

Although most of the variance in adult sexual dysfunctions is explainable by concurrent relational problems, some childhood interpersonal experiences may be viewed as distal contributory causes. Two such issues that are clearly rooted in family socialization are negative attitudes toward sexuality and extreme religious orthodoxy (Kaplan, 1979; Stayton, 1996). Both of these are more psychological than interpersonal constructs. However, each can be viewed as a result of socialization in the family of origin, and each is related to the other. Children who are reared with extremely *orthodox beliefs and values* may view sex as generally inappropriate and improper behavior, unless it is explicitly enacted with the goal of procreation. Armed with such attitudes, some individuals might experience adjustment problems when paired with partners of differing beliefs and values. Related to this are *negative attitudes toward sexuality.* Certain child-rearing practices and family environments may leave a child with a tendency to associate sexuality with feelings of guilt and shame. Other family experiences may lead the child to link sex with disgrace, emotional pain, or betrayal. To the extent that these negative attitudes, often learned in childhood, are durable through the adult years, impairment in sexual functioning is a likely consequence.

Childhood Sexual Abuse

Another early interpersonal experience that can impair adult sexual functioning is *childhood sexual abuse,* especially when this abuse is intrafamilial. Multiple studies show that people who experienced such abuse as children are more likely than those who have not to experience sexual dysfunctions as adults (Mullen, Martin, Anderson, Romans, & Herbison, 1994; Neumann, Houskamp, Pollock, & Briere, 1996; Wilsnack et al., 1997). Two important caveats must be noted, however. First, these same studies show that childhood sexual abuse is situated in a matrix of aversive childhood and family-of-origin experiences (such as excessive conflict, low cohesion, poor boundary regulation, physical abuse, and parental neglect), and that it is associated with a similarly diverse matrix of adult psychosocial problems (such as separation, divorce, relational dissatisfaction, substance abuse, depression, somatization, and anxiety, to name just some). Each of these on its own may be sufficient to interfere with sexual functioning. Disentangling and understanding the effects of sexual abuse in particular continues to be a challenge for mental health research. Second, there is no deterministic relationship between childhood sexual abuse and adult functioning (Watson & Davies, 1997). Some children who experienced sexual abuse go on to develop happy and healthy interpersonal relationships, and are indistinguishable from their nonabused peers. Undoubtedly, this resilience is an amalgamation of personal and social-environmental factors that allows them to minimize and overcome the ill effects of this trauma.

These caveats notwithstanding, childhood sexual abuse is thought to disrupt attachment to caregivers, trust in others, the development of self-esteem, and a sense of mastery (Mullen et al., 1994; Wilsnack et al., 1997). When a survivor of such abuse is confronted with new developmental tasks, such as management and negotiation of adult sexuality, these liabilities may be manifested in a variety of psychosocial problems—including sexual dysfunctions.

Comorbidity of Sexual Dysfunctions with Other Mental Health Problems

Psychogenic sexual dysfunctions tend to coexist with other mental health problems that also have an obvious interpersonal basis. However, unlike problems such as depression or schizophrenia, for example, the comorbidity of sexual dysfunctions has not been as thoroughly researched. This is perhaps due in part to the difficulty of accurately assessing and diagnosing these problems and the fact that such assessment requires ruling out physiological origins.

Studies of people identified as having a psychogenic sexual dysfunction reveal a 30% to 35% incidence of other psychological problems (Catalan, Hawton, & Day, 1990; Fagan, Schmidt, Wise, & Derogatis, 1988). One common problem that is concomitant to sexual dysfunction is depression. As an example, the odds ratio for erectile dysfunction has been estimated at 1.82 in the presence versus absence of depressive symptoms (Araujo, Durante, Feldman, Goldstein, & McKinley, 1998). A study of couples seeking therapy for sexual dysfunction indicated that rates of depression, anxiety disorders, and eating disorders were all elevated in contrast to those in the general population (van Lankveld & Grotjohann, 2000). Lifetime rates of affective disorders (major depression, dysthymia, and bipolar disorder) among the participants in this study were 21.5% and 38.3% for men and women, respectively. Associated rates of anxiety disorders were 19.9% and 37.3% respectively. Thus, problems like depression and anxiety are evident in the backgrounds of about one third of those seeking treatment for sexual dysfunction.

Like personality disorders, sexual dysfunctions tend to be comorbid with other sexual dysfunctions. In a large-sample, multisite pharmaceutical study, 40% of those with hypoactive sexual desire disorder were also diagnosed with a second sexual dysfunction (Segraves & Segraves, 1991).

In view of the ill effects of anxiety on performance and depression on sexual desire, the comorbidity of these problems with sexual dysfunctions is easily understood. However, it is equally evident that these problems are interconnected in at least some cases by interpersonal problems and stressors. When close relationships become distressed and/or when people have a history of interpersonal maltreatment, both depression and sexual dysfunction are likely consequences. Similarly, people who experience a great deal of anxiety in interpersonal contexts, perhaps because of poor social skills, may experience sexual dysfunctions that are secondary to that excessive anxiety.

Conclusion

Psychogenic sexual dysfunctions appear to be every bit as much problems with couple relationships and a psychological sense of intimacy, as problems with the psychophysiology of human sexuality. People with psychogenic sexual dysfunctions often have intimacy problems that extend far beyond just sexual intimacy and include poor social and recreational intimacy with their partners as well (McCabe, 1997). Psychogenic sexual dysfunctions may serve as regulative devices for addressing unresolved conflict and a lack of intimacy. Like those of other mental health problems, the symptoms of psychogenic sexual dysfunctions may draw attention away from more substantial underlying interpersonal problems that a couple is unable or unwilling to address openly. They may also serve as a means of communicating distress indirectly. In either case, sexual dysfunctions may be indices of more pervasive interpersonal/relational problems.

A number of relational themes are evident in studies of sexually dysfunctional couples. These include open conflict, as well as passivity, discouragement, a lack of agreement and understanding, and hostility that is often not expressed directly and openly. Some of these phenomena are even evident through observations of brief laboratory interactions between partners.

Notwithstanding the associations between sexual dysfunctions and current relational problems, some interpersonal childhood experiences may be distal contributory causes of adult sexual dysfunctions. When children are socialized with strict orthodox religious beliefs and values, and/or when they learn negative attitudes toward sexuality, they are predisposed to experience psychogenic sexual dysfunctions as adults. A history of childhood sexual abuse is also more common among those with psychogenic sexual dysfunction, compared to their well-functioning counterparts. Such abuse may set the stage for views of sexuality as coercive, hostile, and motivated by malfeasance.

Both somatoform disorders and psychogenic sexual dysfunctions involve the experience and expression of physical symptoms in the absence of any obvious medical or physiological cause. Each of these disorders is a sign of intrapersonal and interpersonal distress, and serves a communicative value. The interpersonal pathogenesis of somatoform disorders can be primarily located in family-of-origin experiences; although such experiences do play a role in psychogenic sexual dysfunctions, these dysfunctions more strongly signal troubles with family-of-orientation relationships.

10

The Interpersonal Paradigm
in Mental Health

An examination of the scientific literature on interpersonal processes and mental health problems shows that *mental illness* and *interpersonal illness* are inseparable concepts. There are cases of psychological disorders whose origins clearly lie in problematic interpersonal relationships. At the same time, it is apparent that many and perhaps most forms of psychopathology have serious interpersonal ramifications that are unfortunately negative in nature. People with psychological problems, of whatever specific type, will often find that their personal relationships are not what they were during their premorbid state. This deterioration of interpersonal well-being undoubtedly complicates the course of psychosocial problems, and thus afflicted individuals often wind up in a vicious cycle of interpersonal and psychological problems that perpetuate each other.

COMPONENTS OF THE INTERPERSONAL PARADIGM

The analysis of interpersonal issues in mental health problems has thus far been presented in the context of particular problems. At this juncture, it is instructive to move up a level of abstraction to identify interpersonal motifs that cut across multiple mental health problems. These phenomena constitute the building blocks of a more general interpersonal paradigm in mental health.

One of the most fundamental, yet controversial, functions of research programs or paradigms is the stipulation of what count as data. Paradigms focus attention on phenomena of interest, and away from variables that are not central to the key assumptions embedded within the paradigm. The fundamental components of the interpersonal paradigm in mental health can be extrapolated from the available research literature on various psychological problems. This is an admittedly inductive method for defining the interpersonal paradigm. As noted in Chapter 1, the interpersonal paradigm was developed over many decades by a loosely organized collection of theorists and researchers. Unlike other paradigms in mental health with an identifiable starting point and scripture, the components of the interpersonal paradigm must be inferred from an analysis of what the researchers working within this tradition have identified and accepted as central constructs.

For ease of reference, the interpersonal phenomena associated with various mental health problems are summarized in Table 10.1. The contents of Table 10.1 are best interpreted as *highlights*, not as an exhaustive catalog, of the fundamental interpersonal bases of psychological problems. In fact, there are many more interpersonal antecedents, concomitants, and consequences of such problems than what appear in Table 10.1, and even more are sure to be documented through future research. A comparison of the research on different psychological problems, focused on different interpersonal issues, indicates four general domains of inquiry: (1) experiences in the family of origin, occurring during early childhood as well as adulthood; (2) experiences in the family of orientation, namely marriage and parenthood; (3) general personal relationships, such as dating relationships, work relationships, friendships, and even interactions with strangers; and (4) characteristic styles of interpersonal communication. A general summary of common themes within each of these four areas is presented next.

Family-of-Origin Experiences

Social and behavioral scientists have for a long time appreciated the fact that early childhood experiences in the family of origin will set the stage for later adult functioning. Within certain schools of thought, the influence of early childhood experiences has, frankly, been taken too far. Coyne (1999) has used the metaphor of a woolly mammoth to characterize the function of early childhood experiences postulated by psychoanalytic theory. Coyne is critical of the assumption that our interpersonal and psychological constitutions are frozen in ice, forever preserved, once our childhoods are over. It is essential to bear in mind that scientists have yet to isolate any *deterministic* relationships between childhood interpersonal experiences and later adult psychosocial functioning. The implications of experiences within the family of origin for later mental health must be interpreted with this caveat in mind.

TABLE 10.1. Interpersonal Phenomena Associated with Psychological Problems

Problem	Family-of-origin experiences	Family-of-orientation experiences	General relational issues	Interpersonal communication
Depression	Abuse Neglect Low parental care Parental overinvolvement Rejection	Marital distress Parenting problems	Rejection Emotional contagion Distressed/unavailable personal relationships Loneliness	Social skills deficits Excessive reassurance seeking
Social anxiety	Low adaptability High cohesion Low parental care Parental overinvolvement Abuse Parental modeling of dysfunctional attitudes/behaviors Isolation		Rejection Distressed/unavailable personal relationships Loneliness	Social skills deficits Negative expectations for social interactions Self-doubt about making desired impression
Schizophrenia	Communication deviance (CD) Expressed emotion (EE) Negative affective style (AS)		Interpersonal conflict Low social support Rejection	Social skills deficits Poor social cue recognition
Bipolar disorder	EE CD Negative AS Battles for control	Marital distress Parenting problems	Agitated by interpersonal stress	Social skills deficits
Personality disorders	Insecure attachment Approach–avoidance conflicts Abuse Excessive parental attention Low parental care Parental overinvolvement Family chaos Inconsistent parenting	Marital distress (if patients marry at all)	Unstable personal relationships Loneliness Interpersonal conflict Rejection	Attention seeking

Eating disorders	Low cohesion Extreme adaptability EE Inappropriate parental pressure Low parental care Parental overinvolvement Battles for control Parental modeling of dysfunctional attitudes/behaviors Abuse	Marital distress	Distressed/unavailable personal relationships Rejection	Social skills deficits (resulting from sexual abuse)
Alcoholism and other substance use problems	Parental modeling of dysfunctional attitudes/behaviors Low cohesion Excessive adaptability Abuse	"Solution" to a systems problem Poor distance regulation Parenting problems Interpersonal conflict Marital distress	Interpersonal conflict	Social skills deficits
Somatoform disorders	"Solution" to a systems problem Low parental care Parental overinvolvement Interpersonal conflict Abuse Parental modeling of dysfunctional attitudes/behaviors Disrupted attachment	"Solution" to a systems problem	Symptoms as a means of securing support	Indirect communication attempts Alexithymia Symptoms as idioms of distress in certain cultures
Psychogenic sexual dysfunctions	Parental modeling of dysfunctional attitudes/behaviors Abuse	Marital distress Interpersonal conflicts	"Solution" to a systems problem	Interpersonal conflict

To turn to some of the interpersonal problems that are common to multiple mental disorders, issues in the family of origin figure prominently. It is widely understood and accepted that *parental neglect and abuse* are precursors to numerous mental health problems, including alcoholism, depression, loneliness, personality disorders, eating disorders, somatoform disorders, and psychogenic sexual dysfunctions, to name just some. A brief perusal of Table 10.1 will show that abuse or some form of neglect (e.g., low parental care) has been conclusively identified as either a contributory factor, or a phenomenon that occurs with remarkable prevalence, in the vast majority of psychological problems examined.

The data that link childhood physical and sexual abuse to later adult psychosocial problems are virtually overwhelming (e.g., Dinwiddie et al., 2000; Downs & Miller, 1998; Neumann et al., 1996; Polusny & Follette, 1995; Saunders et al., 1992). What are particularly impressive are both the range and severity of problems occurring in the wake of such noxious interpersonal maltreatment. One might speculate that children, even those at a very young age, understand and desire the caregiving role and behavior of their parents. When a provider of care and support turns on a child through either neglect or more overt abuse, a corrupted interpersonal architecture is produced that in many cases will never support the construction of functional and satisfying personal relationships in the future.

Polusny and Follette (1995) have conceptualized the sequelae of childhood abuse from the perspective of emotional avoidance. The avoidance or alleviation of unpleasant internal states becomes a dominant goal for people who have experienced such abuse. Many of the psychosocial problems that follow, such as substance use disorders, bulimia nervosa, dissociation, social phobia, sexual dysfunctions, and somatoform disorders, could be interpreted as a mechanism for escape or distraction from memories of such painful experiences, and perhaps a means for reducing the likelihood of further abuse. Polusny and Follette's conceptualization is consistent with that of Heatherton and Baumeister (1991), who argued that binge eating offers an escape from self-awareness by narrowing attention to the immediate stimulus (i.e., food). It is plausible to assume that many of the other destructive behaviors implicated in the eating disorders, such as drug and alcohol consumption, could similarly serve as mechanisms for escape from self-awareness (Baumeister, 1992). Unfortunately, for many people, a sad feature of the maladjustment that follows childhood maltreatment is a propensity to be situated in interpersonal contexts in which further maltreatment is likely (e.g., socializing with drug-using peers).

It is a lesser-known fact that *excessive parental attention and care-*

giving may have equally devastating consequences for later personal relationships and mental health. When parents fail to maintain the delicate balance between a secure, nurturant environment and a healthy dose of reality and responsibility, the child may develop a self-image that simply cannot be sustained by future relational partners. A gross failure to develop a sense of altruism is a potential consequence. Once again, the blueprints for disaster, ultimately manifested in problems such as loneliness and personality disorders, may well be drawn before a child even leaves the home.

A family-of-origin pattern every bit as dominant as abuse in the mental health literature is an absolutely corrosive combination of parenting behaviors: *parental overinvolvement or overprotectiveness coupled with lack of parental care.* When parents are overly intrusive in the lives of their children, but at the same time emotionally distant, there is a high potential for serious psychosocial consequences that can include depression, eating disorders, schizophrenia, personality disorders, and social anxiety. The ubiquity of this parenting pattern in the mental health literature is as remarkable as the range of problems with which it appears to be associated.

This pattern of parenting may stem from serious problems with boundary regulation and ambivalence about parenthood. Overinvolvement and overprotection reflect a form of boundary dysregulation that may adversely affect a child's ego development and sense of self in relation to other people. A person exposed to parental overinvolvement may form either unrealistic expectations for care that simply cannot be met during later adulthood, or a preoccupation with and fear of interpersonal intrusion. In either case, relational problems are likely to follow, contributing to any of a variety of psychological symptoms. A lack of parental care reflects a parent's ambivalence about or rejection of his or her role. Even young children have an extraordinary aptitude for detecting acceptance or rejection from a caregiver. A lack of parental care sends messages such as "You are not worthy" and "I do not value my relationship with you" to a child. When this is coupled with overinvolvement, a child's (or even an adult's) ability to make sense of these interpersonal experiences may be taxed beyond its limits. The bewilderment, confusion, self-blame, and damaged self-esteem produced by such childhood experiences surely contribute to later psychosocial problems.

One of the primary means by which children learn attitudes and behaviors is modeling. No agents are more readily available and credible than parents. Many of the behaviors and cognitions that constitute mental disorders may in fact be socially learned. *Parental modeling of dysfunctional attitudes and behaviors* has been implicated in such problems as social anxiety, eating disorders, alcoholism and other substance use problems, somatoform disorders, and psychogenic sexual dysfunctions.

In all cases, evidence indicates that children may learn maladaptive behaviors and cognitions that later come back to cause them substantial
distress in their adult lives.

Critics who are sympathetic to the biological paradigm might prefer
to explain parent–child similarities in psychological symptoms with a genetic hypothesis. Indeed, it is difficult to disentangle the effects of genes
and the social environment, as they come from the same source—the
family of origin. However, it is now becoming clear that genes can only
explain a portion of this concordance. Furthermore, such problems as
somatoform disorders and psychogenic sexual dysfunctions are at least
assumed, by definition, to have nonbiological bases (i.e., if such a problem could be explained by biological factors, a person could not receive
the diagnosis). In such cases, it appears that people learn the attitudes
and behaviors underlying these problems through parental modeling, at
least in part.

The effects of family processes on offspring do not end with adulthood. In reality, many adult psychiatric patients still reside in their families of origin. Particularly among the more profoundly affected individuals, such as those with schizophrenia or bipolar disorder, independent
lives outside their families of origin may simply be unattainable because
of problems with employment, maintaining stable relationships, managing finances, and so on. For such people, caustic family processes can
still devastate psychological well-being, and foreclose the possibility of a
complete recovery and functional independent life.

When adult patients reside in households with a great deal of *expressed emotion* (EE), *negative affective style* (AS), and *communication
deviance* (CD), symptoms become aggravated and relapse becomes accelerated. EE and negative AS reflect a critical and overinvolved orientation between a parent and child. These family processes have been implicated in schizophrenia, bipolar disorder, and eating disorders. Even
many adults are still sensitive and susceptible to the ill effects of parental
criticism. Throughout the animal kingdom, parents either nurture their
offspring or simply leave them alone. Aside from humans, it is difficult
to locate species in which some parents actively meddle with or torment
their young during critical periods of psychosocial development. However, many parents may (albeit subtly and with the best intentions) ag-
gravate their children's mental health through criticism and overinvolvement, even into stages of adulthood. Some parents also communicate
with their family members in ways that are peculiar, splintered, and difficult to grasp. This may create a bizarre template for the construal of social interaction that makes rewarding socialization with other people a
near-impossibility, in the same way that extreme isolation or neglect can
permanently mar the capacity for interpersonal relations.

For most people, interpersonal and psychological development are launched and guided by the family. When normal family processes such as nurturance, education, and self-esteem support go awry, psychological distress often follows. Even well into adulthood, the family of origin has a powerful impact on its offspring's psychological health or illness. Unfortunately, for many people, their means of coping with disordered family processes (e.g., substance misuse, binge eating, somatization, and dissociation) are themselves maladaptive and abrasive to mental health.

Family-of-Orientation Experiences

Most people eventually detach themselves to some degree, both emotionally and physically, from their families of origin. In so doing, people shift their focus from relationships with parents and siblings to relationships with a partner and children. These relationships in the family of orientation consume substantial physical and mental energy. Furthermore, whereas in family-of-origin relations there is a natural progression toward some degree of independence, marriage and parenting are relationships that are pledged for life (at least in principle). Consequently, these relationships have a powerful impact on psychological well-being, and the psychological well-being or illness of an individual in such a family context has a powerful impact on these family relations.

There is an exceptionally robust relationship between mental health problems and *marital distress*. This interpersonal problem can be found among those with depression, bipolar disorder, eating disorders, alcoholism and other substance use disorders, and psychogenic sexual dysfunctions. It is extremely difficult to locate an individual whose spouse has major depression or alcoholism, but who otherwise feels that the two of them have a great marriage. Marital distress would presumably be problematic for many people with social anxiety disorder, schizophrenia, or personality disorders, were they actually able to initiate and maintain marriages.

Scientists and philosophers alike might debate which is the more intimate human bond: parent and child, or husband and wife. A parent–child relationship is one of blood; yet a marriage is a relationship of sustained intimacy until death, at least in theory. When a marriage goes bad, mental health can suffer as a result. In this regard, marital distress may act as a stressor that triggers symptoms of psychopathology. A failing marriage can raise questions of blame, faltered responsibility, self-doubt, feelings of personal failure, and uncertainty about the present and future. The catastrophic and dysphoric feelings that accompany marital distress can exhaust the strongest of egos. In many such cases, psychopathology could be interpreted as a result of marital distress.

An alternative account of the relationship between marital distress and psychopathology sees the deterioration of marriage as affected by symptoms of psychological disorder. To state the case plainly, how enjoyable is marriage to a depressed person? What marriage is strong enough to tolerate and absorb the radical shifts in mood and behavior associated with bipolar disorder? How fulfilling can a marriage be to a wife who is starving herself to death and eschewing sexuality, or to a husband who is drinking himself to death and generally incoherent or belligerent? These symptoms are a burden that even the best marriages often cannot bear. A union between two people that is this close is inevitably upset when the mental health of one member depreciates.

Psychological disorders also appear to generate *parenting problems*. There are few if any interpersonal tasks that require as much energy, effort, and skill as raising children. Effective parenting requires undivided attention and emotional resilience. When a parent's mental balance is tipped by problems such as depression, bipolar disorder, or alcoholism, the possibility for effective parenting declines considerably. For this reason, people with mental health problems often raise children with behavioral or psychological problems of their own. Fortunately, many factors that moderate the relationship between parental mental health and child distress can render a child resilient to the ill effects of troubled parenting.

Some consideration should be granted to the possibility (although it is somewhat speculative at this time) that children's behavioral problems may trigger symptoms of psychopathology in parents. Mental health problems are sensitive to a variety of interpersonal contacts, including those with relative strangers. It is reasonable to assume that a child with conduct, attention, emotional, or behavioral problems may stress a parent, perhaps leading to depression when this "failure" at parenting is internalized, or to alcoholism as a means of coping and escape.

Some interpersonal phenomena, such as conflict, EE, negative AS, and the provision of a "solution" to a systems problem, appear in both family-of-origin and family-of-orientation contexts. Though many scientists often conceptualize and test fairly linear cause–effect relations in these contexts (e.g., family conflict leads to depression, bipolar disorder leads to marital distress), family systems theorists see cause *and* effect in all members of a system. Rohrbaugh and Shean (1987), for example, explain:

> A key assumption is that regardless of how problems originate, they persist as aspects of current, ongoing interaction systems. Cybernetic feedback processes provide a framework for understanding how systems are *maintained*, which is of greater interest than etiological hypotheses, or

linear (historical) notions of cause and effect. It is further assumed that problems occur not so much within people as between them—that psychological "symptoms" and interaction systems are inextricably interwoven. (pp. 76–77)

Thus, from a systems perspective, neither the effect of psychopathology on the family nor the effect of the family on psychopathology is a primary focus. Rather, the concern is with the way in which *all* members of the system maintain the psychological problem. In many situations the psychological problem is functional in some way for the family. Families that structure their lives around alcoholism or eating disorders are collectively maintaining the psychological problem. Therefore, the problem is clearly not an *individual* problem, but a *systems* problem.

General Personal Relationships

One of Harry Stack Sullivan's more notable departures from his psychoanalytic origins was a shift away from exclusive attention to family-of-origin relationships, and toward a consideration of both family and peer relationships on ego development and mental health. Psychological problems are entangled with interpersonal problems beyond those in the family of origin or orientation. This is a point that is sadly overlooked by those who seek to explain psychopathology by looking back to early childhood experiences with parents. For example, young adults who are unmarried place a great deal of importance on dating/romantic relationships and platonic friendships. For such people, social support from family members can do little to minimize their loneliness (e.g., Jones & Moore, 1990); what they seek are rewarding relationships with dating/romantic partners and friends. When these relationships are unavailable or distressed, psychological problems are often evident.

The ill effects of *conflict* on personal relationships are well established. The experience of excessive and hostile conflict can have equally severe intrapersonal consequences. Themes of destructive conflict are evident in the findings on eating disorders, personality disorders, alcoholism, schizophrenia, psychogenic sexual dysfunction, and somatoform disorders. Conflict is an interpersonal phenomenon that appears heightened in both family and other relationships. In a very fundamental way, most people appear to seek and desire some form of harmony with at least a few other people with whom they share their lives. When this harmony is corroded by conflict, mental health problems often emerge. At the same time, the experience of a mental health problem such as alcoholism or a personality disorder can also disrupt the harmony inherent in close personal relationships. This itself has the potential to propagate intense interpersonal conflict.

Interpersonal rejection is a social phenomenon that pursues most mental health problems. Although depression is one of the problems that has focused most attention on interpersonal rejection, thanks to Coyne's (1976a, 197b) interactional theory, this phenomenon is evident among people with schizophrenia, eating disorders, and personality disorders. Human beings can be remarkably intolerant of those who present a less than "normal," competent, or personable image. The social-interactional goals of most people leave little room for significant communication with others who have obvious symptoms of psychopathology. Consequently, psychologically distressed individuals are often shunned and rejected by others—even those with whom they have shared close relationships.

The phenomenon of interpersonal rejection can be devastating to one's sense of self-worth. The realization that others do not like, care for, or want to spend time with the self is profoundly distressing for all but the most pathologically avoidant individuals. The anguish that is perpetuated by interpersonal rejection can exacerbate minor psychological frailty into full-blown mental disorder. Of course, as the symptoms of poor mental health become more prominent, the likelihood of eliciting further rejection is increased. Again, the potential for a vicious cycle between psychological and interpersonal problems is clearly evident.

Interpersonal rejection may play a role in more macroscopic interpersonal issues, such as availability of close relationships. One of the most fundamental and basic interpersonal problems associated with psychopathology is a *lack of general personal relationships*. The social networks of people with schizophrenia, depression, social anxiety, and eating disorders, for example, are notoriously impoverished. Once again, there is reason to suspect that this interpersonal problem is both a cause and a consequence of psychological problems. By their social nature, most humans have a very basic need to seek out and form relationships with others. Mental health appears to deteriorate in parallel with the disappearance of opportunities for experiencing the pleasures of personal relationships.

Like interpersonal rejection, experiencing the unavailability of personal relationships can lead to feelings of worthlessness, despair, and grief. Over time, situational attributions for such a state of affairs may be difficult to sustain and eventually give way to feelings of personal blame and responsibility. A deficiency in personal relationships may be taken as evidence of personal deviance or defectiveness. This mental anguish—coupled with the absence of opportunities to share positive and negative affective states with other people, and to enjoy their company and social support—is a potent recipe for serious psychological problems.

Certain interpersonal processes that have been implicated in mental health problems, such as rejection and conflict, are fairly ubiquitous in that they occur in both family and other relationship contexts. However, other processes, such as unavailability of personal relationships and loneliness, appear to be largely unrelated to family issues. In many cases, these processes are present in the lives of people with psychological problems, maintaining, prolonging, and exacerbating their condition.

Interpersonal Communication

It is impossible to separate how we communicate with other people from how we experience our relationships with them. There is no such thing as a high-quality interpersonal relationship based on bad communication. Effective interpersonal communication allows people to achieve their goals, to share information with other people, and to feel understood. Without effective interpersonal communication, even the most simple interactions with other people become an exercise in frustration—for both parties.

The importance of effective communication skills is underscored by the pervasiveness of *social skills deficits* in the literature on interpersonal relations and mental health. The impact of social skills on interpersonal relationships, and in turn on mental health, simply cannot be overstated. Some very well-developed interpersonal theories of mental health stress the role of poor social skills in contributing to the development and course of such problems as depression, social anxiety, schizophrenia, loneliness, eating disorders, alcoholism, and other substance use problems. At the same time, effective social skills may play a prophylactic role by reducing the likelihood of mental health problems when faced with other stressors in life.

The relationship between social skills deficits and mental health problems is manifold. Some people fail to develop adequate social skills for a variety of reasons, ranging from social isolation and minimal opportunity for the practice and development of such skills, to exposure to poor role models. Such individuals face an uphill struggle to develop rewarding interpersonal relationships, much less to execute successful interpersonal interactions. As a consequence, many of the issues already covered, such as interpersonal rejection, unavailability of personal relationships, loneliness, and perhaps even neglect from parents and others, follow. In this way, poor social skills can precipitate poor mental health. For such individuals, effective treatment of this condition will require at least some attention to their social skills.

Alternatively, the symptoms of many different forms of psychopathology can interfere with effective social behavior, corroding social skills. The psychotic symptoms of schizophrenia or bipolar disorder can seriously damage one's ability to communicate with others in a way that is appropriate and effective. Similarly, the difficulty in concentration, psychomotor retardation, and sad affect of depression; the nervousness and preoccupation with failure in social anxiety; and the emotional liability and blunted cognition associated with substance dependence will all have deleterious effects on social communication skills. Even those with good premorbid social skills are prone to experiencing declines concomitant with episodes of psychopathology. As the symptoms of psychological problems continue to worsen, social skills will atrophy. In such cases, improvements in mental health are often accompanied by improvements in social skills (e.g., Hersen, Bellack, & Himmelhoch, 1980).

Many of the other, more specific problems with interpersonal communication that are evident in the mental health literature—such as *excessive reassurance seeking, self-doubt about making a desired impression on others, attention seeking*, and *indirect attempts at communication*—may all be secondary to social skills deficits, or circumscribed forms of such deficits. Many of these interpersonal phenomena may reflect a deficit in motivation for deploying appropriate social behaviors. People may engage in these behaviors, or have these feelings, because they are otherwise unable to get what they are looking for from other people and from their relationships through more standard means of communication. Those with inadequate social skills may turn to more dramatic or histrionic forms of communication (such as excessive reassurance seeking in depression and attention seeking in personality disorders), or to more subtle means of expression (such as the indirect attempts at communication in somatoform disorders and perhaps eating disorders). Because they may lack the wherewithal for effective and direct interpersonal communication as a means of expressing their concerns, people with eating disorders and somatoform disorders use their symptoms to send "messages" or "signals" to other people.

One final word on the topic of social skills is in order: It is apparent that despite the ubiquity of this topic in the mental health literature, some people with psychological problems may have very well-developed social skills. In fact, their social skills may be so well developed and practiced that patients use them to manipulate and exploit other people. People with paranoid symptoms, certain personality disorders, bipolar disorder, and certain paraphilias often have very good social skills, especially perceptual skills. Such people may hone their social skills toward maladaptive and socially unacceptable ends. In such cases, the problem is not so much a social skills deficit as it is an irresponsible application and utilization of social skills.

EXPLANATIONS AND PREDICTIONS IN THE INTERPERSONAL PARADIGM

Mental health researchers working in the interpersonal tradition hold various assumptions about the relationship between interpersonal communication and relationships on the one hand, and mental health problems on the other. These associations can take a variety of forms. Perhaps the most powerful of these assumptions is that *interpersonal phenomena are causally involved in disrupting mental health*. Although this hypothesis has not often been tested directly, it is a deeply held conviction among many theorists and researchers. In some cases of psychopathology, interpersonal issues appear to be the dominant antecedent factor. For example, when marital distress or dissolution immediately precedes an episode of major depression, the development of alcohol dependence, or a somatoform disorder, the disruption of interpersonal relationships is assumed to be the primary cause of the psychological symptoms and distress.

Research evidence in some areas (e.g., personality disorders, eating disorders, and depression) suggests that these interpersonal antecedents to mental health problems need not always be proximal to the onset of the disorders. An intriguing possibility is that certain interpersonal events create dispositions that lie dormant until later adulthood, or that the effects of characteristic styles of communication and relating to other people accumulate over time, until they pass some threshold that then initiates an episode of mental illness. For example, some of the most profound effects of childhood abuse and neglect may not be evident until a child reaches adulthood and attempts to initiate intimate relationships with other adults and/or to raise children of his or her own. Similarly, a child with poor social skills may not experience the full implications of this problem with interpersonal communication until, as an adult, he or she leaves the supportive family context and moves out into the world to establish close relationships with other people.

In addition to being a proximal cause and a distal cause of psychological problems, *interpersonal phenomena may also function as a vulnerability factor in the disruption of mental health*. At least some interpersonal processes, such as parental neglect and overinvolvement, poor social skills, and unavailable personal relationships, may create a vulnerability to the development of psychosocial problems. This conceptualization of the interpersonal origins of mental health problems fits well with diathesis–stress models. In diathesis–stress models of illness, a predisposition or preexisting factor (the diathesis) lies somewhat idle until the person experiences stress, at which time full-blown distress and illness result. For many if not most people, interpersonal issues such as relational distress, maltreatment by parents, and conflict can act as stressors that interact with preexisting temperamental, cognitive, psychological, or biological predispositions to produce episodes of mental illness.

What remain rather mysterious are how and why various interpersonal phenomena lead to vastly differing mental health outcomes in different people. The reasons why the same vulnerability factor, such as parental neglect, may lead to one type of psychopathology in one individual but a different problem in another are not yet well understood. Some people who are abused as children develop major depression later in life. Others develop eating disorders, still others personality disorders, and yet others substance abuse or dependence. And then there are the myriad of people who have experienced vulnerability factors (abuse, parental alcoholism, family conflict, etc.), but who have no symptoms of psychopathology at all. Such people are characterized as "resilient," and present anomalies in need of explanation. These resilient cases are reminders that the relationship between interpersonal distress and psychological distress is probabilistic, not deterministic. The current search for moderating and mediating variables in this context holds great promise for answers to such questions, and is an imperative for future research in the interpersonal paradigm.

Another primary assumption in the interpersonal paradigm is that *interpersonal dysfunction is a consequence of mental health problems.* This assumption has been scientifically proven beyond any reasonable doubt. When people experience episodes of psychopathology—be it depression, schizophrenia, social anxiety, substance abuse or dependence, eating disorders, personality disorders, somatoform disorders, or psychogenic sexual dysfunctions—the quality of their interpersonal relationships and communication is bound to change. Usually this change is for the worse. Part of the reason for this deterioration in interpersonal relations, secondary to poor mental health, is the social behavior of the afflicted individual. Psychological problems can alter the most basic components of verbal and nonverbal communication. People with such problems may not be able or willing to express themselves clearly and openly to other people. Their discourse may be dominated by particular themes and concerns, or may show no coherence or pattern at all in the case of more profound illnesses. Furthermore, psychopathology can alter the way afflicted individuals view and experience relationships with other people. Social relationships that were once experienced as rewarding can become frightening, distressing, and confusing for psychiatric patients.

The disrupted social behavior of the distressed individual is only half the reason for interpersonal deterioration following psychological disorder. A true interpersonal analysis must also consider the reactions of other people. Research studies have repeatedly shown that people react to others with depression, social anxiety, schizophrenia, a personality disorder, or an eating disorder with interpersonal rejection. It is a harsh reality that most people are repelled by those who exhibit signs of psychopathology. People with psychological problems violate our expectations for appropriate and rewarding social interaction. Consequently, most people ultimately prefer to keep their distance from such individuals. The inevitable outcome to this interpersonal pattern is a marked deterioration of social relationships for the person suffering from psychological disorder.

Closely related to the consequence assumption is the belief that *interpersonal interactions will maintain mental health problems*. Within the interpersonal paradigm, many research programs explore how interpersonal interactions maintain poor mental health once it is started. There is an implicit recognition in such research that mental health problems may have numerous origins. Regardless of how a problem was initiated, it is clear that interpersonal interactions can maintain and prolong psychological problems. By analogy, there are multiple causal origins of physical illnesses, such as influenza and the common cold. Regardless of how one contracts such illnesses, diet and rest can affect their course, despite having no straightforward connection to the cause of the illness. One can look at mental health problems from this same perspective. Even in cases where psychological problems may be caused by noninterpersonal agents, the quality of interpersonal relations will often significantly affect the course of the problems. For example, in the area of depression, interpersonal rejection from others may maintain the disorder. Similarly, CD, EE, and negative AS in family members of patients with schizophrenia can prolong the active state of the disorder and precipitate relapse. Interpersonal conflicts and stressors can also activate episodes of substance misuse and disordered eating. These patterns have been conclusively documented, and appear to operate regardless of the actual "cause" of each disorder.

A more radical version of the interpersonal maintenance hypothesis can be found in the faction of the interpersonal school known as *family systems*. Traditional family systems theorists eschew the search for "causal" agents in psychopathology in the traditional linear sense (e.g., *A* causes *B*). Rather, they see cause and effect as inseparable, and they see all components of an interpersonal system as acting on and being acted on all other components. To a systems theorist, what "causes" a disorder is what keeps that disorder alive.

Research in certain areas of mental health (e.g., eating disorders, schizophrenia, substance dependence, and somatoform disorders) clearly illustrates the systems notions of mutual influence or interdependence. In such cases, it is clear that something is not quite right in the social fabric of the patient's interpersonal system. Family members may be hypercritical and overly involved; spouses and friends may be combative and prone to conflict; and parents may exhibit and model behavior that is itself indicative of questionable mental health. Presumably this disturbed interpersonal milieu is abrasive and leads to symptoms of poor mental health. However, at the same time, it is clear that living with an individual who has a psychosocial problem is itself taxing. The presence of a disturbed family member, for instance, will fundamentally alter the interpersonal communication and relationships in that family. Members may change their style of relating both to the "ill" member as well as to each other. People may feel shame, stigma, or burden associated with the presence of mental illness in their family or immediate interpersonal network. These changes in social behavior then go on to affect the person with the psychological problem, and suddenly the attribution of "cause" and "effect" becomes nearly impossible. Systems research showing that families of individuals with alcoholism literally structure their lives around drinking, and that families of patients with eating disorders exhibit preoccupation with food, dieting, and exercise, obfuscate conventional notions of cause and effect or action and reaction. Indeed, the popular terms "alcoholic family" and "eating-disordered family" reflect the key assumption that the disorder is not located within the individual, but rather within the larger social system that maintains and sustains it.

It is important to note that these interpersonal processes in psychological problems, be they causal, consequential, or maintaining factors, apply not only to clinical cases of these problems, but to subclinical instances at well. What has come to be known as the *continuity hypothesis* holds that subclinical and clinical cases of a particular problem differ in degree, not in kind. Although this hypothesis has drawn some controversy, most of the research evidence in the interpersonal domain is supportive of the continuity hypothesis (e.g., Gotlib, Lewinsohn, & Seeley, 1995; Lewinsohn, Solomon, Seeley, & Zeiss, 2000). People with subclinical levels of depression, anxiety, and eating disorders, for example, often experience and exhibit many of the same interpersonal difficulties as those with full-blown clinical cases of these same problems. Often the only difference between the two, interpersonally, is in the *magnitude* of the problems. Indeed, a portion of the research results examined in this book came from studies of subclinical syndromes, and these studies are generally consistent with those of clinically diagnosed cases. Therefore, one of the particularly useful aspects of the interpersonal paradigm in mental health is its explanatory and predictive power for both clinical and subclinical versions of different psychological problems.

INTEGRATION OF THE INTERPERSONAL PARADIGM
WITH OTHER SCHOOLS OF THOUGHT IN MENTAL HEALTH

I have mentioned earlier that paradigms focus attention on what variables are important for explaining a phenomenon. At the same time, these ideologies can divert attention away from other phenomena that are assumed to be unimportant in the etiology and course of a disorder. For this reason, proponents of various schools of thought may dismiss or ignore concepts from differing schools of thought. In more extreme cases, theorists become critical of other perspectives and see them as competing.

As noted in Chapter 1, the interpersonal paradigm in mental health is not a competing or alternative perspective to other well-recognized paradigms, such as the cognitive, behavioral, biological, or psychodynamic schools. In fact, many of the essential constructs in these schools of thought can easily be traced to interpersonal issues. From this perspective, the interpersonal paradigm is complementary to other academic schools of thought.

Some of the key constructs in the cognitive perspective on mental health include *attributions*, *expectations*, and *evaluations*. The maladaptive forms taken by these cognitive processes constitute a fundamental aspect of many forms of psychopathology. However, where do these attributions and expectations come from? One obvious answer to the question lies in interpersonal interactions. Joiner (2001) has noted that "attributions do not occur in an interpersonal vacuum" (p. 131). Common interpersonal processes in depression such as reassurance seeking may be interpreted as a way of gathering information for the formation of attributions. Joiner (2001) has also argued that the hopelessness common to depression may generate interpersonal stressors. Other types of expectations may also be closely linked to interpersonal processes. A child who is abused or neglected may come to expect other people to neglect or abandon him or her. A depressed individual who experiences a great deal of interpersonal rejection is likely to expect further rejection from other people. Parents who pressure their children for inappropriate levels of achievement may inadvertently teach perfectionist attitudes to their children, who then become prone to eating disorders as a maladaptive means of achieving these standards. In cases such as these, the distorted cognitive processes that contribute to the psychological problems have interpersonal origins.

The tradition of behaviorism places the focus not on the internal "unobservable" cognitive processes, but rather on the observable behaviors and the resultant rewards or punishments that they receive from the environment. With a moment's thought, it ought to be apparent that many of the maladaptive behaviors that contribute to and even *define* psychopathology are interpersonal behaviors. Similarly, the behaviors whose extinction can be implicated in the development of psychological problems also tend to be interpersonal in nature. Perhaps most prominently, the sources of reward and punishment are typically found in the *social* environment. If a person becomes lonely and depressed because he or she no longer finds pleasure in relations with other people, and therefore withdraws, his or her feeling of reward or punishment tells only half of the story. The other half concerns what other people do or fail to do to create that sense of reward or punishment. Admittedly, not all behaviors that play a role in poor mental health are interpersonal in nature. However, the behaviors with the greatest capability for producing feelings of reward or punishment tend to be inherently social, involving a transaction between two or more people.

Advances in the medical sciences have brought a tremendous amount of attention to the potential for understanding psychopathology through such biological mechanisms as genetics, neurochemical agents, and neurophysiological structures and functions. The identification of numerous such agents in most of the problems discussed in this book, coupled with the documented efficacy of pharmacological treatments for them, has brought great acclaim to the biological paradigm. How could an interpersonal paradigm possibly be integrated into a biological perspective on mental illness?

The ultimate resolution of the mind–body debate is that biology affects psychology and psychology affects biology. It can now be stated with equal certainty that *interpersonal interaction affects biological functions.* When rats are reared in social isolation, there are clear biological consequences. In one study, experimenters assigned rats to conditions of social isolation or group housing for a period of 7 days, after which they administered a tracer dose of diprenorphine (Vanderschuren, Stein, Wiegant, & Van Ree, 1995). *In vivo* radiographic analysis of brain functions showed an increase in opiate receptor binding in the medial prefrontal cortex for the socially isolated rats. This neurological change was produced with a single week of social isolation. Rats reared in isolation for a period of 60 days had lower brain weights than those reared in a socially enriched environment (Das, Das, & Banamali, 1987; Riege, 1971). Male rats exposed to aggressive behavior from another rat over a period of only 4 days, for 4 hours per day, exhibited adrenal hypertrophy and an increase in basal corticosterone (Haller, Fuchs, Halasz, & Makara, 1999). These biological signs of stress indicate that exposure to aggressive interpersonal behavior can affect physiological structure and neurochemical action. Early adverse experiences (e.g., exposure to maternal depression, inadequate parenting) in neonates produce changes in corticotrophin-releasing-factor containing neurons and the sympathetic nervous system; these changes may be immediately protective, but are detrimental in the long run by creating an increased sensitivity to stress (Graham, Heim, Goodman, Miller, & Nemeroff, 1999). Adults who experience marital distress exhibit a variety of immunosuppressive effects and changes in endocrine function (Kennedy, Kiecolt-Glaser, & Glaser, 1988; Kiecolt-Glaser et al., 1996). These are only a few of the findings that unequivocally establish a connection between interpersonal experiences and subsequent changes in biological structures and functions.

There is considerable plasticity in both human and nonhuman brains well into the lifespan. One of the agents responsible for changes in brain development, as well as other neurological actions, is interpersonal interaction. Therefore, when a biological agent or action is identified in association with a particular psychological disorder, it is essential to bear in mind that interpersonal experiences may be partially or largely responsible for the biological disturbance that some are tempted to conclude "caused" the problem.

Finally, the psychodynamic paradigm seeks to explain psychopathology through largely unconscious motivations and drives that are imbalanced or otherwise maladaptive. As noted in Chapter 1, several key components in this school of thought are inherently interpersonal in nature. Early experiences with the mother and father, as well as siblings, projection, and transference, all figure prominently in psychodynamic explanations. Various factions of the psychodynamic school, such as object relations theorists and attachment theory, are even more explicitly interpersonal in their orientation. Indeed, the "object" in object relations is "people." The "attachment" in attachment theory is attachment to a caregiver (i.e., another person). Although the interpersonal paradigm takes a more behavioral perspective, and the psychodynamic paradigm is more psychological in its orientation, the two actually share many similar interests when it comes to explaining psychopathology.

Over the past 25 years, a new perspective has begun to emerge in the medical and psychological sciences: the *biopsychosocial model* (Engel, 1977). This paradigm is an attempt to encompass virtually all of the models and factors outlined above. It is an explicit recognition that biology, cognition, affect, and social behavior are mutually influential. A complete understanding of any health problem, whether physical or psychological, cannot be attained without granting attention to biological, psychological, and social factors, according to this model. This intelligent recognition is long overdue, and should be something of a wake-up call to advocates of a monolithic paradigm in mental health. Though the interpersonal paradigm has its own core assumptions, explanations, and predictions that are distinct from other schools of thought, its components fit well within the superordinate biopsychosocial model.

CONCLUSION

Historically, scientific inquiry into mental health problems has emanated from a variety of perspectives. Psychodynamic approaches stress unconscious drives and early relationships with parents. Biological approaches emphasize the role of genes, neuroendocrine problems, and neurotransmitter malfunction. Cognitive theories illustrate how dysfunctional schemas and attributional styles can precipitate different types of psychopathology, whereas behavioral theories explain how patterns of reinforcement and punishment can affect mental health. Although not as immediately recognizable and coherently organized, the interpersonal paradigm in psychopathology highlights the role of interpersonal communication processes and close relationships as they may cause or be caused by mental health problems. The science of interpersonal relations and psychopathology has come of age.

Theorists and researchers working in the interpersonal paradigm take as their data interpersonal experiences in the family of origin, the family of orientation, and general personal relationships, along with styles, forms, and functions of interpersonal communication behavior. Their focus is not just on the behavior, cognition, and affect of the afflicted individual, but on the reactions of and relationships with other people who come into contact with the afflicted individual. In this paradigm, interpersonal interactions are assumed to play a causal role in mental health. Interpersonal issues are also recognized as vulnerability factors that make people susceptible to the ill effects of stress, as well as potential stressors themselves. Disturbances in interpersonal relations are viewed as inevitable consequences of most psychological problems. Finally, interpersonal interactions are known to maintain psychopathology and to have a significant impact on the course and outcome of mental disorders.

Along with the knowledge produced by the cognitive, behavioral, biological, and psychodynamic schools, the interpersonal paradigm provides another useful and powerful tool for understanding psychopathology. Its position alongside these other orientations is as well deserved as it is well established by hundreds of research studies indicating that problematic interpersonal relationships and mental health problems are inextricably entwined.

References

Adler, R. H., Zamboni, P., Hofer, T., Hemmeler, W., Hurny, C., Minder, C., Radvila, A., & Zlot, S. I. (1997). How not to miss a somatic needle in the haystack of chronic pain. *Journal of Psychosomatic Research, 42,* 499–506.

Adler, R. H., Zlot, S., Hurny, C., & Minder, C. (1989). Engel's "Psychogenic pain and the pain-prone patient": A retrospective, controlled clinical study. *Psychosomatic Medicine, 51,* 87–101.

Adrian, C., & Hammen, C. (1993). Stress exposure and stress generation in children of depressed mothers. *Journal of Consulting and Clinical Psychology, 61,* 354–359.

Ahmad, S., Waller, G., & Verduyn, C. (1994). Eating attitudes among Asian schoolgirls: The role of perceived parental control. *International Journal of Eating Disorders, 15,* 91–97.

Akhtar, S., & Thomson, J. A. (1982). Overview: Narcissistic personality disorder. *American Journal of Psychiatry, 139,* 12–20.

Akiskal, H. S., Khani, M. K., & Scott-Strauss, A. (1979). Cyclothymic temperament disorders. *Psychiatric Clinics of North America, 2,* 527–554.

Alden, L. E., & Phillips, N. (1990). An interpersonal analysis of social anxiety and depression. *Cognitive Therapy and Research, 14,* 499–513.

Alden, L. E., & Wallace, S. T. (1995). Social phobia and social appraisal in successful and unsuccessful social interactions. *Behaviour Research and Therapy, 33,* 497–505.

Alloy, L. B., & Abramson, L. Y. (1979). Judgment of contingency in depressed and nondepressed students: Sadder but wiser? *Journal of Experimental Psychology: General, 108,* 441–485.

Alloy, L. B., & Abramson, L. Y. (1988). Depressive realism: Four theoretical perspectives. In L. B. Alloy (Ed.), *Cognitive processes in depression* (pp. 223–265). New York: Guilford Press.

Altorfer, A., Goldstein, M. J., Miklowitz, D. J., & Nuechterlein, K. H. (1992). Stress-indicative patterns of non-verbal behaviour: Their role in family interactions. *British Journal of Psychiatry, 161*(Suppl. 18), 103–113.

American Psychiatric Association. (2000). *Diagnostic and statistical manual of mental disorders* (4th ed., Text rev.). Washington, DC: Author.

Amin, N., Foa, E. B., & Coles, M. E. (1998). Negative interpretation bias in social phobia. *Behaviour Research and Therapy, 36*, 945–957.

Amstutz, D. K., & Kaplan, M. F. (1987). Depression, physical attractiveness, and interpersonal acceptance. *Journal of Social and Clinical Psychology, 5*, 365–377.

Anderson, C. M., Reiss, D. J., & Hogarty, G. E. (1986). *Schizophrenia and the family.* New York: Guilford Press.

Andersson, L., Mullins, L. C., & Johnson, D. P. (1990). Parental intrusion versus social isolation: A dichotomous view of the sources of loneliness. In M. Hojat & R. Crandall (Eds.), *Loneliness: Theory, research, and applications* (pp. 125–134). Newbury Park, CA: Sage.

Andrews, B. (1995). Bodily shame as a mediator between abusive experiences and depression. *Journal of Abnormal Psychology, 104*, 277–285.

Apt, C., & Hurlbert, D. F. (1994). The sexual attitudes, behavior, and relationships of women with histrionic personality disorder. *Journal of Sex and Marital Therapy, 20*, 125–133.

Araujo, A. B., Durante, R., Feldman, H. A., Goldstein, I., & McKinlay, J. B. (1988). The relationship between depressive symptoms and male erectile dysfunction: Cross-sectional results from the Massachusetts Male Aging Study. *Psychosomatic Medicine, 60*, 458–465.

Arkowitz, H., Hinton, R., Perl, J., & Himadi, W. (1978). Treatment strategies for dating anxiety in college men based on real-life practice. *Counseling Psychologist, 7*, 41–46.

Arnold, M. E., & Thompson, B. (1996). Love style perceptions in relation to personality function. *Journal of Social Behavior and Personality, 11*, 425–438.

Attie, I., & Brooks-Gunn, J. (1989). Development of eating problems in adolescent girls: A longitudinal study. *Developmental Psychology, 25*, 70–79.

Badger, T. A. (1996a). Family members' experiences living with members with depression. *Western Journal of Nursing Research, 18*, 149–171.

Badger, T. A. (1996b). Living with depression: Family members' experiences and treatment needs. *Journal of Psychosocial Nursing, 34*, 21–29.

Bahr, S. J., Hawks, R. D., & Wang, G. (1993). Family and religious influences on adolescent substance abuse. *Youth and Society, 24*, 443–465.

Baker, D. E., & Stephenson, L. A. (1995). Personality characteristics of adult children of alcoholics. *Journal of Clinical Psychology, 51*, 695–702.

Baker, J. D., Capron, E. W., & Azorlosa, J. (1996). Family environment characteristics of persons with histrionic and dependent personality disorders. *Journal of Personality Disorders, 10*, 82–87.

Ballenger, J. C., Davidson, J. R. T., Lecrubier, Y., Nutt, D. J., Bobes, J., Beidel, D. C., Ono, Y., & Westenberg, H. G. M. (1998). Consensus statement on social anxiety disorder from the International Consensus Group on Depression and Anxiety. *Journal of Clinical Psychiatry, 59*(Suppl. 17), 54–60.

Bandura, A. (1977). *Social learning theory.* Englewood Cliffs, NJ: Prentice-Hall.

Bandura, A. (1986). *Social foundations of thought and action.* Englewood Cliffs, NJ: Prentice-Hall.

Bandura, A. (1999). Social cognitive theory of personality. In L. A. Pervin & O. P. John (Eds.), *Handbook of personality* (2nd ed., pp. 154–196). New York: Guilford Press.

Banmen, J., & Vogel, N. A. (1985). The relationship between marital quality and interpersonal sexual communication. *Family Therapy, 12,* 45–58.

Barbato, N., & Hafner, R. J. (1998). Comorbidity of bipolar and personality disorder. *Australian and New Zealand Journal of Psychiatry, 32,* 276–280.

Barnes, G., Farrell, M., & Cairns, A. (1986). Parental socialization factors and adolescent drinking behaviors. *Journal of Marriage and the Family, 48,* 27–36.

Barrera, M., & Stice, E. (1998). Parent–adolescent conflict in the context of parental support: Families with alcoholic and nonalcoholic fathers. *Journal of Family Psychology, 12,* 195–208.

Barsky, A. J., & Klerman, G. L. (1983). Overview: Hypochondriasis, bodily complaints, and somatic styles. *American Journal of Psychiatry, 140,* 273–283.

Barsky, A. J., Wool, C., Barnett, M. C., & Cleary, P. D. (1994). Histories of childhood trauma in adult hypochondriacal patients. *American Journal of Psychiatry, 151,* 397–401.

Bartels, S. J., Mueser, K. T., & Miles, K. M. (1997). Functional impairments in elderly patients with schizophrenia and major affective illness in the community: Social skills, living skills, and behavior problems. *Behavior Therapy, 28,* 43–63.

Basco, M. R., Prager, K. J., Pite, J. M., Tamir, L. M., & Stephens, J. J. (1992). Communication and intimacy in the marriages of depressed patients. *Journal of Family Psychology, 6,* 184–194.

Bass, C., & Murphy, M. (1995). Somatoform and personality disorders: Syndromal comorbidity and overlapping developmental pathways. *Journal of Psychosomatic Research, 39,* 403–427.

Bateson, G., Jackson, D., Haley, J., & Weakland, J. (1956). Toward a theory of schizophrenia. *Behavioral Science, 1,* 252–264.

Bauman, K. E., & Ennett, S. T. (1994). Peer influence on adolescent drug use. *American Psychologist, 49,* 820–822.

Baumeister, R. F. (1992). Neglected aspects of self theory: Motivation, interpersonal aspects, culture, escape, and existential value. *Psychological Inquiry, 3,* 21–25.

Baumrind, D. (1991). The influence of parenting style on adolescent competence and substance use. *Journal of Early Adolescence, 11,* 56–95.

Beach, S. R. H., Jouriles, E. N., & O'Leary, K. D. (1985). Extramarital sex: Impact on depression and commitment in couples seeking marital therapy. *Journal of Sex and Marital Therapy, 11,* 99–108.

Beach, S. R. H., & O'Leary, K. D. (1993). Marital discord and dysphoria: For whom does the marital relationship predict depressive symptomatology? *Journal of Social and Personal Relationships, 10,* 405–420.

Beach, S. R. H., Sandeen, E. E., & O'Leary, K. D. (1990). *Depression and marriage.* New York: Guilford Press.

Beattie, H. J. (1988). Eating disorders and the mother–daughter relationship. *International Journal of Eating Disorders, 7,* 453–460.

Bebbington, P., & Kuipers, L. (1994). The predictive utility of expressed emotion in schizophrenia: An aggregate analysis. *Psychological Medicine, 24,* 707–718.

Beck, A. T., Rush, A. J., Shaw, B. F., & Emery, G. (1979). *Cognitive therapy of depression.* New York: Guilford Press.

Beck, M. (1983). Double bind is not a theory of schizophrenia. *Australian Journal of Family Therapy, 4,* 251–254.

Beckfield, D. F. (1985). Interpersonal competence among college men hypothesized to be at risk for schizophrenia. *Journal of Abnormal Psychology, 94,* 397–404.

Bedell, J., Lennox, S. S., Smith, A. D., & Rabinowicz, E. F. (1998). Evaluation of problem solving and communication skills of persons with schizophrenia. *Psychiatry Research, 78,* 197–206.

Beidel, D. C., Turner, S. M., & Dancu, C. V. (1985). Physiological, cognitive and behavioral aspects of social anxiety. *Behaviour Research and Therapy, 23,* 109–117.

Beisecker, A. E. (1991). Interpersonal approaches to drug abuse prevention. In L. Donohew, H. E. Sypher, & W. J. Bukoski (Eds.), *Persuasive communication and drug abuse prevention* (pp. 229–238). Hillsdale, NJ: Erlbaum.

Bellack, A. S., Morrison, R. L., Mueser, K. T., & Wade, J. (1989). Social competence in schizoaffective disorder, bipolar disorder, and negative and non-negative schizophrenia. *Schizophrenia Research, 2,* 391–401.

Bellack, A. S., Morrison, R. L., Wixted, J. T., & Mueser, K. T. (1990). An analysis of social competence in schizophrenia. *British Journal of Psychiatry, 156,* 809–818.

Belsher, G., & Costello, C. G. (1991). Do confidants of depressed women provide less social support than confidants of nondepressed women? *Journal of Abnormal Psychology, 100,* 516–525.

Benazon, N. R. (2000). Predicting negative spousal attitudes toward depressed persons: A test of Coyne's interpersonal model. *Journal of Abnormal Psychology, 109,* 550–554.

Benazon, N. R., & Coyne, J. C. (2000). Living with a depressed spouse. *Journal of Family Psychology, 14,* 71–79.

Benjamin, L. S. (1974). Structural Analysis of Social Behavior. *Psychological Review, 81,* 392–425.

Benjamin, L. S. (1992). An interpersonal approach to the diagnosis of borderline personality disorder. In J. F. Clarkin, E. Marziali, & H. Munroe-Blum (Eds.), *Borderline personality disorder: Clinical and empirical perspectives* (pp. 161–196). New York: Guilford Press.

Benjamin, L. S. (1996). *Interpersonal diagnosis and treatment of personality disorders* (2nd ed.). New York: Guilford Press.

Benjamin, L. S., & Wonderlich, S. A. (1994). Social perceptions and borderline personality disorder: The relation to mood disorders. *Journal of Abnormal Psychology, 103,* 610–624.

Bensley, L. S., Spieker, S. J., & McMahon, R. J. (1994). Parenting behavior of adolescent children of alcoholics. *Addiction, 89,* 1265–1276.

Berenbaum, H. (1992). Posed facial expressions of emotion in schizophrenia and depression. *Psychological Medicine, 22,* 927–937.

Berger, A. (1965). A test of the double bind hypothesis of schizophrenia. *Family Process, 4*, 198–205.

Berkowitz, A., & Perkins, W. H. (1988). Personality characteristics of children of alcoholics. *Journal of Consulting and Clinical Psychology, 56*, 206–209.

Biglan, A., Hops, H., Sherman, L., Friedman, L. S., Arthur, J., & Osteen, V. (1985). Problem-solving interactions of depressed women and their husbands. *Behavior Therapy, 16*, 431–451.

Billings, A., Kessler, M., Gomberg, C., & Weiner, S. (1979). Marital conflict-resolution of alcoholic and nonalcoholic couples during sobriety and experimental drinking. *Journal of Studies on Alcohol, 3*, 183–195.

Blackburn, R. (1998). Relationship of personality disorders to observer ratings of interpersonal style in forensic psychiatric patients. *Journal of Personality Disorders, 12*, 77–85.

Blackson, T. C., Tarter, R. E., Loeber, R., Ammerman, R. T., & Windle, M. (1996). The influence of paternal substance abuse and difficult temperament in fathers and sons on sons' disengagement from family to deviant peers. *Journal of Youth and Adolescence, 25*, 389–409.

Blakar, R. M. (1982). Schizophrenia and communication: A paradox of theory and research. *International Journal of Family Psychiatry, 3*, 209–214.

Blaustein, J. P., & Tuber, S. B. (1998). Knowing the unspeakable: Somatization as an expression of disruptions in affective-relational functioning. *Bulletin of the Menninger Clinic, 62*, 351–365.

Blouin, A. G., Zuro, C., & Blouin, J. H. (1990). Family environment in bulimia nervosa: The role of depression. *International Journal of Eating Disorders, 9*, 649–658.

Blumberg, S. R., & Hokanson, J. E. (1983). The effects of another person's response style on interpersonal behavior in depression. *Journal of Abnormal Psychology, 92*, 196–209.

Boney-McCoy, S., & Finkelhor, D. (1996). Is youth victimization related to trauma symptoms and depression after controlling for prior symptoms and family relationships? A longitudinal, prospective study. *Journal of Consulting and Clinical Psychology, 64*, 1406–1416.

Bornstein, R. F. (1992). The dependent personality: Developmental, social, and clinical perspectives. *Psychological Bulletin, 112*, 3–23.

Bornstein, R. F. (1999). Histrionic personality disorder, physical attractiveness, and social adjustment. *Journal of Psychopathology and Behavioral Assessment, 21*, 79–94.

Bouhuys, A. L., Geerts, E., Mersch, P. P. A., & Jenner, J. A. (1996). Nonverbal interpersonal sensitivity and persistence of depression: Perceptions of emotions in schematic faces. *Psychiatry Research, 64*, 193–203.

Boyce, P., Harris, M., Silove, D., Morgan, A., Wilhelm, K., & Hadzi-Pavlovic, D. (1998). Psychosocial factors associated with depression: A study of socially disadvantaged women with young children. *Journal of Nervous and Mental Disease, 186*, 3–11.

Brage, D., & Meredith, W. (1994). A causal model of adolescent depression. *Journal of Psychology, 128*, 455–468.

230   References

Brage, D., Meredith, W., & Woodward, J. (1993). Correlates of loneliness among Midwestern adolescents. *Adolescence, 28,* 685–693.

Braginsky, B. M., Holzberg, J. D., Finison, L., & Ring, K. (1967). Correlates of the mental patient's acquisition of hospital information. *Journal of Personality, 35,* 323–342.

Braginsky, B. M., Holzberg, J. D., Ridley, D., & Braginsky, D. D. (1968). Patient styles of adaptation to a mental hospital. *Journal of Personality, 36,* 282–298.

Braucht, G. N., Brakarsh, D., Follingstad, D., & Berry, K. L. (1973). Deviant drug use in adolescence: A review of psychological correlates. *Psychological Bulletin, 79,* 92–106.

Breuer, J., & Freud, S. (1960). *Studies in hysteria.* Boston, MA: Beacon. (Original work published 1895)

Breznitz, Z. (1992). Verbal indicators of depression. *Journal of General Psychology, 199,* 351–363.

Breznitz, Z., & Sherman, T. (1987). Speech patterning of natural discourse of well and depressed mothers and their young children. *Child Development, 58,* 395–400.

Brink, T. L., & Niemeyer, L. (1993). Hypochondriasis, loneliness, and social functioning. *Psychological Reports, 72,* 1241–1242.

Briscoe, C. W., Smith, J. B., Robins, E., Marten, S., & Gaskin, F. (1973). Divorce and psychiatric disease. *Archives of General Psychiatry, 29,* 119–125.

Brodsky, C. M. (1984). Sociocultural and interactional influences on somatization. *Psychosomatics, 25,* 673–680.

Brokaw, D. W., & McLemore, C. W. (1991). Interpersonal models of personality and psychopathology. In D. G. Gilbert & J. J. Connolly (Eds.), *Personality, social skills, and psychopathology: An individual differences approach* (pp. 49–83). New York: Plenum Press.

Brookings, J. B., & Wilson, J. F. (1994). Personality and family-environment predictors of self-reported eating attitudes and behaviors. *Journal of Personality Assessment, 63,* 313–326.

Brooner, R. K., King, V. L., Kidorf, M., Schmidt, C. W., & Bigelow, G. E. (1997). Psychiatric and substance use comorbidity among treatment-seeking opiod abusers. *Archives of General Psychiatry, 54,* 71–79.

Brown, G. W., & Harris, T. (1978). *Social origins of depression.* New York: Free Press.

Brown, G. W., Monck, E. M., Carstairs, G. M., & Wing, J. K. (1962). Influence of family life on the course of schizophrenic illness. *British Journal of Preventative and Social Medicine, 16,* 55–68.

Brown, J., Cohen, P., Johnson, J. G., & Smailes, E. M. (1999). Childhood abuse and neglect: Specificity of effects on adolescent and young adult depression and suicidality. *Journal of the American Academy of Child and Adolescent Psychiatry, 38,* 1490–1496.

Bruch, M. A., & Heimberg, R. G. (1994). Differences in perceptions of parental characteristics between generalized and nongeneralized social phobics. *Journal of Anxiety Disorders, 8,* 155–168.

Buhr, T. A., & Pryor, B. (1988). Communication apprehension and alcohol abuse. *Journal of Social Behavior and Personality, 3,* 237–243.

Bulik, C. M. (1995). Anxiety disorders and eating disorders: A review of their relationship. *New Zealand Journal of Psychology, 24*, 51–62.

Bull, P. E. (1987). *Posture and gesture.* Oxford: Pergamon Press.

Bullock, R. C., Siegel, R., Weissman, M., & Paykel, E. S. (1972). The weeping wife: Marital relations of depressed women. *Journal of Marriage and the Family, 34*, 488–495.

Burns, D. D., Sayers, S. L., & Moras, K. (1994). Intimate relationships and depression: Is there a causal connection? *Journal of Consulting and Clinical Psychology, 62*, 1033–1043.

Burston, D. (1996). *The wing of madness: The life and work of R. D. Laing.* Cambridge, MA: Harvard University Press.

Buss, D. M., & Shackelford, T. K. (1997). Susceptibility to infidelity in the first year of marriage. *Journal of Research in Personality, 31*, 193–221.

Butzlaff, R. L., & Hooley, J. M. (1998). Expressed emotion and psychiatric relapse. *Archives of General Psychiatry, 55*, 547–552.

Calam, R., Waller, G., Slade, P., & Newton, T. (1990). Eating disorders and perceived relationships with parents. *International Journal of Eating Disorders, 9*, 479–485.

Calev, A., Nigal, D., & Chazan, S. (1989). Retrieval from semantic memory using meaningful and meaningless constructs by depressed, stable bipolar and manic patients. *British Journal of Clinical Psychology, 28*, 67–73.

Cappella, J. N. (1985a). Production principles for turn-taking rules in social interaction: Socially anxious vs. socially secure persons. *Journal of Language and Social Psychology, 4*, 193–212.

Cappella, J. N. (1985b). Controlling the floor in conversation. In A. W. Siegman & S. Feldstein (Eds.), *Multichannel integrations of nonverbal behavior* (pp. 69–103). Hillsdale, NJ: Erlbaum.

Carini, M. A., & Nevid, J. S. (1992). Social appropriateness and impaired perspective in schizophrenia. *Journal of Clinical Psychology, 48*, 170–177.

Carroll, L., Corning, F., Morgan, R., & Stevens, D. (1991). Perceived acceptance, psychological functioning, and sex role orientation of narcissistic persons. *Journal of Social Behavior and Personality, 6*, 943–954.

Carroll, L., Hoenigmann-Stovall, N., King, A., Wienhold, J., & Whitehead, G. I. (1998). Interpersonal consequences of narcissistic and borderline personality disorders. *Journal of Social and Clinical Psychology, 17*, 38–49.

Carroll, L., Hoenigmann-Stovall, N., & Whitehead, G. (1997). Self-narcissism and interpersonal attraction to narcissistic others. *Psychological Reports, 81*, 547–550.

Carson, R. C. (1969). *Interaction concepts of personality.* Chicago: Aldine.

Carson, R. C. (1983). The social-interactional viewpoint. In M. Hersen, A. E. Kazdin, & A. S. Bellack (Eds.), *The clinical psychology handbook* (pp. 143–153). New York: Pergamon Press.

Carson, R. C. (1996). Seamlessness in personality and its derangements. *Journal of Personality Assessment, 66*, 240–247.

Caster, J. B., Inderbitzen, H. M., & Hope, D. (1999). Relationship between youth and parent perceptions of family environment and social anxiety. *Journal of Anxiety Disorders, 13*, 237–251.

Catalan, J., Hawton, K., & Day, A. (1990). Couples referred to a sexual dysfunction clinic: Psychological and physical morbidity. *British Journal of Psychology, 156*, 61–67.

Chadda, R. K., Bhatia, M. S., Shome, S., & Thakur, K. N. (1993). Psychosocial dysfunction in somatizing patients. *British Journal of Psychiatry, 163*, 510–513.

Chafetz, M. E., Blane, H. T., & Hill, M. J. (1971). Children of alcoholics: Observations in a child guidance clinic. *Quarterly Journal of Studies on Alcohol, 32*, 687–698.

Chansky, T. E., & Kendall, P. C. (1997). Social expectancies and self-perceptions in anxiety-disordered children. *Journal of Anxiety Disorders, 11*, 347–363.

Chassin, L., Pitts, S. C., DeLucia, C., & Todd, M. (1999). A longitudinal study of children of alcoholics: Predicting young adult substance use disorders, anxiety, and depression. *Journal of Abnormal Psychology, 108*, 106–119.

Cheek, J. M., & Buss, A. H. (1981). Shyness and sociability. *Journal of Personality and Social Psychology, 41*, 330–339.

Cherulnik, P. D., Neely, W. T., Flanagan, M., & Zachau, M. (1978). Social skill and visual interaction. *Journal of Social Psychology, 104*, 263–270.

Chiariello, M. A., & Orvaschel, H. (1995). Patterns of parent–child communication: Relationship to depression. *Clinical Psychology Review, 15*, 395–407.

Christensen, A. J., Dornink, R., Ehlers, S. L., & Schultz, S. K. (1999). Social environment and longevity in schizophrenia. *Psychosomatic Medicine, 61*, 141–145.

Clair, D. J., & Genest, M. (1992). The Children of Alcoholics Screening Test: Reliability and relationships to family environment, adjustment, and alcohol-related stressors of adolescent offspring of alcoholics. *Journal of Clinical Psychology, 48*, 414–420.

Claridge, G., Davis, C., Bellhouse, M., & Kaptein, S. (1998). Borderline personality, nightmares, and adverse life events in the risk for eating disorders. *Personality and Individual Differences, 25*, 339–351.

Clulow, C. (1984). Sexual dysfunction and interpersonal stress: The significance of the presenting complaint in seeking and engaging help. *British Journal of Medical Psychology, 57*, 371–380.

Cohn, J. F., Campbell, S. B., Matias, R., & Hopkins, J. (1990). Face-to-face interactions of postpartum depressed and nondepressed mother–infant pairs at 2 months. *Developmental Psychology, 26*, 15–23.

Cole, D. A., Lazarick, D. L., & Howard, G. S. (1987). Construct validity and the relation between depression and social skill. *Journal of Counseling Psychology, 34*, 315–321.

Cole, D. A., & Milstead, M. (1989). Behavioral correlates of depression: Antecedents or consequences? *Journal of Counseling Psychology, 36*, 408–416.

Cole, R. E., Grolnick, W., Kane, C. F., Zastowny, T., & Lehman, A. (1993). Expressed emotion, communication, and problem solving in the families of chronic schizophrenic young adults. In R. E. Cole & D. Reiss (Eds.), *How do families cope with chronic illness?* (pp. 141–172). Hillsdale, NJ: Erlbaum.

Conger, A. J., & Farrell, A. D. (1981). Behavioral components of heterosocial skills. *Behavior Therapy, 12*, 41–55.

Connolly, J., Geller, S., Marton, P., & Kutcher, S. (1992). Peer responses to social interaction with depressed adolescents. *Journal of Clinical Child Psychiatry, 21*, 365–370.

Connors, M. E., & Morse, W. (1993). Sexual abuse and eating disorders: A review. *International Journal of Eating Disorders, 13*, 1–11.

Cooke, R. G., Young, L. T., Mohri, L., Blake, P., & Joffe, R. T. (1999). Family-of-origin characteristics in bipolar disorder: A controlled study. *Canadian Journal of Psychiatry, 44*, 379–381.

Coovert, D. L., Kinder, B. N., & Thompson, J. K. (1989). The psychosexual aspects of anorexia nervosa and bulimia nervosa: A review of the literature. *Clinical Psychology Review, 9*, 169–180.

Corrigan, E. (1980). *Alcoholic women in treatment.* New York: Oxford University Press.

Corrigan, P. W. (1997). The social perceptual deficits of schizophrenia. *Psychiatry, 60*, 309–326.

Corrigan, P. W., & Nelson, D. R. (1998). Factors that affect social cue recognition in schizophrenia. *Psychiatry Research, 78*, 189–196.

Corrigan, P. W., & Toomey, R. (1995). Interpersonal problem solving and information processing in schizophrenia. *Schizophrenia Bulletin, 21*, 395–403.

Corrigan, P. W., Wallace, C. J., & Green, M. F. (1992). Deficits in social schemata in schizophrenia. *Schizophrenia Research, 8*, 129–135.

Corruble, E., Ginestet, D., & Guelfi, J. D. (1996). Comorbidity of personality disorders and unipolar major depression: A review. *Journal of Affective Disorders, 37*, 157–170.

Coryell, W., Scheftner, W., Keller, M., Endicott, J., Maser, J., & Klerman, G. L. (1993). The enduring psychosocial consequences of mania and depression. *American Journal of Psychiatry, 150*, 720–727.

Cosoff, S. J., & Hafner, R. J. (1998). The prevalence of comorbid anxiety in schizophrenia, schizoaffective disorder and bipolar disorder. *Australian and New Zealand Journal of Psychiatry, 32*, 67–72.

Costello, C. G. (1982). Social factors associated with depression: A retrospective community study. *Psychological Medicine, 12*, 329–339.

Coyne, J. C. (1976a). Toward an interactional description of depression. *Psychiatry, 39*, 28–40.

Coyne, J. C. (1976b). Depression and the response of others. *Journal of Abnormal Psychology, 85*, 186–193.

Coyne, J. C. (1990). Interpersonal processes in depression. In G. I. Keitner (Ed.), *Depression and families* (pp. 31–54). Washington, DC: American Psychiatric Press.

Coyne, J. C. (1999). Thinking interactionally about depression: A radical restatement. In T. Joiner & J. C. Coyne (Eds.), *The interactional nature of depression* (pp. 365–392). Washington, DC: American Psychological Association.

Coyne, J. C., Burchill, S. A. L., & Stiles, W. B. (1990). An interactional perspective on depression. In C. R. Snyder & D. R. Forsyth (Eds.), *Handbook of social and clinical psychology* (pp. 327–349). New York: Pergamon Press.

Coyne, J. C., & DeLongis, A. (1986). Going beyond social support: The role of social relationships in adaptation. *Journal of Consulting and Clinical Psychology, 54*, 454–460.

Coyne, J. C., Downey, G., & Boergers, J. (1992). Depression in families: A systems perspective. In D. Cicchetti & S. L. Toth (Eds.), *Developmental perspectives on depression* (pp. 211–249). Rochester, NY: University of Rochester Press.

Coyne, J. C., Kahn, J., & Gotlib, I. H. (1987). Depression. In T. Jacob (Ed.), *Family interaction and psychopathology* (pp. 509–533). New York: Plenum Press.

Coyne, J. C., Kessler, R. C., Tal, M., Turnbull, J., Wortman, C. B., & Greden, J. F. (1987). Living with a depressed person. *Journal of Consulting and Clinical Psychology, 55*, 347–352.

Craddock, A. E. (1983). Family cohesion and adaptability as factors in the aetiology of social anxiety. *Australian Journal of Sex, Marriage and Family, 4*, 181–190.

Craig, T. K. J., Boardman, A. P., Mills, K., Daly-Jones, O., & Drake, H. (1993). The south London somatization study: I. Longitudinal course and the influence of early life experiences. *British Journal of Psychiatry, 163*, 579–588.

Crisp, A. H. (1988). Some possible approaches to prevention of eating and body weight/shape disorders, with particular reference to anorexia nervosa. *International Journal of Eating Disorders, 7*, 1–17.

Cummins, R. (1990). Social insecurity, anxiety, and stressful events as antecedents of depressive symptoms. *Behavioral Medicine, 13*, 161–164.

Cupach, W. R., & Comstock, J. (1990). Satisfaction with sexual communication in marriage: Links to sexual satisfaction and dyadic adjustment. *Journal of Social and Personal Relationships, 7*, 179–186.

Curran, J. P., Wallander, J. L., & Fischetti, M. (1980). The importance of behavioral and cognitive factors in heterosexual–social anxiety. *Journal of Personality, 48*, 285–292.

Curran, P. J., & Chassin, L. (1996). A longitudinal study of parenting as a protective factor for children of alcoholics. *Journal of Studies on Alcohol, 57*, 305–313.

Cutting, L. P., & Docherty, N. M. (2000). Schizophrenia outpatients' perceptions of their parents: Is expressed emotion a factor? *Journal of Abnormal Psychology, 109*, 266–272.

Dalley, M. B., Bolocofsky, D. N., & Karlin, N. J. (1994). Teacher-ratings and self-ratings of social competency in adolescents with low- and high-depressive symptoms. *Journal of Abnormal Child Psychology, 22*, 477–485.

Daly, J. A., Vangelisti, A. L., & Lawrence, S. G. (1989). Self-focused attention and public speaking anxiety. *Personality and Individual Differences, 10*, 903–913.

Daly, S. (1978). Behavioral correlates of social anxiety. *British Journal of Social and Clinical Psychology, 17*, 117–120.

Darby, J. K., Simmons, N., & Berger, P. A. (1984). Speech and voice parameters of depression: A pilot study. *Journal of Communication Disorders, 17*, 75–85.

Dare, C., Le Grange, D., Eisler, I., & Rutherford, J. (1994). Redefining the psychosomatic family: Family process of 26 eating disorder families. *International Journal of Eating Disorders, 16*, 211–226.

Das, M., Das, M., & Banamali, M. (1987). Enriched rearing and repeated electroconvulsive shocks: Effects on brain weight and behavior in rats. *Journal of Psychological Research, 31,* 93–99.

David, D., Giron, A., & Mellman, T. A. (1995). Panic-phobic patients and developmental trauma. *Journal of Clinical Psychiatry, 56,* 113–117.

Davidson, K. P., & Pennebaker, J. W. (1996). Social psychosomatics. In E. T. Higgins & A. W. Kruglanski (Eds.), *Social psychology: Handbook of basic principles* (pp. 102–130). New York: Guilford Press.

Davidson, P. S., Frith, C. D., Harrison-Read, P. E., & Johnstone, E. C. (1996). Facial and other nonverbal communicative behaviour in chronic schizophrenia. *Psychological Medicine, 26,* 707–713.

Davila, J. (2001). Paths to unhappiness: The overlapping courses of depression and romantic dysfunction. In S. R. H. Beach (Ed.), *Marital and family processes in depression: A scientific foundation for clinical practice* (pp. 71–87). Washington, DC: American Psychological Association.

Davila, J., Cobb, R., & Lindberg, N. (2001). *Depressive symptoms, personality pathology, and early romantic dysfunction among young individuals: A test of a romantic stress generation model.* Unpublished manuscript, State University of New York at Buffalo.

de Gruy, F. V., Dickinson, P., Dickinson, L., Mullins, H. C., Baker, W., & Blackmon, D. (1989). The families of patients with somatization disorder. *Family Medicine, 21,* 438–442.

DePaulo, B. M., Epstein, J. A., & LeMay, C. S. (1990). Responses of the socially anxious to the prospect of interpersonal evaluation. *Journal of Personality, 58,* 623–640.

DePaulo, B. M., & Friedman, H. S. (1998). Nonverbal communication. In D. T. Gilbert, S. T. Fiske, & G. Lindzey (Eds.), *The handbook of social psychology* (4th ed., Vol. 2, pp. 3–40). Boston: McGraw-Hill.

DePaulo, B. M., & Tang, J. (1994). Social anxiety and social judgment: The example of detecting deception. *Journal of Research in Personality, 28,* 142–153.

Dill, J. C., & Anderson, C. A. (1999). Loneliness, shyness, and depression: The etiology and interrelationships of everyday problems in living. In T. Joiner & J. C. Coyne (Eds.), *The interactional nature of depression* (pp. 93–125). Washington, DC: American Psychological Association.

Dinning, W. D., & Berk, L. A. (1989). The Children of Alcoholics Screening Test: Relationship to sex, family environment, and social adjustment in adolescents. *Journal of Clinical Psychology, 45,* 335–339.

Dinwiddie, S., Heath, A. C., Dunne, M. P., Bucholz, K. K., Madden, P. A. F., Slutske, W. S., Bierut, L. J., Statham, D. B., & Martin, N. G. (2000). Early sexual abuse and lifetime psychopathology: A co-twin–control study. *Psychological Medicine, 30,* 41–52.

Dittmann, A. T. (1987). Body movements as diagnostic cues in affective disorders. In J. D. Maser (Ed.), *Depression and expressive behavior* (pp. 17–36). Hillsdale, NJ: Erlbaum.

Doane, J. A., & Becker, D. F. (1993). Changes in family expressed emotion climate and course of psychiatric illness in hospitalized young adults and adolescents. *New Trends in Experimental and Clinical Psychiatry, 9,* 63–77.

Doane, J. A., Goldstein, M. J., Miklowitz, D. M., & Falloon, I. R. H. (1986). The impact of individual and family treatment on the affective climate of families of schizophrenics. *British Journal of Psychiatry, 148,* 279–287.

Doane, J. A., West, K. L., Goldstein, M. J., Rodnick, E. H., & Jones, J. E. (1981). Parental communication deviance and affective style: Predictors of subsequent schizophrenia spectrum disorders. *Archives of General Psychiatry, 38,* 679–685.

Docherty, N. M. (1995). Expressed emotion and language disturbances in parents of stable schizophrenia patients. *Schizophrenia Bulletin, 21,* 411–418.

Docherty, N. M., DeRosa, M., & Andreasen, N. C. (1996). Communication disturbances in schizophrenia and mania. *Archives of General Psychiatry, 53,* 358–364.

Docherty, N. M., Hall, M. J., & Gordinier, S. W. (1998). Affective reactivity of speech in schizophrenia patients and their nonschizophrenic relatives. *Journal of Abnormal Psychology, 107,* 461–467.

Dodge, C. S., Heimberg, R. G., Nyman, D., & O'Brian, G. T. (1987). Daily interactions of high and low socially anxious college students: A diary study. *Behavior Therapy, 18,* 90–96.

Dolan, B. M., Lieberman, S., Evans, C., & Lacey, J. H. (1990). Family features associated with normal body weight bulimia. *International Journal of Eating Disorders, 9,* 639–647.

Domenico, D., & Windle, M. (1993). Intrapersonal and interpersonal functioning among middle-aged female adult children of alcoholics. *Journal of Consulting and Clinical Psychology, 61,* 659–666.

Dougherty, F. E., Bartlett, E. S., & Izard, C. E. (1974). Responses of schizophrenics to expressions of the fundamental emotions. *Journal of Clinical Psychology, 30,* 243–246.

Dow, M. G., & Craighead, W. E. (1987). Social inadequacy and depression: Overt behavior and self-evaluation processes. *Journal of Social and Clinical Psychology, 5,* 99–113.

Downey, G., & Coyne, J. C. (1990). Children of depressed parents: An integrative review. *Psychological Bulletin, 108,* 50–76.

Downey, G., Feldman, S., Khuri, J., & Friedman, S. (1994). Maltreatment and childhood depression. In W. M. Reynolds & H. F. Johnson (Eds.), *Handbook of depression in children and adolescents* (pp. 481–508). New York: Plenum Press.

Downs, W. R., & Miller, B. A. (1998). Relationships between experiences of parental violence during childhood and women's psychiatric symptomatology. *Journal of Interpersonal Violence, 13,* 438–455.

Ducharme, J., & Bachelor, A. (1993). Perception of social functioning in dysphoria. *Cognitive Therapy and Research, 17,* 53–70.

du Fort, G. G., Kovess, V., & Boivin, J. F. (1994). Spouse similarity for psychological distress and well-being: A population study. *Psychological Medicine, 24,* 431–447.

Dunn, N. J., Jacob, T., Hummon, N., & Seilhamer, R. A. (1987). Marital stability in alcoholic–spouse relationships as a function of drinking pattern and location. *Journal of Abnormal Psychology, 96,* 99–107.

Dworkin, R. H., Lewis, J. A., Cornblatt, B. A., & Erlenmeyer-Kimling, L. (1994).

Social competence deficits in adolescents at risk for schizophrenia. *Journal of Nervous and Mental Disease, 182,* 103–108.

Dykman, B. M., Horowitz, L. M., Abramson, L. Y., & Usher, M. (1991). Schematic and situational determinants of depressed and nondepressed students' interpretation of feedback. *Journal of Abnormal Psychology, 100,* 45–55.

Edison, J. D., & Adams, H. E. (1992). Depression, self-focus, and social interaction. *Journal of Psychopathology and Behavioral Assessment, 14,* 1–19.

Edwards, D. H., & Kravitz, E. A. (1997). Serotonin, social status and aggression. *Current Opinion in Neurobiology, 7,* 812–819.

Egeland, J. A., & Hostetter, A. M. (1983). Amish study: I. Affective disorders among the Amish, 1976–1980. *American Journal of Psychiatry, 140,* 56–61.

Eiden, R. D., Chavez, F., & Leonard, K. E. (1999). Parent–infant interactions among families with alcoholic fathers. *Development and Psychopathology, 11,* 745–762.

Ekman, P., & Friesen, W. V. (1972). Hand movements. *Journal of Communication, 22,* 353–374.

Ekman, P., & Friesen, W. V. (1974). Nonverbal behavior and psychopathology. In R. J. Friedman & M. M. Mintz (Eds.), *The psychology of depression* (pp. 203–224). Washington, DC: Winston.

Ellgring, H. (1986). Nonverbal expression of psychological states in psychiatric patients. *European Archives of Psychiatry and Neurological Sciences, 236,* 31–34.

Ellgring, H., & Scherer, K. R. (1996). Vocal indicators of mood change in depression. *Journal of Nonverbal Behavior, 20,* 83–110.

Ellgring, H., Wagner, H., & Clarke, A. H. (1980). Psychopathological states and their effects on speech and gaze behavior. In H. Giles, W. P. Robinson, & P. M. Smith (Eds.), *Language: Social psychological perspectives* (pp. 267–273). Oxford: Pergamon Press.

Elliott, T. R., MacNair, R. R., Herrick, S. M., Yoder, B., & Byrne, C. A. (1991). Interpersonal reactions to depression and physical disability in dyadic interactions. *Journal of Applied Social Psychology, 21,* 1293–1302.

Engel, G. L. (1977). The need for a new medical model: A challenge for biomedicine. *Science, 196,* 129–136.

Erickson, D. H., Beiser, M., & Iaacono, W. G. (1998). Social support predicts 5-year outcome in first episode schizophrenia. *Journal of Abnormal Psychology, 107,* 681–685.

Erickson, D. H., Beiser, M., Iaacono, W. G., Fleming, J. A. E., & Lin, T. (1989). The role of social relationships in the course of first-episode schizophrenia and affective psychosis. *American Journal of Psychiatry, 146,* 1456–1461.

Ernst, J. M., & Cacioppo, J. T. (1999). Lonely hearts: Psychological perspectives on loneliness. *Applied and Preventive Psychology, 8,* 1–22.

Espelage, D. L. (1998). Comparing social competence in women with and without eating disorders using a behavior-analytic approach. *Dissertation Abstracts International, 58,* 5113B.

Essau, C. A., Conradt, J., & Petermann, F. (1999). Prevalence, comorbidity and psychosocial impairment of somatoform disorders in adolescents. *Psychology, Health and Medicine, 4,* 169–180.

Evans, J., & Le Grange, D. (1995). Body size and parenting in eating disorders: A comparative study of the attitudes of mothers towards their children. *International Journal of Eating Disorders, 18*, 39–48.

Evans, L., & Wertheim, E. H. (1998). Intimacy patterns and relationship satisfaction of women with eating problems and the mediating effects of depression, trait anxiety and social anxiety. *Journal of Psychodynamic Research, 44*, 355–365.

Exline, R. V., Ellyson, S. L., & Long, B. (1975). Visual behavior as an aspect of power role relationships. In P. Pliner, L. Krames, & T. Alloway (Eds.), *Nonverbal communication of aggression* (Vol. 2, pp. 21–52). New York: Plenum Press.

Fagan, P. J., Schmidt, C. W., Wise, T. N., & Derogatis, L. R. (1988). Sexual dysfunction and dual psychiatric diagnoses. *Comprehensive Psychiatry, 29*, 278–284.

Fairburn, C. G., Norman, P. A., Welch, S. L., O'Connor, M. E., Doll, H. A., & Peveler, R. C. (1995). A prospective study of outcome in bulimia nervosa and the long-term effects of three psychological treatments. *Archives of General Psychiatry, 52*, 304–312.

Farabee, D. J., Holcom, M. L., Ramsey, S. L., & Cole, S. G. (1993). Social anxiety and speaker gaze in a persuasive atmosphere. *Journal of Research in Personality, 27*, 365–376.

Faravelli, C., Zucchi, T., Viviani, B., Salmoria, R., Perone, A., Paionni, A., Scarpato, A., Vigliaturo, D., Rosi, S., D'adamo, D. Bartolozzi, C., Cecchi, C., & Abrardi, L. (2000). Epidemiology of social phobia: A clinical approach. *European Psychiatry, 15*, 17–24.

Faucett, J. A., & Levine, J. D. (1991). The contributions of interpersonal conflict to chronic pain in the presence or absence of organic pathology. *Pain, 44*, 35–43.

Ferroni, P., & Taffe, J. (1997). Women's emotional well-being: The importance of communicating sexual needs. *Sexual and Marital Therapy, 12*, 127–138.

Field, T. (1984). Early interactions between infants and their post-partum depressed mothers. *Infant Behavior and Development, 7*, 517–522.

Fincham, F. D., Beach, S. R. H., Harold, G. T., & Osborne, L. N. (1997). Marital satisfaction and depression: Different causal relationships for men and women? *Psychological Science, 8*, 351–357.

Fingeret, A. L., Monti, P. M., & Paxson, M. A. (1985). Social perception, social performance, and self-perception: A study with psychiatric and nonpsychiatric groups. *Behavior Modification, 9*, 345–356.

Finkelhor, D., Hotaling, G., Lewis, I. A., & Smith, C. (1990). Sexual abuse in a national survey of adult men and women: Prevalence, characteristics, and risk factors. *Child Abuse and Neglect, 14*, 19–28.

Finn, P. R., Sharkansky, E. J., Brandt, K. M., & Turcotte, N. (2000). The effects of familial risk, personality, and expectancies on alcohol use and abuse. *Journal of Abnormal Psychology, 109*, 122–133.

Fiscalini, J. (1993). The psychoanalysis of narcissism: An interpersonal view. In J. Fiscalini & A. L. Grey (Eds.), *Narcissism and the interpersonal self* (pp. 318–348). New York: Columbia University Press.

Fiscella, K., Franks, P., & Shields, C. G. (1997). Received family criticism and primary care utilization: Psychosocial and biomedical pathways. *Family Process, 36,* 25–41.

Fischetti, M., Curran, J. P., & Wessberg, H. W. (1977). A sense of timing. *Behavior Modification, 1,* 179–194.

Fiske, V., & Peterson, C. (1991). Love and depression: The nature of depressive romantic relationships. *Journal of Social and Clinical Psychology, 10,* 75–90.

Fitzpatrick, M. A. (1988). *Between husbands and wives: Communication in marriage.* Newbury Park, CA: Sage.

Fleck, S., Lidz, T., & Cornelison, A. R. (1963). Comparison of parent–child relations of male and female schizophrenic patients. *Archives of General Psychiatry, 8,* 1–7.

Flint, A. J., Black, S. E., Campbell-Taylor, I., Gailey, G. F., & Levinton, C. (1993). Abnormal speech articulation, psychomotor retardation, and subcortical dysfunction in major depression. *Journal of Psychiatric Research, 27,* 309–319.

Ford, C. V. (1986). The somatizing disorders. *Psychosomatics, 27,* 327–337.

Ford, C. V. (1995). Dimensions of somatization and hypochondriasis. *Neurologic Clinics, 13,* 241–253.

Forehand, R., & Smith, K. A. (1986). Who depressed whom?: A look at the relationship of adolescent mood to maternal and paternal depression. *Child Study Journal, 16,* 19–23.

Fossati, A., Madeddu, F., & Maffei, C. (1999). Borderline personality disorder and childhood sexual abuse: A meta-analytic study. *Journal of Personality Disorders, 13,* 268–280.

Fossi, L., Faravelli, C., & Paoli, M. (1984). The ethological approach to the assessment of depressive disorders. *Journal of Nervous and Mental Disease, 172,* 332–341.

Foy, D. W., Massey, F. H., Duer, J. D., Ross, J. M., & Wooten, L. S. (1979). Social skills training to improve alcoholics' vocational interpersonal competency. *Journal of Counseling Psychology, 26,* 128–132.

Franck, N., Daprati, E., Michel, F., Saoud, M., Dalery, J., Marie-Cardine, M., & Georgieff, N. (1998). Gaze discrimination is unimpaired in schizophrenia. *Psychiatry Research, 81,* 67–75.

Frank, E., Targum, S. D., Gershon, E. S., Anderson, C., Stewart, B. D., Davenport, Y., Ketchum, K. L., & Kupfer, D. J. (1981). A comparison of nonpatient and bipolar patient–well spouse couples. *American Journal of Psychiatry, 138,* 764–768.

Freud, S. (1966). *Introductory lectures on psychoanalysis* (J. Strachey, Ed. and Trans). New York: Norton. (Original work published 1917)

Friedlander, M. L., & Siegel, S. M. (1990). Separation–individuation difficulties and cognitive-behavioral indicators of eating disorders among college women. *Journal of Counseling Psychology, 37,* 74–78.

Fromm-Reichmann, F. (1960). *Principles of intensive psychotherapy.* Chicago: Phoenix Books.

Fydrich, T., Chambless, D. L., Perry, K. J., Buergener, F., & Beazley, M. B. (1998). Behavioural assessment of social performance: A rating system for social phobia. *Behaviour Research and Therapy, 36,* 995–1010.

Gabbard, G. O. (1989). Two subtypes of narcissistic personality disorder. *Bulletin of the Menninger Clinic, 53,* 527–532.

Gaebel, W., & Wolwer, W. (1992). Facial expression and emotional face recognition in schizophrenia and depression. *European Archives of Psychiatry and Clinical Neuroscience, 242,* 46–52.

Gambrill, E. (1996). Loneliness, social isolation, and social anxiety. In M. A. Mattaini & B. A. Thyer (Eds.), *Finding solutions to social problems: Behavioral strategies for change* (pp. 345–371). Washington, DC: American Psychological Association.

Ganchrow, J. R., Steiner, J. E., Kleiner, M., & Edelstein, E. L. (1978). A multidisciplinary approach to the expression of pain in psychotic depression. *Perceptual and Motor Skills, 47,* 379–390.

Garbarino, C., & Strange, C. (1993). College adjustment and family environments of students reporting parental alcohol problems. *Journal of College Student Development, 34,* 261–266.

Gard, K. A., Gard, G. C., Dossett, D., & Turone, R. (1982). Accuracy in nonverbal communication as affected by trait and state anxiety. *Perceptual and Motor Skills, 55,* 747–753.

Garfinkel, P. E., Garner, D. M., Rose, J., Darby, P. L., Brandes, J. S., O'Hanlon, J., & Walsh, N. (1983). A comparison of characteristics in families of patients with anorexia nervosa and normal controls. *Psychological Medicine, 13,* 821–828.

Garland, M., & Fitzgerald, M. (1998). Social skills correlates of depressed mood in normal young adolescents. *Irish Journal of Psychological Medicine, 15,* 19–21.

Geerts, E., Bouhuys, N., & Van den Hoofdakker, R. H. (1996). Nonverbal attunement between depressed patients and an interviewer predicts subsequent improvement. *Journal of Affective Disorders, 40,* 15–21.

Gelfand, D. M., & Teti, D. M. (1990). The effects of maternal depression on children. *Clinical Psychology Review, 10,* 329–353.

Geller, J., Cockell, S. J., Hewitt, P. L., Goldner, E. M., & Flett, G. L. (2000). Inhibited expression of negative emotions and interpersonal orientation in anorexia nervosa. *International Journal of Eating Disorders, 28,* 8–19.

Gerlsma, C., Emmelkamp, P. M. G., & Arrindell, W. A. (1990). Anxiety, depression, and perception of early parenting: A meta-analysis. *Clinical Psychology Review, 10,* 251–277.

Giannini, A. J., Folts, D. J., & Fiedler, R. C. (1990). Enhanced encoding of nonverbal cues in bipolar illness in males. *Journal of Psychology, 124,* 557–562.

Gibbons, F. X. (1987). Mild depression and self-disclosure intimacy: Self and others' perceptions. *Cognitive Therapy and Research, 11,* 361–380.

Giesler, R. B., & Swann, W. B. (1999). Striving for confirmation: The role of self-verification in depression. In T. E. Joiner & J. C. Coyne (Eds.), *The interactional nature of depression* (pp. 189–217). Washington, DC: American Psychological Association.

Gillberg, I. C., Rastam, M., & Gillberg, C. (1994). Anorexia nervosa outcome: Six-year controlled longitudinal study of 51 cases including a population cohort. *Journal of the American Academy of Child and Adolescent Psychiatry, 33,* 729–739.

Ginsburg, G. S., La Greca, A. M., & Silverman, W. K. (1998). Social anxiety in children with anxiety disorders: Relation with social and emotional functioning. *Journal of Abnormal Child Psychology, 26,* 175–185.

Giunta, C. T., & Compas, B. E. (1994). Adult daughters of alcoholics: Are they unique? *Journal of Studies on Alcohol, 55,* 600–606.

Glaister, J., Feldstein, S., & Pollack, H. (1980). Chronographic speech patterns of acutely psychotic patients: A preliminary note. *Journal of Nervous and Mental Disease, 168,* 219–223.

Glassner, B., & Haldipur, C. V. (1985). A psychosocial study of early-onset bipolar disorder. *Journal of Nervous and Mental Disease, 173,* 387–394.

Glick, M., & Zigler, E. (1986). Premorbid social competence and psychiatric outcome in male and female nonschizophrenic patients. *Journal of Consulting and Clinical Psychology, 54,* 402–403.

Glick, M., Zigler, E., & Zigler, B. (1985). Developmental correlates of age at first hospitalization in nonschizophrenic psychiatric patients. *Journal of Nervous and Mental Disease, 173,* 677–684.

Goldman, L., & Haaga, D. A. F. (1995). Depression and the experience and expression of anger in marital and other relationships. *Journal of Nervous and Mental Disease, 183,* 505–509.

Goldstein, M. J. (1981). Family factors associated with schizophrenia and anorexia nervosa. *Journal of Youth and Adolescence, 10,* 385–405.

Goldstein, M. J. (1984). Family affect and communication related to schizophrenia. In A. B. Doyle & D. S. Moskowitz (Eds.), *Children and families under stress* (pp. 47–62). San Francisco: Jossey-Bass.

Goldstein, M. J. (1985). Family factors that antedate the onset of schizophrenia and related disorders: The results of a fifteen year prospective longitudinal study. *Acta Psychiatrica Scandinavica, 71*(Suppl. 319), 7–18.

Goldstein, M. J. (1987). Family interaction patterns that antedate the onset of schizophrenia and related disorders: A further analysis of data from a longitudinal, prospective study. In K. Hahlweg & M. J. Goldstein (Eds.), *Understanding major mental disorder: The contribution of family interaction research* (pp. 11–32). New York: Family Process Press.

Goldstein, M. J. (1999). New directions in family intervention programs for psychotic patients: Implications from expressed emotion research. In D. S. Janowsky (Ed.), *Psychotherapy indications and outcomes* (pp. 323–339). Washington, DC: American Psychiatric Press.

Goldstein, M. J., Rea, M., & Miklowitz, D. J. (1996). Family factors related to the course and outcome of bipolar disorder. In C. Mundt, M. J. Goldstein, K. Hahlweg, & P. Fiedler (Eds.), *Interpersonal factors in the origin and course of affective disorders* (pp. 193–203). London: Gaskell.

Goldstein, M. J., & Strachan, A. M. (1987). The family and schizophrenia. In T. Jacob (Ed.), *Family interaction and psychopathology: Theories, methods, and findings* (pp. 481–508). New York: Plenum Press.

Goldstein, M. J., Talvoic, S. A., Nuechterlein, K. H., Fogelson, D. L., Subotnik, K. L., & Asarnow, R. F. (1992). Family interaction vs. individual psychopathology: Do they indicate the same processes in the families of schizophrenics? *British Journal of Psychiatry, 161,* 97–102.

Goodwin, F. K., & Jamison, K. R. (1990). *Manic–depressive illness*. New York: Oxford University Press.

Gorad, S. (1971). Communicational styles and interaction of alcoholics and their wives. *Family Process, 10,* 475–489.

Gotlib, I. H. (1982). Self-reinforcement and depression in interpersonal interaction: The role of performance level. *Journal of Abnormal Psychology, 91,* 3–13.

Gotlib, I. H. (1983). Perception and recall of interpersonal feedback: Negative bias in depression. *Cognitive Therapy and Research, 7,* 399–412.

Gotlib, I. H., & Beatty, M. E. (1985). Negative responses to depression: The role of attributional style. *Cognitive Therapy and Research, 9,* 91–103.

Gotlib, I. H., & Lee, C. M. (1989). The social functioning of depressed patients: A longitudinal assessment. *Journal of Social and Clinical Psychology, 8,* 223–237.

Gotlib, I. H., Lewinsohn, P. M., & Seeley, J. R. (1995). Symptoms versus a diagnosis of depression: Differences in psychosocial functioning. *Journal of Consulting and Clinical Psychology, 63,* 90–100.

Gotlib, I. H., Lewinsohn, P. M., & Seeley, J. R. (1998). Consequences of depression during adolescence: Marital status and marital functioning in early adulthood. *Journal of Abnormal Psychology, 107,* 686–690.

Gotlib, I. H., & Meltzer, S. J. (1987). Depression and the perception of social skills in dyadic interaction. *Cognitive Therapy and Research, 11,* 41–54.

Gotlib, I. H., Mount, J. H., Cordy, N. I., & Whiffen, V. E. (1988). Depression and perceptions of early parenting: A longitudinal investigation. *British Journal of Psychiatry, 152,* 24–27.

Gotlib, I. H., & Robinson, L. A. (1982). Responses to depressed individuals: Discrepancies between self-report and observer-rated behavior. *Journal of Abnormal Psychology, 91,* 231–240.

Gotlib, I. H., & Whiffen, V. E. (1989). Depression and marital functioning: An examination of specificity and gender differences. *Journal of Abnormal Psychology, 98,* 23–30.

Grabow, R. W., & Burkhart, B. R. (1986). Social skill and depression: A test of cognitive and behavioral hypotheses. *Journal of Clinical Psychology, 42,* 21–27.

Graham, Y. P., Heim, C., Goodman, S. H., Miller, A., & Nemeroff, C. B. (1999). The effects of neonatal stress on brain development: Implications for psychopathology. *Development and Psychopathology, 11,* 545–565.

Greden, J. F., Albala, A. A., Smokler, I. A., Gardner, R., & Carroll, B. J. (1981). Speech pause time: A marker of psychomotor retardation among endogenous depressives. *Biological Psychiatry, 16,* 851–859.

Greden, J. F., & Carroll, B. J. (1980). Decrease in speech pause times with treatment of endogenous depression. *Biological Psychiatry, 15,* 575–587.

Greden, J. F., Genero, N., Price, L., Feinberg, M., & Levine, S. (1986). Facial electromyography in depression. *Archives of General Psychiatry, 43,* 269–274.

Greenberg, J., Pyszczynski, T., & Stine, P. (1985). Social anxiety and anticipation of future interaction as determinants of the favorability of self-presentation. *Journal of Research in Personality, 19,* 1–11.

Greenberg, J. R., & Mitchell, S. A. (1983). *Object relations in psychoanalytic theory*. Cambridge, MA: Harvard University Press.

Grissett, N. I., & Norvell, N. K. (1992). Perceived social support, social skills, and quality of relationships in bulimic women. *Journal of Consulting and Clinical Psychology, 60*, 293–299.

Grossman, L. S., & Harrow, M. (1996). Interactive behavior in bipolar manic and schizophrenic patients and its link to thought disorder. *Comprehensive Psychiatry, 37*, 245–252.

Gunderson, J. G., Kerr, J., & Englund, D. W. (1980). The families of borderlines. *Archives of General Psychiatry, 37*, 27–33.

Gunderson, J. G., & Zanarini, M. C. (1987). Current overview of the borderline diagnosis. *Journal of Clinical Psychiatry, 48*, 5–11.

Gurtman, M. B. (1987). Depressive affect and disclosures as factors in interpersonal rejection. *Cognitive Therapy and Research, 11*, 87–100.

Haber, J. R., & Jacob, T. (1997). Marital interactions of male versus female alcoholics. *Family Process, 36*, 385–402.

Hadley, J. A., Holloway, E. L., & Mallinckrodt, B. (1993). Common aspects of object relations and self-presentations in offspring from disparate dysfunctional families. *Journal of Counseling Psychology, 40*, 348–356.

Hafner, H., Loffler, W., Maurer, K., Hambrecht, M., & an der Heiden, W. (1999). Depression, negative symptoms, social stagnation and decline in the early course of schizophrenia. *Acta Psychiatrica Scandinavica, 100*, 105–118.

Hale, W. W., Jansen, J. H. C., Bouhuys, A. L., Jenner, J. A., & van der Hoofdakker, R. H. (1997). Non-verbal behavioral interactions of depressed patients with partners and strangers: The role of behavioral social support and involvement in depression persistence. *Journal of Affective Disorders, 44*, 111–122.

Haley, W. E. (1985). Social skills deficits and self-evaluation among depressed and nondepressed psychiatric inpatients. *Journal of Clinical Psychology, 41*, 162–168.

Halford, W. K., & Hayes, R. L. (1995). Social skills in schizophrenia: Assessing the relationship between social skills, psychopathology and community functioning. *Social Psychiatry and Psychiatric Epidemiology, 30*, 14–19.

Hall, R. C. W., Tice, L., Beresford, T. P., Wooley, B., & Hall, A. K. (1989). Sexual abuse in patients with anorexia nervosa and bulimia. *Psychosomatics, 30*, 73–79.

Haller, J., Fuchs, E., Halasz, J., & Makara, G. B. (1999). Defeat is a major stressor in males while social instability is stressful mainly for females: Towards the development of a social stress model in female rats. *Brain Research Bulletin, 50*, 33–39.

Hamid, P. N. (1989). Contact and intimacy patterns of lonely students. *New Zealand Journal of Psychology, 18*, 84–86.

Hamilton, E. B., Jones, M., & Hammen, C. (1993). Maternal interaction style in affective disordered, physically ill, and normal women. *Family Process, 32*, 329–340.

Hammen, C. L. (1991). Generation of stress in the course of unipolar depression. *Journal of Abnormal Psychology, 100*, 555–561.

Hammen, C. L., Burge, D., & Adrian, C. (1991). Timing of mother and child depression in a longitudinal study of children at risk. *Journal of Consulting and Clinical Psychology, 59*, 341–345.

Hammen, C. L., Burge, D., Burney, E., & Adrian, C. (1990). Longitudinal study of diagnoses in children of women with unipolar and bipolar affective disorder. *Archives of General Psychiatry, 47*, 1112–1117.

Hammen, C. L., Ellicott, A., & Gitlin, M. (1992). Stressors and sociotropy/autonomy: A longitudinal study of their relationship to the course of bipolar disorder. *Cognitive Therapy and Research, 16*, 409–418.

Hammen, C. L., Ellicott, A., Gitlin, M., & Jamison, K. R. (1989). Sociotropy/autonomy and vulnerability to specific life events in patients with unipolar depression and bipolar disorders. *Journal of Abnormal Psychology, 98*, 154–160.

Hammen, C. L., Gordon, D., Burge, D., Adrian, C., Janicke, C., & Hiroto, D. (1987). Communication patterns of mothers with affective disorders and their relationship to children's status and social functioning. In K. Hahlweg & M. J. Goldstein (Eds.), *Understanding major mental disorder* (pp. 103–119). New York: Family Process Press.

Hammen, C. L., & Peters, S. D. (1977). Differential responses to male and female depressive reactions. *Journal of Consulting and Clinical Psychology, 45*, 994–1001.

Hammen, C. L., & Peters, S. D. (1978). Interpersonal consequences of depression: Responses to men and women enacting a depressed role. *Journal of Abnormal Psychology, 87*, 322–332.

Harbach, R. L., & Jones, W. P. (1995). Family beliefs among adolescents at risk for substance abuse. *Journal of Drug Education, 25*, 1–9.

Hardy, P., Jouvent, R., & Widlocher, D. (1984). Speech pause time and the Retardation Rating Scale for Depression (ERD): Towards a reciprocal validation. *Journal of Affective Disorders, 6*, 123–127.

Harrington, C. M., & Metzler, A. E. (1997). Are adult children of dysfunctional families with alcoholism different from adult children of dysfunctional families without alcoholism?: A look at committed, intimate relationships. *Journal of Counseling Psychology, 44*, 102–107.

Harrison, K. (1997). Does interpersonal attraction to thin media personalities promote eating disorders? *Journal of Broadcast and Electronic Media, 41*, 478–500.

Harrison, K., & Cantor, J. (1997). The relationship between media consumption and eating disorders. *Journal of Communication, 47*, 40–67.

Hart, T. A., Turk, C. L., Heimberg, R. G., & Liebowitz, M. R. (1999). Relation of marital status to social phobia severity. *Depression and Anxiety, 10*, 28–32.

Harter, S. L. (2000). Psychosocial adjustment of adult children of alcoholics: A review of the recent empirical literature. *Clinical Psychology Review, 20*, 311–337.

Harter, S. L., & Taylor, T. L. (2000). Parental alcoholism, child abuse, and adult adjustment. *Journal of Substance Abuse, 11*, 31–44.

Hartman, L. M. (1980). The interface between sexual dysfunction and marital conflict. *American Journal of Psychiatry, 137*, 576–579.

Hautzinger, M., Linden, M., & Hoffman, N. (1982). Distressed couples with and without a depressed partner: An analysis of their verbal interaction. *Journal of Behavior Therapy and Experimental Psychiatry, 13,* 307–314.

Havey, J. M., & Dodd, D. K. (1993). Variables associated with alcohol abuse among self-identified collegiate COAs and their peers. *Addictive Behaviors, 18,* 567–575.

Hawkins, J. D., Catalano, R. F., & Miller, J. Y. (1992). Risk and protective factors for alcohol and other drug problems in adolescence and early adulthood: Implications for substance abuse prevention. *Psychological Bulletin, 112,* 64–105.

Hays, J. C., Landerman, L. R., George, L. K., Flint, E. P., Koenig, H. G., Land, K. C., & Blazer, D. G. (1998). Social correlates of the dimensions of depression in the elderly. *Journals of Gerontology, 53B,* P31–P39.

Head, S. B., & Williamson, D. A. (1990). Association of family environment and personality disturbances in bulimia nervosa. *International Journal of Eating Disorders, 9,* 667–674.

Heatherton, T. F., & Baumeister, R. F. (1991). Binge eating as escape from self-awareness. *Psychological Bulletin, 110,* 86–108.

Heavey, A., Parker, Y., Bhat, A. V., Crisp, A. H., & Gowers, S. G. (1989). Anorexia nervosa and marriage. *International Journal of Eating Disorders, 8,* 275–284.

Heimberg, R. G., Acerra, M. C., & Holstein, A. (1985). Partner similarity mediates interpersonal anxiety. *Cognitive Therapy and Research, 9,* 443–453.

Heinssen, R. K., & Glass, C. R. (1990). Social skills, social anxiety, and cognitive factors in schizophrenia. In H. Leitenberg (Ed.), *Handbook of social and evaluation anxiety* (pp. 325–355). New York: Plenum Press.

Heller, K., Sher, K. J., & Benson, C. S. (1982). Problems associated with risk overprediction in studies of offspring of alcoholics: Implications for prevention. *Clinical Psychology Review, 2,* 183–200.

Henderson, M. C., Albright, J. S., Kalichman, S. C., & Dugoni, B. (1994). Personality characteristics of young adult offspring of substance abusers: A study highlighting methodological issues. *Journal of Personality Assessment, 63,* 117–134.

Henwood, P. G., & Solano, C. H. (1994). Loneliness in young children and their parents. *Journal of Genetic Psychology, 155,* 35–45.

Herman, J. L., Perry, C., & van der Kolk, B. A. (1989). Childhood trauma in borderline personality disorder. *American Journal of Psychiatry, 146,* 490–495.

Hersen, M., Bellack, A. S., & Himmelhoch, J. M. (1980). Treatment of unipolar depression with social skills training. *Behavior Modification, 4,* 547–556.

Herzog, D. B., Pepose, M., Norman, D. K., & Rigotti, N. A. (1985). Eating disorders and social maladjustment in female medical students. *Journal of Nervous and Mental Disease, 173,* 734–737.

Hewitt, P. L., & Flett, G. L. (1991a). Dimensions of perfectionism in unipolar depression. *Journal of Abnormal Psychology, 100,* 98–101.

Hewitt, P. L., & Flett, G. L. (1991b). Perfectionism in the self and social contexts: Conceptualization, assessment, and association with psychopathology. *Journal of Personality and Social Psychology, 60,* 456–470.

Hewitt, P. L., & Flett, G. L. (1993). Dimensions of perfectionism, daily stress, and depression: A test of the specific vulnerability hypothesis. *Journal of Abnormal Psychology, 102*, 58–65.

Higley, J. D., King, S. T., Hasert, M. F., Champoux, M., Suomi, S. J., & Linnoila, M. (1996). Stability of interindividual differences in serotonin function and its relationship to severe aggression and competent social behavior in rhesus macaque females. *Neuropsychopharmacology, 14*, 67–76.

Hill, A., Weaver, C., & Blundell, J. E. (1990). Dieting concerns of 10-year-old girls and their mothers. *British Journal of Clinical Psychology, 29*, 346–348.

Hiller, W., Rief, W., & Fichter, M. M. (1997). How disabled are patients with somatoform disorders? *General Hospital Psychiatry, 19*, 432–438.

Hinchliffe, M. K., Hooper, D., & Roberts, F. J. (1978). *The melancholy marriage*. New York: Wiley.

Hinchliffe, M. K., Hooper, D., Roberts, F. J., & Vaughan, P. W. (1978). The melancholy marriage: An inquiry into the interaction of depression. IV. Disruptions. *British Journal of Medical Psychology, 51*, 15–24.

Hinchliffe, M. K., Lancashire, M., & Roberts, F. J. (1970). Eye-contact and depression: A preliminary report. *British Journal of Psychiatry, 117*, 571–572.

Hinchliffe, M. K., Lancashire, M., & Roberts, F. J. (1971a). Depression: Defence mechanisms in speech. *British Journal of Psychiatry, 118*, 471–472.

Hinchliffe, M. K., Lancashire, M., & Roberts, F. J. (1971b). A study of eye-contact changes in depressed and recovered psychiatric patients. *British Journal of Psychiatry, 119*, 213–215.

Hinchliffe, M. K., Vaughan, P. W., Hooper, D., & Roberts, F. J. (1978). The melancholy marriage: An inquiry into the interaction of depression. III. Responsiveness. *British Journal of Medical Psychology, 51*, 1–13.

Hinson, R. C., Becker, L. S., Handal, P. J., & Katz, B. M. (1993). The heterogeneity of children of alcoholics: Emotional needs and help-seeking propensity. *Journal of College Student Development, 34*, 47–52.

Hirschfeld, R. M. A., Klerman, G. L., Keller, M. B., Andreasen, N. C., & Clayton, P. J. (1986). Personality of recovered patients with bipolar affective disorder. *Journal of Affective Disorders, 11*, 81–89.

Hoffman, G. M. A., Gonze, J. C., & Mendlewicz, J. (1985). Speech pause time as a method for the evaluation of psychomotor retardation in depressive illness. *British Journal of Psychiatry, 146*, 535–538.

Hokanson, J. E., & Butler, A. C. (1992). Cluster analysis of depressed college students' social behaviors. *Journal of Personality and Social Psychology, 62*, 273–280.

Hokanson, J. E., Hummer, J. T., & Butler, A. C. (1991). Interpersonal perceptions by depressed college students. *Cognitive Therapy and Research, 15*, 443–457.

Hokanson, J. E., Rubert, M. P., Welker, R. A., Hollander, G. R., & Hedeen, C. (1989). Interpersonal concomitants and antecedents of depression among college students. *Journal of Abnormal Psychology, 98*, 209–217.

Hooley, J. M. (1985). Expressed emotion: A review of the critical literature. *Clinical Psychology Review, 5*, 119–139.

Hooley, J. M. (1998). Expressed emotion and psychiatric illness: From empirical data to clinical practice. *Behavior Therapy, 29*, 631–646.

Hooley, J. M., & Hiller, J. B. (1997). Family relationships and major mental disorder: Risk factors and preventive strategies. In S. Duck (Ed.), *Handbook of personal relationships* (2nd ed., pp. 621–648). Chichester, UK: Wiley.

Hooley, J. M., & Hiller, J. B. (1998). Expressed emotion and the pathogenesis of relapse in schizophrenia. In M. F. Lenzenweger & R. H. Dworkin (Eds.), *Origins and development of schizophrenia* (pp. 447–468). Washington, DC: American Psychological Association.

Hooley, J. M., Richters, J. E., Weintraub, S., & Neale, J. M. (1987). Psychopathology and marital distress: The positive side of positive symptoms. *Journal of Abnormal Psychology, 96*, 27–33.

Hooper, D., Vaughan, P. W., Hinchliffe, M. K., & Roberts, J. (1978). The melancholy marriage: An inquiry into the interaction of depression. V. Power. *British Journal of Medical Psychology, 51*, 387–398.

Hoover, C. F., & Fitzgerald, R. G. (1981a). Marital conflict of manic–depressive patients. *Archives of General Psychiatry, 38*, 65–67.

Hoover, C. F., & Fitzgerald, R. G. (1981b). Dominance in the marriages of affective patients. *Journal of Nervous and Mental Disease, 169*, 624–628.

Hope, D. A., Sigler, K. D., Penn, D. L., & Meier, V. (1998). Social anxiety, recall of interpersonal information, and social impact on others. *Journal of Cognitive Psychotherapy: An International Quarterly, 12*, 303–322.

Hops, H., Biglan, A., Sherman, L., Arthur, J., Friedman, L., & Osteen, V. (1987). Home observations of family interactions of depressed women. *Journal of Consulting and Clinical Psychology, 55*, 341–346.

Horesh, N., Apter, A., Ishai, J., Danziger, Y., Miculincer, M., Stein, D., Lepkifker, E., & Minouni, M. (1996). Abnormal psychosocial situations and eating disorders in adolescence. *Journal of the American Academy of Child and Adolescent Psychiatry, 35*, 921–927.

Horowitz, J. A. (1978). Sexual difficulties as indicators of broader personal and interpersonal problems. *Perspectives in Psychiatric Care, 16*, 66–69.

Hover, S., & Gaffney, L. R. (1991). The relationship between social skills and adolescent drinking. *Alcohol and Alcoholism, 26*, 207–214.

Howard, M. C. (1992). Adolescent substance abuse: A social learning theory perspective. In G. W. Lawson & A. W. Lawson (Eds.), *Adolescent substance abuse: Etiology, treatment, and prevention* (pp. 29–40). Gaithersburg, MD: Aspen.

Hsu, L. K. G. (1989). The gender gap in eating disorders: Why are the eating disorders more common among women? *Clinical Psychology Review, 9*, 393–407.

Hudson, J. L., & Rapee, R. M. (2000). The origins of social phobia. *Behavior Modification, 24*, 102–129.

Hughes, A. M., Medley, I., Turner, G. N., & Bond, M. R. (1987). Psychogenic pain: A study of marital adjustment. *Acta Psychiatrica Scandinavica, 75*, 166–170.

Humphrey, L. L. (1986). Family relations in bulimic–anorexic and nondistressed families. *International Journal of Eating Disorders, 5*, 223–232.

Humphrey, L. L. (1989). Observed family interactions among subtypes of eating disorders using structural analysis of social behavior. *Journal of Consulting and Clinical Psychology, 57*, 206–214.

Hurrelmann, K., Engel, U., Holler, B., & Nordlohne, E. (1988). Failure in school, family conflicts, and psychosomatic disorders in adolescence. *Journal of Adolescence, 11*, 237–249.

Hyronemus, G., Penn, D. L., Corrigan, P. W., & Martin, J. (1998). Social perception and social skill in schizophrenia. *Psychiatry Research, 80*, 275–286.

Ikebuchi, E., Nakagome, K., & Takahashi, N. (1999). How do early stages of information processing influence social skills in patients with schizophrenia? *Schizophrenia Research, 35*, 255–262.

Inskip, H. M., Harris, C. E., & Barraclough, B. (1998). Lifetime risk of suicide for affective disorder, alcoholism, and schizophrenia. *British Journal of Psychiatry, 172*, 35–37.

Jacob, T., Dunn, N. J., Leonard, K., & Davis, P. (1985). Alcohol-related impairments in male alcoholics and the psychiatric symptoms of their spouses: An attempt to replicate. *American Journal of Drug and Alcohol Abuse, 11*, 55–67.

Jacob, T., Haber, J. R., Leonard, K. E., & Rushe, R. (2000). Home interactions of high and low antisocial male alcoholics and their families. *Journal of Studies on Alcohol, 61*, 72–80.

Jacob, T., & Johnson, S. L. (1997). Parenting influences on the development of alcohol abuse and dependence. *Alcohol Health and Research World, 21*, 204–209.

Jacob, T., & Johnson, S. L. (1999). Family influences on alcohol and substance abuse. In P. J. Ott, R. E. Tarter, & R. T. Ammerman (Eds.), *Sourcebook on substance abuse: Etiology, epidemiology, assessment, and treatment* (pp. 166–174). Boston: Allyn & Bacon.

Jacob, T., Krahn, G. L., & Leonard, K. (1991). Parent–child interactions in families with alcoholic fathers. *Journal of Consulting and Clinical Psychology, 59*, 176–181.

Jacob, T., & Leonard, K. (1986). Psychosocial functioning in children of alcoholic fathers, depressed fathers and control fathers. *Journal of Studies on Alcohol, 47*, 373–380.

Jacob, T., & Leonard, K. (1988). Alcoholic–spouse interaction as a function of alcoholism subtype and alcohol consumption interaction. *Journal of Abnormal Psychology, 97*, 231–237.

Jacob, T., & Leonard, K. (1992). Sequential analysis of marital interactions involving alcoholic, depressed, and nondistressed men. *Journal of Abnormal Psychology, 101*, 647–656.

Jacob, T., Ritchey, D., Cvitkovic, J., & Blane, H. (1981). Communication styles of alcoholic and nonalcoholic families when drinking and not drinking. *Journal of Studies on Alcohol, 42*, 466–482.

Jacob, T., & Seilhamer, R. A. (1987). Alcoholism and family interaction. In T. Jacob (Ed.), *Family interaction and psychopathology: Theories, methods, and findings* (pp. 535–580). New York: Plenum Press.

Jacob, T., Windle, M., Seilhamer, R. A., & Bost, J. (1999). Adult children of alcoholics: Drinking, psychiatric, and psychosocial status. *Psychology of Addictive Behaviors, 13*, 3–21.

Jacobs, J., & Wolin, S. J. (1989). Alcoholism and family factors: A critical review.

In M. Galanter (Ed.), *Recent developments in alcoholism* (Vol. 7, pp. 147–164). New York: Plenum Press.

Jacobson, N. S., & Anderson, E. A. (1982). Interpersonal skill and depression in college students: An analysis of the timing of self-disclosures. *Behavior Therapy, 13,* 271–282.

Janowsky, D. S., Leff, M., & Epstein, R. S. (1970). Playing the manic game. *Archives of General Psychiatry, 22,* 252–261.

Jarvis, T. J., Copeland, J., & Walton, L. (1998). Exploring the nature of the relationship between child sexual abuse and substance use among women. *Addiction, 93,* 865–875.

Jennison, K. M., & Johnson, K. A. (1997). Resilience to drinking vulnerability in women with alcoholic parents: The moderating effects of dyadic cohesion in marital communication. *Substance Use and Misuse, 32,* 1461–1489.

Johnson, J. G., Rabkin, J. G., Williams, J. B. W., Remien, R. H., & Gorman, J. M. (2000). Difficulties in interpersonal relationships associated with personality disorders and Axis I disorders: A community-based longitudinal investigation. *Journal of Personality Disorders, 14,* 42–56.

Johnson, R. L., & Glass, C. R. (1989). Heterosocial anxiety and direction of attention in high school boys. *Cognitive Therapy and Research, 13,* 509–526.

Johnson, S. L., & Jacob, T. (2000). Sequential interactions in the marital communication of depressed men and women. *Journal of Consulting and Clinical Psychology, 68,* 4–12.

Johnson, S. L., Winett, C. A., Meyer, B., Greenhouse, W. J., & Miller, I. (1999). Social support and the course of bipolar disorder. *Journal of Abnormal Psychology, 108,* 558–566.

Johnson, V., & Pandina, R. J. (1991). Effects of the family environment on adolescent substance use, delinquency, and coping styles. *American Journal of Drug and Alcohol Abuse, 17,* 71–88.

Joiner, T. E. (1994). Contagious depression: Existence, specificity to depressive symptoms, and the role of reassurance seeking. *Journal of Personality and Social Psychology, 67,* 287–296.

Joiner, T. E. (1995). The price of soliciting and receiving negative feedback: Self-verification theory as a vulnerability to depression theory. *Journal of Abnormal Psychology, 104,* 364–372.

Joiner, T. E. (1996). Depression and rejection: On strangers and friends, symptom specificity, length of relationship, and gender. *Communication Research, 23,* 451–471.

Joiner, T. E. (1997). Shyness and low social support as interactive diatheses, with loneliness as mediator: Testing an interpersonal–personality view of vulnerability to depressive symptoms. *Journal of Abnormal Psychology, 106,* 386–394.

Joiner, T. E. (1999). Self-verification and bulimic symptoms: Do bulimic women play a role in perpetuating their own dissatisfaction and symptoms? *International Journal of Eating Disorders, 26,* 145–151.

Joiner, T. E. (2001). Nodes of consilience between interpersonal-psychological theories of depression. In S. R. H. Beach (Ed.), *Marital and family processes in depression: A scientific foundation for clinical practice* (pp. 129–138). Washington, DC: American Psychological Association.

Joiner, T. E., Alfano, M. S., & Metalsky, G. I. (1992). When depression breeds contempt: Reassurance-seeking, self-esteem, and rejection of depressed college students by their roommates. *Journal of Abnormal Psychology, 101,* 165–173.

Joiner, T. E., & Coyne, J. C. (Eds.). (1999). *The interactional nature of depression: Advances in interpersonal approaches.* Washington, DC: American Psychological Association.

Joiner, T. E., Coyne, J. C., & Blalock, J. (1999). On the interpersonal nature of depression: Overview and synthesis. In T. E. Joiner & J. C. Coyne (Eds.), *The interactional nature of depression: Advances in interpersonal approaches* (pp. 3–19). Washington, DC: American Psychological Association.

Joiner, T. E., Heatherton, T. F., Rudd, M. D., & Schmidt, N. B. (1997). Perfectionism, perceived weight status, and bulimic symptoms: Two studies testing a diathesis–stress model. *Journal of Abnormal Psychology, 106,* 145–153.

Joiner, T. E., & Katz, J. (1999). Contagion of depressive symptoms and mood: Meta-analytic review and explanations from cognitive, behavioral, and interpersonal viewpoints. *Clinical Psychology: Science and Practice, 6,* 149–164.

Joiner, T. E., Katz, J., & Lew, A. S. (1997). Self-verification and depression among youth psychiatric inpatients. *Journal of Abnormal Psychology, 106,* 608–618.

Joiner, T. E., Katz, J., & Lew, A. (1999). Harbingers of depressotypic reassurance seeking: Negative life events, increased anxiety, and decreased self-esteem. *Personality and Social Psychology Bulletin, 25,* 630–637.

Joiner, T. E., Metalsky, G. I., Katz, J., & Beach, S. R. H. (1999). Depression and excessive reassurance-seeking. *Psychological Inquiry, 10,* 269–278.

Jones, D. C., & Houts, R. (1992). Parental drinking, parent–child communication, and social skills in young adults. *Journal of Studies on Alcohol, 53,* 48–56.

Jones, I. H., & Pansa, M. (1979). Some nonverbal aspects of depression and schizophrenia occurring during the interview. *Journal of Nervous and Mental Disease, 167,* 402–409.

Jones, J. E. (1977). Patterns of transactional style deviance in the TAT's of parents of schizophrenics. *Family Process, 16,* 327–337.

Jones, W. H., Briggs, S. R., & Smith, T. G. (1986). Shyness: Conceptualization and measurement. *Journal of Personality and Social Psychology, 51,* 629–639.

Jones, W. H., & Carpenter, B. N. (1986). Shyness, social behavior, and relationships. In W. H. Jones, J. M. Cheek, & S. Briggs (Eds.), *Shyness: Perspectives on research and treatment* (pp. 227–238). New York: Plenum Press.

Jones, W. H., Hobbs, S. A., & Hockenbury, D. (1982). Loneliness and social skill deficits. *Journal of Personality and Social Psychology, 42,* 682–689.

Jones, W. H., & Moore, T. L. (1990). Loneliness and social support. In M. Hojat & R. Crandall (Eds.), *Loneliness: Theory, research, and applications* (pp. 145–156). Newbury Park, CA: Sage.

Jones, W. H., Rose, J., & Russell, D. (1990). Loneliness and social anxiety. In H. Leitenberg (Ed.), *Handbook of social and evaluation anxiety* (pp. 247–266). New York: Plenum Press.

Joyce, P. R. (1984). Parental bonding in bipolar affective disorder. *Journal of Affective Disorders, 7*, 319–324.

Judd, L. J., Akiskal, H. S., Zeller, P. J., Paulus, M., Leon, A. C., Maser, J. D., Endicott, J., Coryell, W., Kunovac, J. L., Mueller, T. I., Rice, J. P., & Keller, M. B. (2000). Psychosocial disability during the long-term course of unipolar major depressive disorder. *Archives of General Psychiatry, 57*, 375–380.

Kahn, J., Coyne, J. C., & Margolin, G. (1985). Depression and marital disagreement: The social construction of despair. *Journal of Social and Personal Relationships, 2*, 447–461.

Kandel, D. B. (1973). Adolescent marijuana use: Role of parents and peers. *Science, 181*, 1067–1070.

Kandel, D. B. (1978). Convergences in prospective longitudinal surveys of drug use in normal populations. In D. B. Kandel (Ed.), *Longitudinal research on drug use: Empirical findings and methodological issues* (pp. 3–38). Washington, DC: Hemisphere.

Kandel, D. B., & Andrews, K. (1987). Process of adolescent socialization by parents and peers. *International Journal of the Addictions, 22*, 319–342.

Kandel, D. B., Johnson, J. G., Bird, H. R., Weissman, M. M., Goodman, S. H., Lahey, B. B., Regier, D. A., & Schwab-Stone, M. E. (1999). Psychiatric comorbidity among adolescents with substance use disorders: Findings from the MECA study. *Journal of the American Academy of Child and Adolescent Psychiatry, 38*, 693–699.

Kaplan, H. S. (1979). *Disorders of sexual desire.* New York: Brunner/Mazel.

Karney, B. R. (2001). Depressive symptoms and marital satisfaction in the early years of marriage: Narrowing the gap between theory and research. In S. R. H. Beach (Ed.), *Marital and family processes in depression: A scientific foundation for clinical practice* (pp. 45–68). Washington, DC: American Psychological Association.

Katz, J., & Beach, S. R. H. (1997). Romance in the crossfire: When do women's depressive symptoms predict partner relationship dissatisfaction? *Journal of Social and Clinical Psychology, 16*, 243–258.

Katz, J., Beach, S. R. H., & Joiner, T. E. (1998). When does partner devaluation predict emotional distress?: Prospective moderating effects of reassurance-seeking and self-esteem. *Personal Relationships, 5*, 409–421.

Katz, J., Beach, S. R. H., & Joiner, T. E. (1999). Contagious depression in dating couples. *Journal of Social and Clinical Psychology, 18*, 1–13.

Kaufman, G., & Krupka, J. (1973). Integrating one's sexuality. *International Journal of Group Psychotherapy, 23*, 445–464.

Kay, J. H., Altshuler, L. L., Ventura, J., & Mintz, J. (1999). Prevalence of Axis II comorbidity in bipolar patients with and without alcohol use disorders. *Annals of Clinical Psychiatry, 11*, 187–195.

Kazdin, A. E., Sherick, R. B., Esveldt-Dawson, K., & Rancurello, M. D. (1985). Nonverbal behavior and childhood depression. *Journal of the American Academy of Child Psychiatry, 24*, 303–309.

Kellam, S. G., Brown, C. H., Rubin, B. R., & Ensminger, M. E. (1983). Path leading to teenage psychiatric symptoms and substance use: Developmental epidemiological studies in Woodlawn. In S. B. Guze, F. J. Earls, & J. E. Barrett

(Eds.), *Childhood psychopathology and development* (pp. 17–51). New York: Raven Press.

Kendler, K. S., Gallagher, T. J., Abelson, J. M., & Kessler, R. C. (1996). Lifetime prevalence, demographic risk factors and diagnostic validity of nonaffective psychosis as assessed in a U. S. community sample: The National Comorbidity Survey. *Archives of General Psychiatry, 53,* 1022–1031.

Kendler, K., MacLean, C., Neale, M., Kessler, R., Heath, A., & Eaves, L. (1991). The genetic epidemiology of bulimia nervosa. *American Journal of Psychiatry, 148,* 1627–1637.

Kendler, K. S., Karkowski, L. M., Neale, M. C., & Prescott, C. A. (2000). Illicit psychoactive substance use, heavy use, abuse, and dependence in a US population-based sample of male twins. *Archives of General Psychiatry, 57,* 261–269.

Kennedy, S., Kiecolt-Glaser, & Glaser, R. (1988). Immunological consequences of acute and chronic stressors: Mediating role of interpersonal relationships. *British Journal of Medical Psychology, 61,* 77–85.

Kennedy, S., Thompson, R., Stancer, H. C., Roy, A., & Persad, E. (1983). Life events precipitating mania. *British Journal of Psychiatry, 142,* 398–403.

Kernberg, O. F. (1975). *Borderline conditions and pathological narcissism.* New York: Aronson.

Kessler, R. C., McGonagle, K. A., Shanyang, Z., Nelson, C., Hughes, M., Eshleman, S., Wittchen, H. U., & Kendler, K. S. (1994). Lifetime and 12-month prevalence of DSM-III-R psychiatric disorders in the United States. *Archives of General Psychiatry, 51,* 8–19.

Kiecolt-Glaser, J. K., Newton, T., Cacioppo, J. T., MacCallum, R. C., Glaser, R., & Malarkey, W. B. (1996). Marital conflict and endocrine function: Are men really more physiologically affected than women? *Journal of Consulting and Clinical Psychology, 64,* 324–332.

Kiesler, D. J. (1983). The 1982 interpersonal circle: A taxonomy for complementarity in human transactions. *Psychological Review, 90,* 185–214.

Kiesler, D. J. (1996). *Contemporary interpersonal theory and research: Personality, psychopathology, and psychotherapy.* New York: Wiley.

Kiesler, D. J., van Denburg, T. D., Sikes-Nova, V. E., Larus, J. P., & Goldston, C. S. (1990). Interpersonal behavior profiles of eight cases of DSM-III personality disorders. *Journal of Clinical Psychology, 46,* 440–453.

Kilpatrick, D. G., Acierno, R., Saunders, B., Resnick, H. S., Best, C. L., & Schnurr, P. P. (2000). Risk factors for adolescent substance abuse and dependence: Data from a national sample. *Journal of Consulting and Clinical Psychology, 68,* 19–30.

Kinzl, J. F., Traweger, C., & Biebl, W. (1995). Family background and sexual abuse associated with somatization. *Psychotherapy and Psychosomatics, 64,* 82–87.

Kinzl, J. F., Traweger, C., Guenther, V., & Biebl, W. (1994). Family background and sexual abuse associated with eating disorders. *American Journal of Psychiatry, 151,* 1127–1131.

Kirmayer, L. J., Dao, T. H. T., & Smith, A. (1998). Somatization and psychologization: Understanding cultural idioms of distress. In S. O. Okpaku (Ed.),

Clinical methods in transcultural psychiatry (pp. 233–265). Washington, DC: American Psychiatric Press.

Kirmayer, L. J., & Young, A. (1998). Culture and somatization: Clinical, epidemiological, and ethnographic perspectives. *Psychosomatic Medicine, 60,* 420–430.

Kisely, S., Goldberg, D., & Simon, G. (1997). A comparison between somatic symptoms with and without clear organic cause: Results of an international study. *Psychological Medicine, 27,* 1011–1019.

Klerman, G. L. (1986). Historical perspectives on contemporary schools of psychopathology. In T. Millon & G. L. Klerman (Eds.), *Contemporary directions in psychopathology: Toward the DSM-IV* (pp. 3–28). New York: Guilford Press.

Koenig, J. E., Sachs-Ericsson, N., & Miklowitz, D. J. (1997). How do psychiatric patients experience interactions with their relatives? *Journal of Family Psychology, 11,* 251–256.

Koenigsberg, H. W., Kaplan, R. D., Gilmore, M. M., & Cooper, A. M. (1985). The relation between syndrome and personality disorder in DSM III: Experience with 2,412 patients. *American Journal of Psychiatry, 142,* 207–212.

Kog, E., & Vandereycken, W. (1985). Family characteristics of anorexia nervosa and bulimia: A review of the research literature. *Clinical Psychology Review, 5,* 159–180.

Kohut, H. (1968). The psychoanalytic treatment of narcissistic personality disorders. *Psychoanalytic Study of the Child, 23,* 86–113.

Kuhn, T. S. (1970). *The structure of scientific revolutions* (2nd ed.). Chicago: University of Chicago Press.

Kuiper, N. A., & MacDonald, M. R. (1983). Schematic processing in depression: The self-based consensus bias. *Cognitive Therapy and Research, 7,* 469–484.

Kuiper, N. A., & McCabe, S. B. (1985). The appropriateness of social topics: Effects of depression and cognitive vulnerability on self and other judgments. *Cognitive Therapy and Research, 9,* 371–379.

Kuny, S., & Stassen, H. H. (1993). Speaking behavior and voice sound characteristics in depressive patients during recovery. *Journal of Psychiatric Research, 27,* 289–307.

Lacey, J. H. (1990). Incest, incestuous fantasy and indecency: A clinical catchment area study of normal weight bulimic women. *British Journal of Psychiatry, 157,* 399–403.

La Greca, A. M., & Lopez, N. (1998). Social anxiety among adolescents: Linkages with peer relations and friendships. *Journal of Abnormal and Child Psychology, 26,* 83–94.

Laing, R. D. (1959). *The divided self: An existential study in sanity and madness.* London: Tavistock.

Laing, R. D. (1965). Mystification, confusion, and conflict. In I. Boszormenyi-Nagy & J. L. Framo (Eds.), *Intensive family therapy* (pp. 343–363). New York: Harper.

Laing, R. D. (1967). *The politics of experience.* Harmondsworth, UK: Penguin Press.

Laing, R. D. (1971). *The politics of the family.* New York: Vintage Press.

Laing, R. D., & Esterson, A. (1964). *Sanity, madness and the family.* London: Tavistock.

Lake, E. A., & Arkin, R. M. (1985). Reactions to objective and subjective interpersonal evaluation: The influence of social anxiety. *Journal of Social and Clinical Psychology, 3,* 143–160.

Lane, J. D., & DePaulo, B. M. (1999). Completing Coyne's cycle: Dysphorics' ability to detect deception. *Journal of Research in Personality, 33,* 311–329.

Lasègue, E. C. (1873). On hysterical anorexia. *Medical Times and Gazette, 2,* 367–369.

Leary, M. R. (1983a). Social anxiousness: The construct and its measurement. *Journal of Personality Assessment, 47,* 66–75.

Leary, M. R. (1983b). The conceptual distinctions are important: Another look at communication apprehension and related constructs. *Human Communication Research, 10,* 305–312.

Leary, M. R., & Atherton, S. C. (1986). Self-efficacy, social anxiety, and inhibition in interpersonal encounters. *Journal of Social and Clinical Psychology, 4,* 256–267.

Leary, M. R., & Dobbins, S. E. (1983). Social anxiety, sexual behavior, and contraceptive use. *Journal of Personality and Social Psychology, 45,* 1347–1354.

Leary, M. R., Knight, P. D., & Johnson, K. A. (1987). Social anxiety and dyadic conversation: A verbal response mode analysis. *Journal of Social and Clinical Psychology, 5,* 34–50.

Leary, M. R., & Kowalski, R. M. (1995a). *Social anxiety.* New York: Guilford Press.

Leary, M. R., & Kowlaski, R. M. (1995b). The self-presentational model of social phobia. In R. G. Heimberg, M. R. Liebowitz, D. A. Hope, & F. R. Schneier (Eds.), *Social phobia: Diagnosis, assessment, and treatment* (pp. 94–112). New York: Guilford Press.

Leary, M. R., Kowalski, R. M., & Campbell, C. D. (1988). Self-presentational concerns and social anxiety: The role of generalized impression expectations. *Journal of Research in Personality, 22,* 308–321.

Leary, T. (1955). The theory and measurement methodology of interpersonal communication. *Psychiatry, 18,* 147–161.

Leary, T. (1957). *Interpersonal diagnosis of personality.* New York: Ronald Press.

Leary, T. (1969). The effects of consciousness-expanding drugs on prisoner rehabilitation. *Psychedelic Review, 10,* 29–45.

Leary, T. (1996). Commentary. *Journal of Personality Assessment, 66,* 301–307.

Lecrubier, Y., Wittchen, H. U., Faravelli, C., Bobes, J., Patel, A., & Knapp, M. (2000). A European perspective on social anxiety disorder. *European Psychiatry, 15,* 5–16.

Lee, C. M., & Gotlib, I. H. (1991). Adjustment of children of depressed mothers: A 10-month follow-up. *Journal of Abnormal Psychology, 100,* 473–477.

Lee, S. (1997). A Chinese perspective of somatoform disorders. *Journal of Psychosomatic Research, 43,* 115–119.

Le Grange, D., Eisler, I., Dare, D., & Hodes, M. (1992). Family criticism and self-starvation: A study of expressed emotion. *Journal of Family Therapy, 14,* 177–192.

Le Poire, B. A. (1992). Does the codependent encourage substance-dependence behavior?: Paradoxical injunctions in the codependent relationship. *International Journal of the Addictions, 27,* 1465–1474.

Le Poire, B. A. (1994). Inconsistent nurturing as control theory: Implications for communication-based research and treatment programs. *Journal of Applied Communication Research, 22,* 60–74.

Le Poire, B. A., Erlandson, K. T., & Hallett, J. S. (1998). Punishing versus reinforcing strategies of drug discontinuance: Effect of persuaders' drug use. *Health Communication, 10,* 293–316.

Le Poire, B. A., Hallett, J. S., & Erlandson, K. T. (2000). An initial test of inconsistent nurturing as control theory: How partners of drug abusers assist their partners' sobriety. *Human Communication Research, 26,* 432–457.

Lesser, L. M., Ford, C. V., & Friedman, C. T. H. (1979). Alexithymia in somatization patients. *General Hospital Psychiatry, 1,* 256–261.

Levin, S., Hall, J. A., Knight, R. A., & Alpert, M. (1985). Verbal and nonverbal expression of affect in speech of schizophrenic and depressed patients. *Journal of Abnormal Psychology, 94,* 487–497.

Levine, P. (1996). Eating disorders and their impact on family systems. In F. W. Kaslow (Ed.), *Handbook of relational diagnosis and dysfunctional family patterns* (pp. 463–476). New York: Wiley.

Lewinsohn, P. M. (1974). A behavioral approach to depression. In R. J. Friedman & M. M. Katz (Eds.), *The psychology of depression: Contemporary theory and research* (pp. 157–185). Washington, DC: Winston–Wiley.

Lewinsohn, P. M. (1975). The behavioral study and treatment of depression. In M. Hersen, R. M. Eisler, & P. M. Miller (Eds.), *Progress in behavior modification* (Vol. 1, pp. 19–64). New York: Academic Press.

Lewinsohn, P. M., Hoberman, H. M., & Rosenbaum, M. (1988). A prospective study of risk factors for unipolar depression. *Journal of Abnormal Psychology, 97,* 251–264.

Lewinsohn, P. M., Hoberman, H., Teri, L., & Hautzinger, M. (1985). An integrative theory of depression. In S. Reiss & R. R. Bootzin (Eds.), *Theoretical issues in behavior therapy* (pp. 331–359). New York: Academic Press.

Lewinsohn, P. M., Mischel, W., Chaplin, W., & Barton, R. (1980). Social competence and depression: The role of illusory self-perceptions. *Journal of Abnormal Psychology, 89,* 203–212.

Lewinsohn, P. M., Roberts, R. E., Seeley, J. R., Rohde, P., Gotlib, I. H., & Hops, H. (1994). Adolescent psychopathology: II. Psychosocial risk factors for depression. *Journal of Abnormal Psychology, 103,* 302–315.

Lewinsohn, P. M., & Rosenbaum, M. (1987). Recall of parental behavior by acute depressives, remitted depressives, and nondepressives. *Journal of Personality and Social Psychology, 52,* 611–619.

Lewinsohn, P. M., Solomon, A., Seeley, J. R., & Zeiss, A. (2000). Clinical implications of "subthreshold" depressive symptoms. *Journal of Abnormal Psychology, 109,* 345–351.

Lewis, J. M., Rodnick, E. H., & Goldstein, M. J. (1981). Intrafamilial interactive behavior, parental communication deviance, and risk for schizophrenia. *Journal of Abnormal Psychology, 90,* 448–457.

Lidz, T. (1958). Schizophrenia and the family. *Psychiatry, 21*, 21–27.

Lidz, T., Cornelison, A., Fleck, S., & Terry, D. (1957). The intrafamilial environment of schizophrenic patients: 2. Marital schism and marital skew. *American Journal of Psychiatry, 114*, 241–248.

Lieb, R., Pfister, H., Mastaler, M., & Wittchen, H. U. (2000). Somatoform syndromes and disorders in a representative population sample of adolescents and young adults: Prevalence, comorbidity and impairments. *Acta Psychiatrica Scandinavica, 101*, 194–208.

Liebowitz, M. R., Gorman, J. M., Fyer, A. J., & Klein, D. F. (1985). Social phobia: Review of a neglected anxiety disorder. *Archives of General Psychiatry, 42*, 729–736.

Liebowitz, M. R., Heimberg, R. G., Fresco, D. M., Travers, J., & Stein, M. B. (2000). Social phobia or social anxiety disorder: What's in a name? *Archives of General Psychiatry, 57*, 191–192.

Linden, M., Hautzinger, M., & Hoffman, N. (1983). Discriminant analysis of depressive interactions. *Behavior Modification, 7*, 403–422.

Links, P. S. (1992). Family environment and family psychopathology in the etiology of borderline personality disorder. In J. F. Clarkin, E. Marziali, & H. Munroe-Blum (Eds.), *Borderline personality disorder: Clinical and empirical perspectives* (pp. 15–66). New York: Guilford Press.

Links, P. S., & Munroe-Blum, H. (1990). Family environment and borderline personality disorder: Developments of etiological models. In P. S. Links (Ed.), *Family environment and borderline personality disorder* (pp. 27–39). Washington, DC: American Psychiatric Press.

Lively, S., Friedrich, R. M., & Buckwalter, K. C. (1995). Sibling perception of schizophrenia: Impact on relationships, roles, and health. *Issues in Mental Health Nursing, 16*, 225–238.

Lizardi, H., Klein, D. N., Ouimette, P. C., Riso, L. P., Anderson, R. L., & Donaldson, S.K. (1995). Reports of the childhood home environment in early-onset dysthymia and episodic major depression. *Journal of Abnormal Psychology, 104*, 132–139.

Lobdell, J., & Perlman, D. (1986). The intergenerational transmission of loneliness: A study of college freshmen and their parents. *Journal of Marriage and the Family, 48*, 589–595.

Lowe, P. (2000, May 18). Video made before girl's death: "Rebirthing" therapy session was taped; child, 10, died next day and cops investigating. *Rocky Mountain News* [Denver, CO], p. 5A.

Lucas, A. R., Beard, C. M., O'Fallon, W. M., & Kurland, L. T. (1988). Anorexia nervosa in Rochester, Minnesota: A 45-year study. *Mayo Clinic Proceedings, 63*, 433–442.

Luntz, B. K., & Widom, C. S. (1994). Antisocial personality disorder in abuse and neglected children grown up. *American Journal of Psychiatry, 151*, 670–674.

Lyon, M. A., & Seefeldt, R. W. (1995). Failure to validate personality characteristics of adult children of alcoholics: A replication and extension. *Alcoholism Treatment Quarterly, 12*, 69–85.

Lysaker, P. H., Bell, M. D., Zito, W. S., & Bioty, S. M. (1995). Social skills at work:

Deficits and predictors of improvements in schizophrenia. *Journal of Nervous and Mental Disease, 183*, 688–692.

Macdonald, E. M., Jackson, H. J., Hayes, R. L., Baglioni, A. J., & Madden, C. (1998). Social skill as a determinant of social networks and perceived social support in schizophrenia. *Schizophrenia Research, 29*, 275–286.

Maes, H. H. M., Neale, M. C., Kendler, K. S., Hewitt, J. K., Silberg, J. L., Foley, D. L., Meyer, J. M., Rutter, M., Simonoff, E., Pickles, A., & Eaves, L. J. (1998). Assortative mating for major psychiatric diagnoses in two population-based samples. *Psychological Medicine, 28*, 1389–1401.

Magee, W. J. (1999). Effects of negative life experiences on phobia onset. *Social Psychiatry and Psychiatric Epidemiology, 34*, 343–351.

Malkus, B. M. (1994). Family dynamic and structural correlates of adolescent substance abuse: A comparison of families of non-substance abusers and substance abusers. *Journal of Child and Adolescent Substance Abuse, 3*, 39–52.

Mallinckrodt, B., McCreary, B. A., & Robertson, A. K. (1995). Co-occurrence of eating disorders and incest: The role of attachment, family environment, and social competencies. *Journal of Counseling Psychology, 42*, 178–186.

Malow, R. M., & Olson, R. E. (1984). Family characteristics of myofascial pain dysfunction syndrome patients. *Family Systems Medicine, 2*, 428–431.

Mandal, M. K., & Palchoudhury, S. (1985). Decoding of facial affect in schizophrenia. *Psychological Reports, 56*, 651–652.

Mandal, M. K., Pandey, R., & Prasad, A. B. (1998). Facial expression of emotions and schizophrenia: A review. *Schizophrenia Bulletin, 24*, 399–412.

Mandal, M. K., Srivastava, P., & Singh, S. K. (1990). Paralinguistic characteristics of speech in schizophrenics and depressives. *Journal of Psychiatric Research, 24*, 191–196.

Manley, A. (1992). Comorbidity of mental and addictive disorders. *Journal of Health Care for the Poor and Underserved, 3*, 60–72.

Mansell, W., & Clark, D. M. (1999). How do I appear to others?: Social anxiety and processing of the observable self. *Behaviour Research and Therapy, 37*, 419–434.

Marinangeli, M. G., Butti, G., Scinto, A., Di Cicco, L., Petruzzi, C., Daneluzzo, E., & Rossi, A. (2000). Patterns of comorbidity among DSM-III-R personality disorders. *Psychopathology, 32*, 69–74.

Marks, T., & Hammen, C. L. (1982). Interpersonal mood induction: Situational and individual determinants. *Motivation and Emotion, 6*, 387–399.

Marley, J. A. (1998). People matter: Client-reported interpersonal interaction and its impact on symptoms of schizophrenia. *Social Work, 43*, 437–444.

Martin, J. I. (1995). Intimacy, loneliness, and openness to feelings in adult children of alcoholics. *Health and Social Work, 20*, 52–59.

Masia, C. L., & Morris, T. L. (1998). Parental factors associated with social anxiety: Methodological limitations and suggestions for integrated behavioral research. *Clinical Psychology: Science and Practice, 5*, 211–228.

Matussek, P., Luks, O., & Seibt, G. (1986). Partner relationships of depressives. *Psychopathology, 19*, 143–156.

McCabe, M. P. (1994). The influence of quality of relationship on sexual dysfunction. *Australian Journal of Marriage and Family, 15*, 2–8.

McCabe, M. P. (1997). Intimacy and quality of life among sexually dysfunctional men and women. *Journal of Sex and Marital Therapy, 23,* 276–290.

McCabe, S. B., & Gotlib, I. H. (1993). Interactions of couples with and without a depressed spouse: Self-report and observations of problem-solving interactions. *Journal of Social and Personal Relationships, 10,* 589–599.

McCann, C. D. (1990). Social factors in depression: The role of interpersonal expectancies. In C. D. McCann & N. S. Endler (Eds.), *Depression: New directions in theory, research, and practice* (pp. 27–47). Toronto: Wall & Emerson.

McCann, C. D., & LaLonde, R. N. (1993). Dysfunctional communication and depression. *American Behavioral Scientist, 36,* 271–287.

McCroskey, J. C. (1977). Oral communication apprehension: A summary of recent history and research. In M. Burgoon (Ed.), *Human Communication Research, 4,* 78–96.

McCroskey, J. C. (1982). Oral communication apprehension: A reconceptualization. *Communication yearbook* (Vol. 6, pp. 136–170). Beverly Hills, CA: Sage.

McFarlane, W. R., & Beels, C. C. (1988). The family and schizophrenia: Perspectives from contemporary research. In E. W. Nunnally, C. S. Chilman, & F. M. Cox (Eds.), *Mental illness, delinquency, addictions, and neglect* (pp. 17–38). Newbury Park, CA: Sage.

McKay, J. R., Maisto, S. A., Beattie, M. C., Longabaugh, R., & Noel, N. E. (1993). Differences between alcoholics and spouses in their perceptions of family functioning. *Journal of Substance Abuse Treatment, 10,* 17–21.

McLemore, C. W., & Benjamin, L. S. (1979). Whatever happened to interpersonal diagnosis? *American Psychologist, 34,* 17–34.

McNamara, K., & Hackett, G. (1986). Gender, sex-type and cognitive distortion: Self-perceptions of social competence among mild depressives. *Social Behavior and Personality, 14,* 113–121.

McNiel, D. E., Arkowitz, H. S., & Pritchard, B. E. (1987). The response of others to face-to-face interaction with depressed patients. *Journal of Abnormal Psychology, 96,* 341–344.

Medora, N., & Woodward, J. C. (1986). Loneliness among adolescent college students at a Midwestern university. *Adolescence, 82,* 391–402.

Melges, F. T., & Swartz, M. S. (1989). Oscillations of attachment in borderline personality disorder. *American Journal of Psychiatry, 146,* 1115–1120.

Mendlowicz, M. V., & Stein, M. B. (2000). Quality of life in individuals with anxiety disorders. *American Journal of Psychiatry, 157,* 669–682.

Menees, M. M. (1997). The role of coping, social support, and family communication in explaining the self-esteem of adult children of alcoholics. *Communication Reports, 10,* 9–19.

Menees, M. M., & Segrin, C. (2000). The specificity of disrupted processes in families of adult children of alcoholics. *Alcohol and Alcoholism, 35,* 361–367.

Merikangas, K. R. (1984). Divorce and assortative mating among depressed patients. *American Journal of Psychiatry, 141,* 74–76.

Merikangas, K. R., & Spiker, D. G. (1982). Assortative mating among in-patients with primary affective disorder. *Psychological Medicine, 12,* 753–764.

Metz, M. E., & Dwyer, M. (1993). Relationship conflict management patterns among sex dysfunction, sex offender, and satisfied couples. *Journal of Sex and Marital Therapy, 19*, 104–122.

Meyer, E. B., & Hokanson, J. E. (1985). Situational influences on social behaviors of depression-prone individuals. *Journal of Clinical Psychology, 41*, 29–35.

Miklowitz, D. J. (1994). Family risk indicators in schizophrenia. *Schizophrenia Bulletin, 20*, 137–149.

Miklowitz, D. J., & Alloy, L. B. (1999). Psychosocial factors in the course and treatment of bipolar disorder: Introduction to the special section. *Journal of Abnormal Psychology, 108*, 555–557.

Miklowitz, D. J., Goldstein, M. J., Doane, J. A., Nuechterlein, K. H., Strachan, A. M., Snyder, K. S., & Magana-Amato, A. (1989). Is expressed emotion an index of a transactional process?: I. Parents' affective style. *Family Process, 28*, 153–167.

Miklowitz, D. J., Goldstein, M. J., & Nuechterlein, K. H. (1995). Verbal interactions in the families of schizophrenic and bipolar affective patients. *Journal of Abnormal Psychology, 104*, 268–276.

Miklowitz, D. J., Goldstein, M. J., Nuechterlein, K. H., Snyder, K. S., & Doane, J. A. (1987). The family and the course of recent-onset mania. In K. Hahlweg & M. J. Goldstein (Eds.), *Understanding major mental disorder: The contribution of family interaction research* (pp. 195–211). New York: Family Process Press.

Miklowitz, D. J., Goldstein, M. J., Nuechterlein, K. H., Snyder, K. S., & Mintz, J. (1988). Family factors and the course of bipolar affective disorder. *Archives of General Psychiatry, 45*, 225–231.

Miklowitz, D. J., Simoneau, T. L., Sachs-Ericsson, N., Warner, R., & Suddath, R. (1996). Family risk indicators in the course of bipolar affective disorder. In C. Mundt, M. J. Goldstein, K. Hahlweg, & P. Fiedler (Eds.), *Interpersonal factors in the origin and course of affective disorders* (pp. 204–217). London: Gaskell.

Miklowitz, D. J., Stracham, A. M., Goldstein, M. J., Doane, J. A., Snyder, K. S., Hogarty, G. E., & Falloon, I. R. (1986). Expressed emotion and communication deviance in the families of schizophrenics. *Journal of Abnormal Psychology, 95*, 60–66.

Miklowitz, D. J., Velligan, D. I., Goldstein, M. J., Nuechterlein, K. H., Gitlin, M. J., Ranlett, G., & Doane, J. A. (1991). Communication deviance in families of schizophrenic and manic patients. *Journal of Abnormal Psychology, 100*, 163–173.

Miller, R. E., Ranelli, C. J., & Levine, J. M. (1977). Nonverbal communication as an index of depression. In I. Hanin & E. Usdin (Eds.), *Animal models in psychiatry and neurology* (pp. 171–180). New York: Pergamon Press.

Millon, T. (1981). *Disorders of personality: DSM-III, Axis II*. New York: Wiley–Interscience.

Millon, T. (1990). The disorders of personality. In L. A. Pervin (Ed.), *Handbook of personality: Theory and research* (pp. 339–370). New York: Guilford Press.

Millon, T., & Davis, R. (2000). *Personality disorders in modern life*. New York: Wiley.

Minuchin, S., Rosman, B. L., & Baker, L. (1978). *Psychosomatic families: Anorexia nervosa in context*. Cambridge, MA: Harvard University Press.

Mishler, E. G., & Waxler, N. E. (1965). Family interaction processes and schizophrenia: A review of current theories. *Merrill–Palmer Quarterly, 11,* 269–316.

Modestin, J. (1987). Quality of interpersonal relationships: The most characteristic DSM-III BPD criterion. *Comprehensive Psychiatry, 28,* 397–402.

Moltz, D. A. (1993). Bipolar disorder and the family: An integrative model. *Family Process, 32,* 409–423.

Monti, P. M., Corriveau, D. P., & Zwick, W. (1981). Assessment of social skills in alcoholics and other psychiatric patients. *Journal of Studies on Alcohol, 42,* 526–529.

Monti, P. M., & Fingeret, A. L. (1987). Social perception and communication skills among schizophrenics and nonschizophrenics. *Journal of Clinical Psychology, 43,* 197–205.

Moore, D., & Schultz, N. R. (1983). Loneliness at adolescence: Correlates, attributions, and coping. *Journal of Youth and Adolescence, 12,* 95–100.

Moos, R. H., & Moos, B. S. (1984). The process of recovery from alcoholism: III. Comparing functioning in families of alcoholics and matched control families. *Journal of Studies on Alcohol, 45,* 111–118.

Morgan, C. D., Wiederman, M. W., & Pryor, T. L. (1995). Sexual functioning and attitudes of eating-disordered women: A follow-up study. *Journal of Sex and Marital Therapy, 21,* 67–77.

Morrison, H. L. (Ed.). (1983). *Children of depressed parents: Risk, identification, and intervention.* New York: Grune & Stratton.

Morrison, J. (1989). Childhood sexual histories of women with somatization disorder. *American Journal of Psychiatry, 146,* 239–241.

Morrison, R. L., & Bellack, A. S. (1987). Social functioning of schizophrenic patients: Clinical and research issues. *Schizophrenia Bulletin, 13,* 715–725.

Mothersead, P. K., Kivlighan, D. M., & Wynkoop, T. F. (1998). Attachment, family dysfunction, parental alcoholism, and interpersonal distress in late adolescence: A structural model. *Journal of Counseling Psychology, 45,* 196–203.

Mueser, K. T., Bellack, A. S., Douglas, M. S., & Morrison, R. L. (1991). Prevalence and stability of social skill deficits in schizophrenia. *Schizophrenia Research, 5,* 167–176.

Mueser, K. T., Bellack, A. S., Morrison, R. L., & Wixted, J. T. (1990). Social competence in schizophrenia: Premorbid adjustment, social skill, and domains of functioning. *Journal of Psychiatric Research, 24,* 51–63.

Mueser, K. T., Bellack, A. S., Wade, J. H., Sayers, S. L., Tierney, A., & Haas, G. (1993). Expressed emotion, social skill, and response to negative affect in schizophrenia. *Journal of Abnormal Psychology, 102,* 339–351.

Mueser, K. T., Doonan, R., Penn, D. L., Blanchard, J. J., Bellack, A. S., Nishith, P., & DeLeon, J. (1996). Emotion recognition and social competence in chronic schizophrenia. *Journal of Abnormal Psychology, 105,* 271–275.

Mulder, R. T., Joyce, P. R., Sullivan, P. F., & Oakley-Browne, M. A. (1996). Intimate bonds in depression. *Journal of Affective Disorders, 40,* 175–178.

Mullen, P. E., Martin, J. L., Anderson, J. C., Romans, S. E., & Herbison, G. P. (1994). The effect of child sexual abuse on social, interpersonal and sexual function in adult life. *British Journal of Psychiatry, 165,* 35–47.

Murphy, C. M., & O'Farrell, T. J. (1997). Couple communication patterns of maritally aggressive and nonaggressive male alcoholics. *Journal of Studies on Alcohol, 58*, 83–90.

Nash, M. R., Hulsey, T. L., Sexton, M. C., Harralson, T. L., & Lambert, W. (1993). Long-term sequelae of childhood sexual abuse: Perceived family environment, psychopathology, and dissociation. *Journal of Consulting and Clinical Psychology, 61*, 276–283.

Natale, M. (1977a). Effects of induced elation–depression on speech in the initial interview. *Journal of Consulting and Clinical Psychology, 45*, 45–52.

Natale, M. (1977b). Induction of mood states and their effect on gaze behaviors. *Journal of Consulting and Clinical Psychology, 45*, 960.

Natale, M., Entin, E., & Jaffe, J. (1979). Vocal interruption in dyadic communication as a function of speech and social anxiety. *Journal of Personality and Social Psychology, 37*, 865–878.

Neeliyara, T., Nagalakshmi, S. V., & Ray, R. (1989). Interpersonal relationships in alcohol dependent individuals. *Journal of Personality and Clinical Studies, 5*, 199–202.

Nelson, G. M., & Beach, S. R. H. (1990). Sequential interaction in depression: Effects of depressive behavior on spousal aggression. *Behavior Therapy, 21*, 167–182.

Nemiah, J. C. (1977). Alexithymia. *Psychotherapy and Psychosomatics, 28*, 199–206.

Nestadt, G., Romanoski, A. J., Chahal, R., Merchant, A., Folstein, M. F., Gruenberg, E. M., & McHugh, P. R. (1990). An epidemiological study of histrionic personality disorder. *Psychological Medicine, 20*, 413–422.

Neumann, D. A., Houskamp, B. M., Pollock, V. E., & Briere, J. (1996). The long-term sequelae of childhood sexual abuse in women: A meta-analytic review. *Child Maltreatment, 1*, 6–16.

Neumark-Sztainer, D., Story, M., Hannan, P. J., Beuhring, T., & Resnick, M. D. (2000). Disordered eating among adolescents: Associations with sexual/physical abuse and other familial/psychosocial factors. *International Journal of Eating Disorders, 28*, 249–258.

Nezlek, J. B., Imbrie, M., & Shean, G. D. (1994). Depression and everyday social interaction. *Journal of Personality and Social Psychology, 67*, 1101–1111.

Nezlek, J. B., Kowlaski, R. M., Leary, M. R., Blevins, T., & Holgate, S. (1997). Personality moderators of reactions to interpersonal rejection: Depression and trait self-esteem. *Personality and Social Psychology Bulletin, 23*, 1235–1244.

Nichols, W. C. (1996). Persons with antisocial and histrionic personality disorders in relationships. In F. W. Kaslow (Ed.), *Handbook of relational diagnosis and dysfunctional family patterns* (pp. 287–299). New York: Wiley.

Nichter, M. (1998). The mission within the madness: Self-initiated medicalization as expression of agency. In M. Lak & P. Koujert (Eds.), *Pragmatic women and body politics* (pp. 327–353). Cambridge, UK: Cambridge University Press.

Nielsen, S., Moller-Madsen, S., Isager, T., Jorgensen, J., Pagsberg, K., & Theander, S. (1998). Standardized mortality in eating disorders: A quantitative summary of previously published and new evidence. *Journal of Psychosomatic Research, 44*, 413–434.

Nilsonne, A. (1988). Speech characteristics as indicators of depressive illness. *Acta Psychiatrica Scandinavica, 77*, 253–263.

Nisenson, L. G., & Berenbaum, H. (1998). Interpersonal interactions in individuals with schizophrenia: Individual differences among patients and their partners. *Psychiatry, 61*, 2–11.

Noel, N. E., McCrady, B. S., Stout, R. L., & Fisher-Nelson, H. (1991). Gender differences in marital functioning of male and female alcoholics. *Family Dynamics of Addiction Quarterly, 1*, 31–38.

Nordahl, H. M., & Stiles, T. C. (1997). Perceptions of parental bonding in patients with various personality disorders, lifetime depressive disorders, and healthy controls. *Journal of Personality Disorders, 11*, 391–402.

Norden, K. A., Klein, D. N., Donaldson, S. K., Pepper, C. M., & Klein, L. M. (1995). Reports of the early home environment in DSM-III-R personality disorders. *Journal of Personality Disorders, 9*, 213–223.

Norman, R. M. G., & Malla, A. K. (1983). Adolescents' attitudes toward mental illness: Relationship between components and sex differences. *Social Psychiatry, 18*, 45–50.

Notarius, C. I., & Herrick, L. R. (1988). Listener response strategies to a distressed other. *Journal of Social and Personal Relationships, 5*, 97–108.

Ohannessian, C. M., & Hesselbrock, V. M. (1999). Predictors of substance abuse and affective diagnosis: Does having a family history of alcoholism make a difference? *Applied Developmental Science, 3*, 239–247.

Oldham, J. M. (1994). Personality disorders: Current perspectives. *Journal of the American Medical Association, 14*, 1770–1776.

Oliveau, D., & Willmuth, R. (1979). Facial muscle electromyography in depressed and nondepressed hospitalized subjects: A partial replication. *American Journal of Psychiatry, 136*, 548–550.

Oliver, J. M., Handal, P. J., Finn, T., & Herdy, S. (1987). Depressed and nondepressed students and their siblings in frequent contact with thier families: Depression and perceptions of the family. *Cognitive Therapy and Research, 11*, 501–515.

Olson, D. H. (1993). Circumplex model of marital and family systems: Assessing family functioning. In F. Walsh (Ed.), *Normal family processes* (2nd ed., pp. 104–137). New York: Guilford Press.

Olson, D. H., Sprenkle, D. H., & Russell, C. S. (1979). Circumplex model of marital and family systems: I. Cohesion and adaptability dimensions, family types, and clinical applications. *Family Process, 18*, 3–28.

O'Mahony, J. F., & Hollwey, S. (1995). Eating problems and interpersonal functioning among several groups of women. *Journal of Clinical Psychology, 51*, 345–351.

O'Malley, P. M., Johnson, L. D., & Bachman, J. G. (1999). Epidemiology of substance abuse in adolescence. In P. J. Ott, R. E. Tarter, & R. T. Ammerman (Eds.), *Sourcebook on substance abuse: Etiology, epidemiology, assessment, and treatment* (pp. 14–31). Boston: Allyn & Bacon.

Oppenheimer, R., Howells, K., Palmer, R. L., & Chaloner, D. A. (1985). Adverse sexual experience in childhood and clinical eating disorders: A preliminary description. *Journal of Psychiatric Research, 19*, 357–361.

Overholser, J. C. (1996). The dependent personality and interpersonal problems. *Journal of Nervous and Mental Disease, 184*, 8–16.

Oxman, T. E., Rosenberg, S. D., Schnurr, P. P., & Tucker, G. J. (1985). Linguistic dimensions of affect and though in somatization disorder. *American Journal of Psychiatry, 142*, 1150–1155.

Oxman, T. E., Rosenberg, S. D., Schnurr, P. P., & Tucker, G. J. (1988). Somatization, paranoia, and language. *Journal of Communication Disorders, 21*, 33–50.

Palmer, R. L., Oppenheimer, R., & Marshall, P. D. (1988). Eating-disordered patients remember their parents: A study using the Parental Bonding Instrument. *International Journal of Eating Disorders, 7*, 101–106.

Pantano, M., Grave, R. D., Oliosi, M., Bartocci, C., Todisco, P., & Marchi, S. (1997). Family backgrounds and eating disorders. *Psychopathology, 30*, 163–169.

Papsdorf, M., & Alden, L. (1998). Mediators of social rejection in social anxiety: Similarity, self-disclosure, and overt signs of anxiety. *Journal of Research in Personality, 32*, 351–369.

Paris, J. (1994). The etiology of borderline personality disorder: A biopsychosocial approach. *Psychiatry, 57*, 316–325.

Parker, G. (1977). Reported parental characteristics of agoraphobics and social phobics. *British Journal of Psychiatry, 135*, 555–560.

Parker, G. (1983). Parental "affectionless control" as an antecedent to adult depression. *Archives of General Psychiatry, 40*, 856–860.

Patterson, B. R., & Bettini, L. A. (1993). Age, depression, and friendship: Development of a general friendship inventory. *Communication Research Reports, 10*, 161–170.

Patterson, B. W., Parsons, O. A., Schaeffer, K. W., & Errico, A. L. (1998). Interpersonal problem solving in alcoholics. *Journal of Nervous and Mental Disease, 176*, 707–713.

Patterson, M. L. (1977). Interpersonal distance, affect, and equilibrium theory. *Journal of Social Psychology, 101*, 205–214.

Patterson, M. L., Churchill, M. E., & Powell, J. L. (1991). Interpersonal expectations and social anxiety in anticipating interaction. *Journal of Social and Clinical Psychology, 10*, 414–423.

Patterson, M. L., & Ritts, V. (1997). Social and communicative anxiety: A review and meta-analysis. In B. R. Burleson (Ed.), *Communication yearbook* (Vol. 20, pp. 263–303). Thousand Oaks, CA: Sage.

Paxton, S. J., Wertheim, E. H., Gibbons, K., Szmukler, G. I., Hillier, L., & Petrovich, J. L. (1991). Body image satisfaction, dieting beliefs, and weight loss behaviors in adolescent girls and boys. *Journal of Youth and Adolescence, 20*, 361–379.

Penn, D. L., Hope, D. A., Spaulding, W., & Kucera, J. (1994). Social anxiety and schizophrenia. *Schizophrenia Research, 11*, 277–284.

Penn, D. L., Mueser, K. T., Doonan, R., & Nishith, P. (1995). Relations between social skills and ward behavior in chronic schizophrenia. *Schizophrenia Research, 16*, 225–232.

Penn, D. L., Mueser, K. T., Spaulding, W., Hope, D. A., & Reed, D. (1995). Information processing and social competence in chronic schizophrenia. *Schizophrenia Bulletin, 21,* 269–281.

Pentz, M. A. (1985). Social competence and self-efficacy as determinants of substance abuse in adolescence. In S. Shiffman & T. A. Wills (Eds.), *Coping and substance abuse* (pp. 117–232). New York: Academic Press.

Peplau, L. A., & Caldwell, M. A. (1978). Loneliness: A cognitive analysis. *Essence, 2,* 207–220.

Peplau, L. A., Russell, D., & Heim, M. (1979). The experience of loneliness. In I. H. Frieze, D. Bar-Tal, & J. S. Caroll (Eds.), *New approaches to social problems* (pp. 53–78). San Francisco: Jossey-Bass.

Perlick, D., Clarkin, J. F., Sirey, J., Raue, P., Greenfield, S., Struening, E., & Rosenheck, R. (1999). Burden experienced by care-givers of persons with bipolar affective disorder. *British Journal of Psychiatry, 175,* 56–62.

Perris, C., Maj, M., Perris, H., & Eisemann, M. (1985). Perceived parental rearing behaviour in unipolar and bipolar depressed patients: A verification study in an Italian sample. *Acta Psychiatrica Scandinavica, 72,* 172–175.

Persad, S. M., & Polivy, J. (1993). Differences between depressed and non-depressed individuals in the recognition of and response to facial emotional cues. *Journal of Abnormal Psychology, 102,* 358–368.

Perugi, G., Akiskal, H. S., Rossi, L., Paiano, A., Quilici, C., Madaro, D., Musetti, L., & Cassano, G. B. (1998). Chronic mania: Family history, prior course, clinical picture and social consequences. *British Journal of Psychiatry, 173,* 514–518.

Peterson, L., Mullins, L. L., & Ridley-Johnson, R. (1985). Childhood depression: Peer reactions to depression and life stress. *Journal of Abnormal Child Psychology, 13,* 597–609.

Peven, D. E., & Shulman, B. H. (1998). Bipolar disorder and the marriage relationship. In J. Carlson & L. Sperry (Eds.), *The disordered couple* (pp. 13–28). New York: Brunner/Mazel.

Philippot, P., Kornreich, C., Blairy, S., Baert, I., Dulk, A. D., Le Bon, O., Streel, E., Hess, U., Pelc, I., & Verbanck, P. (1999). Alcoholics' deficits in the decoding of emotional facial expression. *Alcoholism: Clinical and Experimental Research, 23,* 1031–1038.

Pierce, J. W., & Wardle, J. (1993). Self-esteem, parental appraisal and body size in children. *Journal of Child Psychology and Psychiatry, 34,* 1125–1136.

Pike, K. M., & Rodin, J. (1991). Mothers, daughters, and disordered eating. *Journal of Abnormal Psychology, 100,* 198–204.

Pini, S., Dell'osso, L., Mastroconque, A., Vignoli, S., Pallanti, S., & Cassano, G. B. (1999). Axis I comorbidity in bipolar disorder with psychotic features. *British Journal of Psychiatry, 175,* 467–471.

Pollack, L. E. (1993). Self-perceptions of interpersonal and sexual functioning in women with mood disorders: A preliminary report. *Issues in Mental Health Nursing, 14,* 201–218.

Pollock, V. E., Schneider, L. S., Garielli, W. F., & Goodwin, D. W. (1987). Sex of parent and offspring in the transmission of alcoholism: A meta-analysis. *Journal of Nervous and Mental Disease, 173,* 668–673.

Polusny, M. A., & Follette, V. M. (1995). Long-term correlates of child sexual abuse: Theory and review of the empirical literature. *Applied and Preventive Psychology, 4,* 143–166.

Pope, B., Blass, T., Siegman, A. W., & Raher, J. (1970). Anxiety and depression in speech. *Journal of Consulting and Clinical Psychology, 35,* 128–133.

Pope, H. G., & Hudson, K. I. (1992). Is childhood sexual abuse a risk factor for bulimia nervosa? *American Journal of Psychiatry, 149,* 455–463.

Potthoff, J. G., Holahan, C. J., & Joiner, T. E. (1995). Reassurance seeking, stress generation, and depressive symptoms: An integrative model. *Journal of Personality and Social Psychology, 68,* 664–670.

Priebe, S., Wildgrube, C., & Muller-Oerlinghausen, B. (1989). Lithium prophylaxis and expressed emotion. *British Journal of Psychiatry, 154,* 396–399.

Prkachin, K. M., Craig, K. D., Papageorgis, D., & Reith, G. (1977). Nonverbal communication deficits and response to performance feedback in depression. *Journal of Abnormal Psychology, 86,* 224–234.

Purine, D. M., & Carey, M. P. (1997). Interpersonal communication and sexual adjustment: The roles of understanding and agreement. *Journal of Consulting and Clinical Psychology, 65,* 1017–1025.

Rabinor, J. R. (1994). Mothers, daughters, and eating disorders: Honoring the mother–daughter relationship. In P. Fallon, M. A. Katzman, & S. Wooley (Eds.), *Feminist perspectives on eating disorders* (pp. 272–286). New York: Guilford Press.

Raciti, M., & Hendrick, S. S. (1992). Relationship between eating disorder characteristics and love and sex attitudes. *Sex Roles, 27,* 553–564.

Ragin, A. B., & Oltmanns, T. F. (1983). Predictability as an index of impaired verbal communication in schizophrenic and affective disorders. *British Journal of Psychiatry, 143,* 578–583.

Ragin, A. B., Pogue-Geile, M., & Oltmanns, T. F. (1989). Poverty of speech in schizophrenia and depression during in-patient and post-hospital periods. *British Journal of Psychiatry, 154,* 52–57.

Ranelli, C. J., & Miller, R. E. (1981). Behavioral predictors of amitriptyline response in depression. *American Journal of Psychiatry, 138,* 30–34.

Rapee, R. M., & Lim, L. (1992). Discrepancy between self- and observer ratings of performance in social phobics. *Journal of Abnormal Psychology, 101,* 728–731.

Regier, D. A., Narrow, W. E., Rae, D. S., Manderscheid, R. W., Locke, B. Z., & Goodwin, F. K. (1993). The de facto US mental and addictive disorders service system: Epidemiologic Catchment Area prospective 1-year prevalence rates of disorders and services. *Archives of General Psychiatry, 50,* 85–94.

Reich, W., Earls, F., Frankel, O., & Shayka, J. J. (1993). Psychopathology in children of alcoholics. *Journal of the American Academy of Child and Adolescent Psychiatry, 32,* 995–1002.

Revenson, T. A., & Johnson, J. L. (1984). Social and demographic correlates of loneliness in late life. *American Journal of Community Psychology, 12,* 71–85.

Rey, J. M., Singh, M., Morris-Yates, A., & Andrews, G. (1997). Referred adolescents as young adults: The relationship between psychosocial functioning and personality disorder. *Australian and New Zealand Journal of Psychiatry, 31,* 219–226.

Rhodes, B., & Kroger, J. (1992). Parental bonding and separation–individuation difficulties among late-adolescent eating disordered women. *Child Psychiatry and Human Development, 22*, 249–263.

Rhodes, J. E., & Jason, L. A. (1990). A social stress model of substance abuse. *Journal of Consulting and Clinical Psychology, 58*, 395–401.

Rhodewalt, F., & Morf, C. C. (1995). Self and interpersonal correlates of the Narcissistic Personality Inventory: A review and new findings. *Journal of Research in Personality, 29*, 1–23.

Rich, A. R., & Bonner, R. L. (1987). Interpersonal moderators of depression among college students. *Journal of College Student Personnel, 28*, 337–342.

Rich, A. R., & Scovel, M. (1987). Causes of depression in college students: A cross-lagged panel correlational analysis. *Psychological Reports, 60*, 27–30.

Richter, J., Richter, G., & Eismann, M. (1990). Parental rearing behaviour, family atmosphere and adult depression: A pilot study with psychiatric inpatients. *Acta Psycitrica Scandinavica, 82*, 219–222.

Riebel, L. K. (1989). Communication skills for eating-disordered clients. *Psychotherapy, 26*, 69–74.

Riege, W. H. (1971). Environmental influences on brain and behavior of year-old rats. *Developmental Psychobiology, 4*, 157–167.

Riggio, R. E. (1986). Assessment of basic social skills. *Journal of Personality and Social Psychology, 51*, 649–660.

Riggio, R. E., Throckmorton, B., & DePaola, S. (1990). Social skills and self-esteem. *Personality and Individual Differences, 11*, 799–804.

Riggio, R. E., Tucker, J., & Throckmorton, B. (1988). Social skills and deception ability. *Personality and Social Psychology Bulletin, 13*, 568–577.

Rodriguez, V. B., Cafias, F., Bayon, C., Franco, B., Salvador, M., Graell, M., & Santo-Domingo, J. (1996). Interpersonal factors in female depression. *European Journal of Psychiatry, 10*, 16–24.

Roffe, M. W., & Britt, B. C. (1981). A typology of marital interaction for sexually dysfunctional couples. *Journal of Sex and Marital Therapy, 7*, 207–222.

Rohde, P., Lewinsohn, P. M., & Seeley, J. R. (1990). Are people changed by the experience of having an episode of depression?: A further test of the scar hypothesis. *Journal of Abnormal Psychology, 99*, 264–271.

Rohrbaugh, M., & Shean, G. D. (1987). Anxiety disorders: An interactional view of agoraphobia. *Journal of Psychotherapy and the Family, 3*, 65–85.

Root, M. P., & Fallon, P. (1988). The incidence of victimization experiences in a bulimic sample. *Journal of Interpersonal Violence, 3*, 161–173.

Root, M. P., Fallon, P., & Friedrich, W. N. (1986). *Bulimia: A systems approach to treatment*. New York: Norton.

Rorty, M., & Yager, J. (1996). Speculations on the role of childhood abuse in the development of eating disorders among women. In M. F. Schwartz & L. Cohn (Eds.), *Sexual abuse and eating disorders* (pp. 23–35). New York: Brunner/Mazel.

Rorty, M., Yager, J., Rossotto, E., & Buckwalter, G. (2000). Parental intrusiveness in adolescence recalled by women with a history of bulimia nervosa and comparison women. *International Journal of Eating Disorders, 28*, 202–208.

Rosenfarb, I. S., Goldstein, M. J., Mintz, J., & Nuechterlein, K. H. (1995). Expressed emotion and subclinical psychopathology observable with the transactions between schizophrenic patients and their family members. *Journal of Abnormal Psychology, 104,* 259–267.

Rosenthal, R., Hall, J. A., DiMatteo, M. R., Rogers, P. L., & Archer, D. (1979). *Sensitivity to nonverbal communication: The PONS test.* Baltimore: Johns Hopkins University Press.

Rosse, R. B., Kendrick, K., Wyatt, R. J., Isaac, A., & Deutsch, S. I. (1994). Gaze discrimination in patients with schizophrenia: Preliminary report. *American Journal of Psychiatry, 151,* 919–921.

Rost, K. M., Akins, R. N., Brown, F. W., & Smith, G. R. (1992). The comorbidity of DSM-III-R personality disorders in somatization disorder. *General Hospital Psychiatry, 14,* 322–326.

Rotenberg, K. J., & Hamel, J. (1988). Social interaction and depression in elderly individuals. *International Journal of Aging and Human Development, 27,* 305–318.

Rothschild, B., Dimson, C., Storaasli, R., & Clapp, L. (1997). Personality profiles of veterans entering treatment for domestic violence. *Journal of Personality Disorders, 12,* 259–274.

Rounsaville, B. J., Klerman, G. L., Weissman, M. M., & Chevron, E. S. (1985). Short-term interpersonal psychotherapy (IPT) for depression. In E. E. Beckham & W. R. Leber (Eds.), *Handbook of depression* (pp. 124–150). Homewood, IL: Dorsey Press.

Rounsaville, B. J., Weissman, M. M., Prusoff, B. A., & Herceg-Baron, R. L. (1979). Marital disputes and treatment outcome in depressed women. *Comprehensive Psychiatry, 20,* 483–490.

Rubinow, D. R., & Post, R. M. (1992). Impaired recognition of affect in facial expression in depressed patients. *Biological Psychiatry, 31,* 947–953.

Rudolph, K. D., Hammen, C., & Burge, D. (1994). Interpersonal functioning and depressive symptoms in childhood: Addressing the issues of specificity and comorbidity. *Journal of Abnormal Child Psychology, 22,* 355–371.

Rund, B. R., Oie, M., Borchgrevink, T. S., & Fjell, A. (1995). Expressed emotion, communication deviance and schizophrenia. *Psychopathology, 28,* 220–228.

Ruscher, S. M., & Gotlib, I. H. (1988). Marital interaction patterns of couples with and without a depressed partner. *Behavior Therapy, 19,* 455–470.

Russek, L. G., Schwartz, G. E., Bell, I. R., & Baldwin, C. M. (1998). Positive perceptions of parental caring are associated with reduced psychiatric and somatic symptoms. *Psychosomatic Medicine, 60,* 654–657.

Russell, G. F. M., Szmukler, G. I., Dare, C., & Eisler, I. (1987). An evaluation of family therapy in anorexia nervosa and bulimia nervosa. *Archives of General Psychiatry, 44,* 1047–1056.

Rust, J., Golombok, S., & Collier, J. (1988). Marital problems and sexual dysfunction: How are they related? *British Journal of Psychiatry, 152,* 629–631.

Rutter, D. R. (1973). Visual interaction in psychiatric patients: A review. *British Journal of Psychiatry, 123,* 193–202.

Rutter, D. R. (1977a). Speech patterning in recently admitted and chronic long-stay schizophrenic patients. *British Journal of Social and Clinical Psychology, 16,* 47–55.

Rutter, D. R. (1977b). Visual interaction and speech patterning in remitted and acute schizophrenic patients. *British Journal of Social and Clinical Psychology, 16*, 357–361.

Rutter, D. R. (1978). Visual interaction in schizophrenic patients: The timing of looks. *British Journal of Social and Clinical Psychology, 17*, 281–282.

Rutter, D. R., & Stephenson, G. M. (1972). Visual interaction in a group of schizophrenic and depressive patients. *British Journal of Social and Clinical Psychology, 11*, 57–65.

Sacco, W. P. (1999). A social-cognitive model of interpersonal processes in depression. In T. E. Joiner & J. C. Coyne (Eds.), *The interactional nature of depression: Advances in interpersonal approaches* (pp. 329–362). Washington, DC: American Psychological Association.

Sacco, W. P., Milana, S., & Dunn, V. K. (1985). Effect of depression level and length of acquaintance on reactions of others to a request for help. *Journal of Personality and Social Psychology, 49*, 1728–1737.

Salem, J. E., & Kring, A. M. (1999). Flat affect and social skills in schizophrenia: Evidence for their independence. *Psychiatry Research, 87*, 159–167.

Salem, J. E., Kring, A. M., & Kerr, S. L. (1996). More evidence for generalized poor performance in facial emotion perception in schizophrenia. *Journal of Abnormal Psychology, 105*, 480–483.

Saunders, B. E., Villeponteaux, L. A., Lipovsky, J. A., Kilpatrick, D. G., & Veronen, L. J. (1992). Child sexual assault as a risk factor for mental disorders among women: A community survey. *Journal of Interpersonal Violence, 7*, 189–204.

Scazufca, M., & Kuipers, E. (1998). Stability of expressed emotion in relatives of those with schizophrenia and its relationship with burden of care and perception of patients' social functioning. *Psychological Medicine, 28*, 453–461.

Scherer, K. R. (1987). Vocal assessment of affective disorders. In J. D. Maser (Ed.), *Depression and expressive behavior* (pp. 57–82). Hillsdale, NJ: Erlbaum.

Schlenker, B. R., & Leary, M. R. (1982). Social anxiety and self-presentation: A conceptualization and model. *Psychological Bulletin, 92*, 641–669.

Schlenker, B. R., & Leary, M. R. (1985). Social anxiety and communication about the self. *Journal of Language and Social Psychology, 4*, 171–192.

Schmaling, K. B., & Jacobson, N. S. (1990). Marital interaction and depression. *Journal of Abnormal Psychology, 99*, 229–236.

Schmidt, N. B., Lerew, D. R., & Jackson, R. J. (1999). Prospective evaluation of anxiety sensitivity in the pathogenesis of panic: Replication and extension. *Journal of Abnormal Psychology, 108*, 532–537

Schmidt, N. B., Lerew, D. R., & Joiner, T. E. (1998). Anxiety sensitivity and pathogenesis of anxiety and depression: Evidence for symptom specificity. *Behaviour Research and Therapy, 36*, 165–177.

Schmidt, U., Humfress, H., & Treasure, J. (1997). The role of general family environment and sexual and physical abuse in the origins of eating disorders. *European Eating Disorders Review, 5*, 184–207.

Schmidt, U., Tiller, J., & Morgan, H. G. (1995). The social consequences of eating disorders. In G. Szmukler, C. Dare, & J. Treasure (Eds.), *Handbook of eating disorders: Theory, treatment and research* (pp. 260–270). Chichester, UK: Wiley.

Schneier, F. R., Heckelman, L. R., Garfinkel, R., Campeas, R. Fallon, B. A., Gitow, A., Street, L., Del Bene, D., & Liebowitz, M. R. (1994). Functional impairment in social phobia. *Journal of Clinical Psychiatry, 55*, 322–331.

Schroeder, J. E. (1995). Self-concept, social anxiety, and interpersonal perception skills. *Personality and Individual Differences, 19*, 955–958.

Schwartz, C. E., Dorer, D. J., Beardslee, W. R., Lavor, P. W., & Keller, M. B. (1990). Maternal expressed emotion and parental affective disorder: Risk for childhood depressive disorder, substance abuse, or conduct disorder. *Journal of Psychiatric Research, 24*, 231–250.

Schwartz, G. E., Fair, P. L., Mandel, M. R., Salt, P., Mieske, M., & Klerman, G. L. (1978). Facial electromyography in the assessment of improvement in depression. *Psychosomatic Medicine, 40*, 355–360.

Schwartz, G. E., Fair, P. L. Salt, P., Mandel, M. R., & Klerman, G. L. (1976a). Facial muscle patterning to affective imagery in depressed and nondepressed subjects. *Science, 192*, 489–491.

Schwartz, G. E., Fair, P. L., Salt, P., Mandel, M. R., & Klerman, G. L. (1976b). Facial expression and imagery in depression: An electromyographic study. *Psychosomatic Medicine, 38*, 337–347.

Schwartz, L., Slater, M. A., & Birchler, G. R. (1994). Interpersonal stress and pain behaviors in patients with chronic pain. *Journal of Consulting and Clinical Psychology, 62*, 861–864.

Schweitzer, R., Wilks, J., & Callan, V. J. (1992). Alcoholism and family interaction. *Drug and Alcohol Review, 11*, 31–34.

Schwenzer, M. (1996). Social fears in hypochondriasis. *Psychological Reports, 78*, 971–975.

Seagraves, K. B., & Seagraves, R. T. (1991). Hypoactive sexual desire disorder: Prevalence and comorbidity in 906 subjects. *Journal of Sex and Marital Therapy, 17*, 55–58.

Segal, B. M. (1990). Interpersonal disorder in borderline patients. In P. S. Links (Ed.), *Family environment and borderline personality disorder* (pp. 27–39). Washington, DC: American Psychiatric Press.

Segrin, C. (1990). A meta-analytic review of social skill deficits in depression. *Communication Monographs, 57*, 292–308.

Segrin, C. (1992). Specifying the nature of social skill deficits associated with depression. *Human Communication Research, 19*, 89–123.

Segrin, C. (1993a). Interpersonal reactions to depression: The role of relationship with partner and perceptions of rejection. *Journal of Social and Personal Relationships, 10*, 83–97.

Segrin, C. (1993b). Social skills deficits and psychosocial problems: Antecedent, concomitant, or consequent? *Journal of Social and Clinical Psychology, 12*, 336–353.

Segrin, C. (1993c). Effects of dysphoria and loneliness on social perceptual skills. *Perceptual and Motor Skills, 77*, 1315–1329.

Segrin, C. (1996). The relationship between social skills deficits and psychosocial problems: A test of a vulnerability model. *Communication Research, 23*, 425–450.

Segrin, C. (1998). Interpersonal communication problems associated with depression and loneliness. In P. A. Anderson & L. A. Guerrero (Eds.), *The handbook of communication and emotion* (pp. 215–242). San Diego: Academic Press.

Segrin, C. (1999). Social skills, stressful life events, and the development of psychosocial problems. *Journal of Social and Clinical Psychology, 18*, 14–34.

Segrin, C. (2000). Social skills deficits associated with depression. *Clinical Psychology Review, 20*, 379–403.

Segrin, C. (2001). Social skills and negative life events: Testing the deficits stress generation hypothesis. *Current Psychology: Developmental, Learning, Personality, Social, 20*, 16–32.

Segrin, C., & Abramson, L. Y. (1994). Negative reactions to depressive behaviors: A communication theories analysis. *Journal of Abnormal Psychology, 103*, 655–668.

Segrin, C., & Allspach, L. (1999). Loneliness. In D. Levinson, J. J. Ponzetti, & P. F. Jorgensen (Eds.), *Encyclopedia of human emotions* (pp. 424–430). New York: Macmillan.

Segrin, C., & Dillard, J. P. (1991). (Non)depressed persons' cognitive and affective reactions to (un)successful interpersonal influence. *Communication Monographs, 58*, 115–134.

Segrin, C., & Dillard, J. P. (1992). The interactional theory of depression: A meta-analysis of the research literature. *Journal of Social and Clinical Psychology, 11*, 43–70.

Segrin, C., & Dillard, J. P. (1993). The complex link between social skill and dysphoria: Conceptualization, perspective, and outcome. *Communication Research, 20*, 76–104.

Segrin, C., & Fitzpatrick, M. A. (1992). Depression and verbal aggressiveness in different marital couple types. *Communication Studies, 43*, 79–91.

Segrin, C., & Flora, J. (1998). Depression and verbal behavior in conversations with friends and strangers. *Journal of Language and Social Psychology, 17*, 494–505.

Segrin, C., & Flora, J. (2000). Poor social skills are a vulnerability factor in the development of psychosocial problems. *Human Communication Research, 26*, 489–514.

Segrin, C., & Givertz, M. (in press). Social skills training. In J. O. Greene & B. R. Burleson (Eds.), *Handbook of communication and social interaction skills*. Mahwah, NJ: Erlbaum.

Segrin, C., & Kinney, T. (1995). Social skills deficits among the socially anxious: Loneliness and rejection from others. *Motivation and Emotion, 19*, 1–24.

Segrin, C., & Menees, M. M. (1996). The impact of coping styles and family communication on the social skills of children of alcoholics. *Journal of Studies on Alcohol, 57*, 29–33.

Seilhamer, R. A., & Jacob, T. (1990). Family factors and adjustment of children of alcoholics. In M. Windle & J. S. Searles (Eds.), *Children of alcoholics: Critical perspectives* (pp. 168–188). New York: Guilford Press.

Seilhamer, R. A., Jacob, T., & Dunn, N. J. (1993). The impact of alcohol consumption on parent–child relationships in families of alcoholics. *Journal of Studies on Alcohol, 54*, 189–198.

Semple, S. J., Patterson, T. L., Shaw, W. S., Grant, I., Moscona, S., & Jeste, D. V.

(1999). Self-perceived interpersonal competence in older schizophrenia patients: The role of patient characteristics and psychosocial factors. *Acta Psychiatrica Scandinavica, 100*, 126–135.

Senchak, M., Greene, B. W., Carroll, A., & Leonard, K. E. (1996). Global, behavioral and self ratings of interpersonal skills among adult children of alcoholic, divorced and control parents. *Journal of Studies on Alcohol, 57*, 638–645.

Shachnow, J., Clarkin, J., DiPalma, C. S., Thurston, F., Hull, J., & Shearin, E. (1997). Biparental psychopathology and borderline personality disorder. *Psychiatry, 60*, 171–181.

Shapira, B., Zislin, J., Gelfin, Y., Osher, Y., Gorfine, M., Souery, D., Mendlewicz, J., & Lerner, B. (1999). Social adjustment and self-esteem in remitted patients with unipolar and bipolar affective disorder: A case-control study. *Comprehensive Psychiatry, 40*, 24–30.

Shean, G. (1978). *Schizophrenia: An introduction to research and theory.* Cambridge, MA: Winthrop.

Shean, G. D., & Heefner, A. S. (1995). Depression, interpersonal style, and communication skills. *Journal of Nervous and Mental Disease, 183*, 485–487.

Shedler, J., & Block, J. (1990). Adolescent drug use and psychological health. *American Psychologist, 45*, 612–630.

Sheffield, M., Carey, J., Patenaude, W., & Lambert, M. J. (1995). An exploration of the relationship between interpersonal problems and psychological health. *Psychological Reports, 76*, 947–956.

Shek, D. T. L. (1998). A longitudinal study of the relations of family factors to adolescent psychological symptoms, coping resources, school behavior, and substance abuse. *International Journal of Adolescent Medicine and Health, 10*, 155–184.

Sher, K. J. (1991). *Children of alcoholics: A critical appraisal of theory and research.* Chicago: University of Chicago Press.

Sher, K. J., Walitzer, K. S., Wood, P. K., & Brent, E. E. (1991). Characteristics of children of alcoholics: Putative risk factors, substance use and abuse, and psychopathology. *Journal of Abnormal Psychology, 100*, 427–448.

Sheridan, M. J. (1995). A proposed intergenerational model of substance abuse, family functioning, and abuse/neglect. *Child Abuse and Neglect, 19*, 519–530.

Sheridan, M. J., & Green, R. G. (1993). Family dynamics and individual characteristics of adult children of alcoholics: An empirical analysis. *Journal of Social Service Research, 17*, 73–97.

Siegel, S. J., & Alloy, L. B. (1990). Interpersonal perceptions and consequences of depressive–significant other relationships: A naturalistic study of college roommates. *Journal of Abnormal Psychology, 99*, 361–373.

Siegman, A. W. (1987). The pacing of speech in depression. In J. D. Maser (Ed.), *Depression and expressive behavior* (pp. 83–102). Hillsdale, NJ: Erlbaum.

Sights, J. R., & Richards, H. C. (1984). Parents of bulemic women. *International Journal of Eating Disorders, 3*, 3–13.

Silverstein, B., & Perlick, D. (1995). *The cost of competence: Why inequality causes depression, eating disorders, and illness in women.* New York: Oxford University Press.

Simon, G. E., & Von Korff, M. (1998). Suicide mortality among patients treated for depression in an insured population. *American Journal of Epidemiology, 147*, 155–160.

Simoneau, T. L., Miklowitz, D. J., Goldstein, M. J., Nuechterlein, K. H., & Richards, J. A. (1996). Nonverbal interactional behavior in the families of persons with schizophrenic and bipolar disorders. *Family Process, 35*, 83–102.

Simons, R. L., Conger, R. D., & Whitbeck, L. B. (1988). A multistage social learning model of the influences of family and peers upon adolescent substance abuse. *Journal of Drug Issues, 18*, 293–315.

Singer, M., & Wynne, L. (1965). Though disorder and family relations of schizophrenics: III. Methodology using projective techniques. *Archives of General Psychiatry, 12*, 187–200.

Singer, M., Wynne, L., & Toohey, M. (1978). Communication disorders and the families of schizophrenics. In L. C. Wynne, R. L. Cromwell, & S. Matthysse (Eds.), *The nature of schizophrenia: New approaches to research and treatment* (pp. 499–511). New York: Wiley.

Skodol, A. E., Oldham, J. M., & Gallaher, P. E. (1999). Axis II comorbidity of substance use disorders among patients referred for treatment of personality disorders. *American Journal of Psychiatry, 156*, 733–738.

Skodol, A. E., Oldham, J. M., Hyler, S. E., Kellman, H. D., Doidge, N., & Davies, M. (1993). Comorbidity of DSM-III-R eating disorders and personality disorders. *International Journal of Eating Disorders, 14*, 403–416.

Slotkin, J. S. (1942). The nature and effects of social interaction in schizophrenia. *Journal of Abnormal and Social Psychology, 37*, 345–368.

Smari, J., Bjarnadottir, A., & Bragadottir, B. (1998). Social anxiety, social skills and expectancy/cost of negative social events. *Scandinavian Journal of Behaviour Therapy, 27*, 149–155.

Snell, W. E. (1989). Willingness to self-disclose to female and male friends as a function of social anxiety and gender. *Personality and Social Psychology Bulletin, 15*, 113–125.

Snyder, D. K., & Berg, P. (1983). Determinance of sexual dissatisfaction in sexually distressed couples. *Archives of Sexual Behavior, 12*, 237–246.

Sobal, J., & Bursztyn, M. (1998). Dating people with anorexia nervosa: Attitudes and beliefs of university students. *Women and Health, 27*, 73–88.

Sobin, C., & Sackeim, H. A. (1997). Psychomotor symptoms of depression. *American Journal of Psychiatry, 154*, 4–17.

Solano, C. H., & Koester, N. H. (1989). Loneliness and communication problems: Subjective anxiety or objective skills. *Personality and Social Psychology Bulletin, 15*, 126–133.

Solovay, M. R., Shenton, M. E., & Holzman, P. S. (1987). Comparative studies of thought disorders: I. Mania and schizophrenia. *Archives of General Psychiatry, 44*, 13–20.

Sonne, S. C., & Brady, K. T. (1999). Substance abuse and bipolar comorbidity. *Psychiatric Clinics of North America, 22*, 609–627.

Spence, S. H., Donovan, C., & Brechman-Toussaint, M. (1999). Social skills, social outcomes, and cognitive features of childhood social phobia. *Journal of Abnormal Psychology, 108*, 211–221.

Spitzberg, B. H., & Canary, D. J. (1985). Loneliness and relationally competent communication. *Journal of Social and Personal Relationships, 2,* 387–402.

Stayton, W. R. (1996). Sexual and gender identity disorders in a relational perspective. In F. W. Kaslow (Ed.), *Handbook of relational diagnosis and dysfunctional family patterns* (pp. 357–370). New York: Wiley.

Stefos, G., Bauwens, F., Staner, L., Pardoen, D., & Mendlewicz, J. (1996). Psychosocial predictors of major affective recurrences in bipolar disorder: A 4-year longitudinal study of patients on prophylactic treatment. *Acta Psychiatrica Scandinavica, 93,* 420–426.

Steiger, H., Puentes-Neuman, G., & Leung, F. Y. K. (1991). Personality and family features of adolescent girls with eating symptoms: Evidence for restricter/binger differences in a nonclinical population. *Addictive Behaviors, 16,* 303–314.

Steiger, H., Stotland, S., Trottier, J., & Ghadirian, A. M. (1996). Familial eating concerns and psychopathological traits: Causal implications of transgenerational effects. *International Journal of Eating Disorders, 19,* 147–157.

Stein, D., Lilenfeld, L. R., Plotnicov, K., Pollice, C., Rao, R., Strober, M., & Kaye, W. H. (1999). Familial aggregation of eating disorders: Results from a controlled family study of bulimia nervosa. *International Journal of Eating Disorders, 26,* 211–215.

Stein, M. B., Walker, J. R., Anderson, G., Hazen, A. L., Ross, C. A., Eldrige, G., & Forde, D. R. (1996). Childhood physical and sexual abuse in patients with anxiety disorders and in a community sample. *American Journal of Psychiatry, 153,* 275–277.

Steinglass, P. (1979). The alcoholic family in the interaction laboratory. *Journal of Nervous and Mental Disease, 167,* 428–436.

Steinglass, P. (1981a). The alcoholic family at home. *Archives of General Psychiatry, 38,* 578–584.

Steinglass, P. (1981b). The impact of alcoholism on the family. *Journal of Studies on Alcohol, 42,* 288–303.

Steinglass, P. (1985). Family systems approaches to alcoholism. *Journal of Substance Abuse Treatment, 2,* 161–167.

Steinglass, P., & Robertson, A. (1983). The alcoholic family. In B. Kissin & H. Begleiter (Eds.), *The biology of alcoholism: Vol. 6. The pathogenesis of alcoholism: Psychosocial factors* (pp. 243–307). New York: Plenum Press.

Steinglass, P., Tislenko, L., & Reiss, D. (1985). Stability/instability in the alcoholic marriage: The interrelationships between course of alcoholism, family process, and marital outcome. *Family Process, 24,* 365–376.

Steinglass, P., Weiner, S., & Mendelson, J. H. (1971). A systems approach to alcoholism: A model and its clinical application. *Archives of General Psychiatry, 24,* 401–408.

Stern, M. I., Herron, W. G., Primavera, L. H., & Kakuma, T. (1997). Interpersonal perceptions of depressed and borderline inpatients. *Journal of Clinical Psychology, 53,* 41–49.

Stone, M. H. (1990). Abuse and abusiveness in borderline personality disorder. In P. S. Links (Ed.), *Family environment and borderline personality disorder* (pp. 133–148). Washington, DC: American Psychiatric Press.

Stone, N. (1993). Parental abuse as a precursor to childhood onset depression and suicidality. *Child Psychiatry and Human Development, 24*, 13–24.

Stopa, L., & Clark, D. M. (2000). Social phobia and interpretation of social events. *Behaviour Research and Therapy, 38*, 273–283.

Strack, S. (1996). Introduction to the special series—Interpersonal theory and the interpersonal circumplex: Timothy Leary's legacy. *Journal of Personality Assessment, 66*, 212–216.

Strahan, E., & Conger, A. J. (1998). Social anxiety and its effects on performance and perception. *Journal of Anxiety Disorders, 12*, 293–305.

Strauss, C. C., Lahey, B. B., Frick, P., Frame, C. L., & Hynd, G. W. (1988). Peer social status of children with anxiety disorders. *Journal of Consulting and Clinical Psychology, 56*, 137–141.

Strickland, D. E., & Pittman, D. J. (1984). Social learning and teenage alcohol use: Interpersonal and observational influences within the sociocultural environment. *Journal of Drug Issues, 14*, 137–150.

Strober, M., & Humphrey, L. L. (1987). Familial contributions to the etiology and course of anorexia nervosa and bulimia. *Journal of Consulting and Clinical Psychology, 55*, 654–659.

Stuart, S., & Noyes, R. (1999). Attachment and interpersonal communication in somatization. *Psychosomatics, 40*, 34–43.

Sullivan, H. S. (1953a). *Conceptions of modern psychiatry.* New York: Norton.

Sullivan, H. S. (1953b). *The interpersonal theory of psychiatry.* New York: Norton.

Suman, L. N., & Nagalakshmi, S. V. (1993). Personality dimensions of alcohol dependent individuals and their spouses. *National Institute of Mental Health and Neurosciences, 11*, 95–98.

Svrakic, D. M. (1986). The real self of narcissistic personalities: A clinical approach. *American Journal of Psychoanalysis, 46*, 219–229.

Swann, W. B. (1990). To be adored or to be known?: The interplay of self-enhancement and self-verification. In E. T. Higgins & R. M. Sorrentino (Eds.), *Handbook of motivation and cognition* (Vol. 2, pp. 408–480). New York: Guilford Press.

Swendsen, J. D., & Merikangas, K. R. (2000). The comorbidity of depression and substance use disorders. *Clinical Psychology Review, 20*, 173–189.

Sylph, J. A., Ross, H. E., & Kendward, H. B. (1977). Social disability in chronic psychiatric patients. *American Journal of Psychiatry, 134*, 1391–1394.

Szabadi, E., Bradshaw, C. M., & Besson, J. A. O. (1976). Elongation of pause-time in speech: A simple, objective measure of motor retardation in depression. *British Journal of Psychiatry, 129*, 592–597.

Talavera, J. A., Saiz-Ruiz, J., & Garcia-Toro, M. (1994). Quantitative measurement of depression through speech analysis. *European Psychiatry, 9*, 185–193.

Tantam, D. (1995). Empathy, persistent aggression and antisocial personality disorder. *Journal of Forensic Psychiatry, 6*, 10–18.

Targum, S. D., Dibble, E. D., Davenport, Y. B., & Gershon, E. S. (1981). The Family Attitudes Questionnaire: Patients' and spouses' views of bipolar illness. *Archives of General Psychiatry, 38*, 562–568.

Taylor, M. A. (1993). *The neuropsychiatric guide to modern everyday psychiatry.* New York: Free Press.

Teasdale, J. D., & Bancroft, J. (1977). Manipulation of thought content as a determinant of mood and corrugator electromyographic activity in depressed patients. *Journal of Abnormal Psychology, 86,* 235–241.

Teasdale, J. D., Fogarty, S. J., & Williams, M. G. (1980). Speech rate as a measure of short-term variation in depression. *British Journal of Social and Clinical Psychology, 19,* 271–278.

Thelen, M. H., Farmer, J., Mann, L. M., & Pruitt, J. (1990). Bulimia and interpersonal relationships: A longitudinal study. *Journal of Counseling Psychology, 37,* 85–90.

Thomas, A. M., & Forehand, R. (1991). The relationship between parental depressive mood and early adolescent parenting. *Journal of Family Psychology, 4,* 260–271.

Thompson, J. M., Whiffen, V. E., & Blain, M. D. (1995). Depressive symptoms, sex, and perceptions of intimate relationships. *Journal of Social and Personal Relationships, 12,* 49–66.

Thompson, K. M., Wonderlich, S. A., Crosby, R. D., & Mitchell, J. E. (1999). The neglected link between eating disturbances and aggressive behavior in girls. *Journal of the American Academy of Child and Adolescent Psychiatry, 38,* 1277–1284.

Todt, E. H., & Howell, R. J. (1980). Vocal cues as indices of schizophrenia. *Journal of Speech and Hearing Research, 23,* 517–526.

Tolkmitt, F., Helfrich, H., Standke, R., & Scherer, K. R. (1982). Vocal indicators of psychiatric treatment effects in depressives and schizophrenics. *Journal of Communicative Disorders, 15,* 209–222.

Tompson, M. C., Rea, M. M., Goldstein, M. J., Miklowitz, D. J., & Weisman, A. G. (2000). Difficulty in implementing a family intervention for bipolar disorder: The predictive role of patient and family attributes. *Family Process, 39,* 105–120.

Toomey, R., Wallace, C. J., Corrigan, P. W., Schuldberg, D., & Green, M. F. (1997). Social processing correlates of nonverbal social perception in schizophrenia. *Psychiatry, 60,* 292–300.

Torgalsboen, A. K. (1999). Comorbidity in schizophrenia: A prognostic study of personality disorders in recovered and non-recovered schizophrenia patients. *Scandinavian Journal of Psychology, 40,* 147–152.

Troisi, A., & Moles, A. (1999). Gender differences in depression: An ethological study of nonverbal behavior during interviews. *Journal of Psychiatric Research, 33,* 243–250.

Trull, T. J., Useda, D., Conforti, K., & Doan, B. (1997). Borderline personality disorder features in nonclinical young adults: 2. Two-year outcome. *Journal of Abnormal Psychology, 106,* 307–314.

Tsai, S. Y., Lee, J. C., & Chen, C. C. (1999). Characteristics and psychosocial problems of patients with bipolar disorder at high risk for suicide attempt. *Journal of Affective Disorders, 52,* 145–152.

Turley, B., Bates, G. W., Edwards, J., & Jackson, H. J. (1992). MCMI-II personality disorder. *Journal of Clinical Psychology, 48,* 320–329.

Turner, S. M., Beidel, D. C., Dancu, C. B., & Keys, D. J. (1986). Psychopathology of social phobia and comparison to avoidant personality disorder. *Journal of Abnormal Psychology, 95*, 389–394.

Turner, S. M., Beidel, D. C., & Townsley, R. M. (1990). Social phobia: Relationship to shyness. *Behaviour Research and Therapy, 28*, 497–505.

Twentyman, C. T., Greenwald, D. P., Greenwood, M. A., Kloss, J. D., Kovaleski, M. E., & Zibung-Hoffman, P. (1982). An assessment of social skill deficits in alcoholics. *Behavioral Assessment, 4*, 317–326.

Twentyman, C. T., & McFall, R. M. (1975). Behavioral training of social skills in shy males. *Journal of Consulting and Clinical Psychology, 43*, 384–395.

Uecok, A., Karaveli, D., Kundakci, T., & Yazici, O. (1998). Comorbidity of personality disorders with bipolar mood disorders. *Comprehensive Psychiatry, 39*, 72–74.

Van Buren, D. J., & Williamson, D. A. (1988). Marital relationships and conflict resolution skills of bulimics. *International Journal of Eating Disorders, 7*, 735–741.

van Furth, E. F., van Strien, D. C., Martina, L. M. L., van Son, M. J. M., Hendrickx, J. J. P., & van Engeland, H. (1996). Expressed emotion and the prediction of outcome in adolescent eating disorders. *International Journal of Eating Disorders, 20*, 19–31.

Vandereycken, W., Kog, E., & Vanderlinden, J. (Eds.). (1989). *The family approach to eating disorders*. Great Neck, NY: Publishers Marketing Association.

Vanderlinden, J., & Vandereycken, W. (1996). Is sexual abuse a risk factor for developing an eating disorder? In M. F. Schwartz & L. Cohn (Eds.), *Sexual abuse and eating disorders* (pp. 17–21). New York: Brunner/Mazel.

Vanderschuren, L. J. M. J., Stein, E. A., Wiegant, V., & Van Ree, J. M. (1995). Social isolation and social interaction alter regional brain opioid receptor binding in rats. *European Neuropsychpharmacology, 5*, 119–127.

Vanger, P. (1987). An assessment of social skill deficiencies in depression. *Comprehensive Psychiatry, 28*, 508–512.

Vanger, P., Summerfield, A. B., Rosen, B. K., & Watson, J. P. (1991). Cultural differences in interpersonal responses to depressives' nonverbal behaviour. *International Journal of Social Psychiatry, 37*, 151–158.

Vanger, P., Summerfield, A. B., Rosen, B. K., & Watson, J. P. (1992). Effects of communication content on speech behavior of depressives. *Comprehensive Psychiatry, 33*, 39–41.

van Lankveld, J. J. D. M., & Grotjohann, Y. (2000). Psychiatric comorbidity in heterosexual couples with sexual dysfunction assessed with the Composite International Diagnostic Interview. *Archives of Sexual Behavior, 29*, 479–498.

Vaughn, C., & Leff, J. P. (1976). The measurement of expressed emotion in the families of psychiatric patients. *British Journal of Clinical and Social Psychology, 15*, 157–165.

Vaughn, C. E., & Leff, J. P. (1981). Patterns of emotional response in relatives of schizophrenic patients. *Schizophrenia Bulletin, 7*, 43–44.

Vaux, A. (1988). Social and emotional loneliness: The role of social and personal characteristics. *Personality and Social Psychology Bulletin, 14*, 722–734.

Velleman, R. (1992). Intergenerational effects—A review of environmentally oriented studies concerning the relationship between parental alcohol problems and family disharmony in the genesis of alcohol and other problems: I. The intergenerational effects of alcohol problems. *International Journal of the Addictions, 27,* 253–280.

Velleman, R., & Orford, J. (1993). The adult adjustment of offspring of parents with drinking problems. *British Journal of Psychiatry, 162,* 503–516.

Velligan, D. I., Funderburg, L. G., Giesecke, S. L., & Miller, A. L. (1995). Longitudinal analysis of communication deviance in the families of schizophrenic patients. *Psychiatry, 58,* 6–19.

Velligan, D. I., Miller, A. L., Eckert, S. L., Funderburg, L. G., True, J. E., Mahurin, R. K., Diamond, P., & Hazelton, B. C. (1996). The relationship between parental communication deviance and relapse in schizophrenia patients in the 1-year period after hospital discharge. *Journal of Nervous and Mental Disease, 184,* 490–496.

Vernberg, E. M., Abwender, D. A., Ewell, K. K., & Beery, S. H. (1992). Social anxiety and peer relationships in early adolescence: A prospective analysis. *Journal of Clinical Child Psychology, 21,* 189–196.

Vitousek, K., & Manke, F. (1994). Personality variables and disorders in anorexia nervosa and bulimia nervosa. *Journal of Abnormal Psychology, 103,* 137–147.

Vittengl, J. R., & Holt, C. S. (1998). Positive and negative affect in social interactions as a function of partner familiarity, quality of communication, and social anxiety. *Journal of Social and Clinical Psychology, 17,* 196–208.

Vohs, K. D., Bardone, A. M., Joiner, T. E., Abramson, L. Y., & Heatherton, T. F. (1999). Perfectionism, perceived weight status, and self-esteem interact to predict bulimic symptoms: A model of bulimic symptom development. *Journal of Abnormal Psychology, 108,* 695–700.

Wagner, A. W., & Linehan, M. M. (1999). Facial expression recognition ability among women with borderline personality disorder: Implications for emotion regulation? *Journal of Personality Disorders, 13,* 329–344.

Wahlberg, K. E., Wynne, L. C., Oja, H., Keskitalo, P., Pykalainen, L., Lahti, I., Moring, J., Naarala, M., Sorru, A., Seitanaa, M., Laksy, K., Lolassa, J., & Tienari, P. (1997). Gene–environment interaction in vulnerability to schizophrenia: Findings from the Finnish adoption family study. *American Journal of Psychiatry, 154,* 355–362.

Walker, L. S., Garber, J., & Greene, J. W. (1994). Somatic complaints in pediatric patients: A prospective study of the role of negative life events, child social and academic competence, and parental somatic symptoms. *Journal of Consulting and Clinical Psychology, 62,* 1213–1221.

Wallace, S. T., & Alden, L. E. (1991). A comparison of social standards and perceived ability in anxious and nonanxious men. *Cognitive Therapy and Research, 15,* 237–254.

Wallace, S. T., & Alden, L. E. (1995). Social anxiety and standard setting following social success or failure. *Cognitive Therapy and Research, 19,* 613–631.

Wallace, S. T., & Alden, L. E. (1997). Social phobia and positive social events: The price of success. *Journal of Abnormal Psychology, 106,* 416–424.

Waller, G. (1994). Borderline personality disorder and perceived family dysfunction in the eating disorders. *Journal of Nervous and Mental Disease, 182,* 541–546.

Waller, G. (1998). Perceived control in eating disorders: Relationship with reported sexual abuse. *International Journal of Eating Disorders, 23,* 213–216.

Waller, G., & Calam, R. (1994). Parenting and family factors in eating problems. In L. Alexander-Mott & D. B. Lumsden (Eds.), *Understanding eating disorders: Anorexia nervosa, bulimia nervosa, and obesity* (pp. 61–76). Philadelphia: Taylor & Francis.

Waller, G., Calam, R., & Slade, P. (1989). Eating disorders and family interaction. *British Journal of Clinical Psychology, 28,* 285–286.

Waller, G., Slade, P., & Calam, R. (1990a). Family adaptability and cohesion: Relation to eating attitudes and disorders. *International Journal of Eating Disorders, 9,* 225–228.

Waller, G., Slade, P., & Calam, R. (1990b). Who knows best? Family interaction and eating disorders. *British Journal of Psychiatry, 156,* 546–550.

Walters, K. S., & Inderbitzen, H. M. (1998). Social anxiety and peer relations among adolescents: Testing a psychobiological model. *Journal of Anxiety Disorders, 12,* 183–198.

Warner, V., Weissman, M. M., Fendrich, M., Wickramaratne, P., & Moreau, D. (1992). The course of major depression in the offspring of depressed parents: Incidence, recurrence, and recovery. *Archives of General Psychiatry, 49,* 795–801.

Watson, D. C., & Sinha, B. K. (1998). Comorbidity of DSM-IV personality disorders in a nonclinical sample. *Journal of Clinical Psychology, 54,* 773–780.

Watson, J. P., & Davies, T. (1997). ABC of mental health: Psychosexual problems. *British Journal of Medicine, 315,* 239–242.

Watts, W. D., & Ellis, A. M. (1992). Drug abuse and eating disorders: Prevention implications. *Journal of Drug Education, 22,* 223–240.

Watzlawick, P., Bavelas, J. B., & Jackson, D. D. (1967). *Pragmatics of human communication.* New York: Norton.

Waxer, P. (1974). Nonverbal cues for depression. *Journal of Abnormal Psychology, 83,* 319–322.

Webb, J. A., & Baer, P. E. (1995). Influence of family disharmony and parental alcohol use on adolescent social skills, self-efficacy, and alcohol use. *Addictive Behaviors, 20,* 127–135.

Webster, J. J., & Palmer, R. L. (2000). The childhood and family background of women with clinical eating disorders: A comparison with women with major depression and women without psychiatric disorder. *Psychological Medicine, 30,* 53–60.

Weeks, D. G., Michela, J. L., Peplau, L. A., & Bragg, M. E. (1980). Relation between loneliness and depression: A structural equation analysis. *Journal of Personality and Social Psychology, 39,* 1238–1244.

Weinberg, N. Z., Rahdert, E., Colliver, J. D., & Glantz, M. D. (1998). Adolescent substance abuse: A review of the past 10 years. *Journal of the American Academy of Child and Adolescent Psychiatry, 37,* 252–261.

Weiner, E. J., & Stephens, L. (1996). Sexual barrier weight: A new approach. In M.

F. Schwartz & L. Cohn (Eds.), *Sexual abuse and eating disorders* (pp. 68–77). New York: Brunner/Mazel.

Weintraub, W., & Aronson, H. (1967). The application of verbal behavior analysis to the study of psychopathological defense mechanisms: IV. Speech pattern associated with depressive behavior. *Journal of Nervous and Mental Disease, 144*, 22–28.

Weiss, K. M., Chapman, H. A., Strauss, M. E., & Gilmore, G. C. (1992). Visual information decoding deficits in schizophrenia. *Psychiatry Research, 44*, 203–216.

Weissman, M. M. (1993). The epidemiology of personality disorders: A 1990 update. *Journal of Personality Disorders, 7*(Suppl. 1), 44–62.

Weissman, M. M., & Klerman, G. L. (1973). Psychotherapy with depressed women: An empirical study of content themes and reflection. *British Journal of Psychiatry, 123*, 55–61.

Weissman, M. M., Markowitz, J. C., & Klerman, G. L. (2000). *Comprehensive guide to interpersonal psychotherapy.* New York: Basic Books.

Wenzlaff, R. M., & Beevers, C. G. (1998). Depression and interpersonal responses to others' moods: The solicitation of negative information about happy people. *Personality and Social Psychology Bulletin, 24*, 386–398.

West, M. O., & Prinz, R. J. (1987). Parental alcoholism and childhood psychopathology. *Psychological Bulletin, 102*, 204–218.

Westen, D. (1990). Psychoanalytic approaches to personality. In L. A. Pervin (Ed.), *Handbook of personality: Theory and research* (pp. 21–65). New York: Guilford Press.

Westman, M., & Vinokur, A. D. (1998). Unraveling the relationship of distress levels within couples: Common stressors, empathic reactions, or crossover via social interaction? *Human Relations, 51*, 137–156.

Whiffen, V. E., & Gotlib, I. H. (1989). Infants of postpartum depressed mothers: Temperament and cognitive status. *Journal of Abnormal Psychology, 98*, 274–279.

Whisman, M. A. (2001). The association between depression and marital dissatisfaction. In S. R. H. Beach (Ed.), *Marital and family processes in depression: A scientific foundation for clinical practice* (pp. 3–24). Washington, DC: American Psychological Association.

White, J. H. (1992). Women and eating disorders: Part II. Developmental, familial, and biological risk factors. *Health Care for Women International, 13*, 363–373.

Whittaker, J. F., Connell, J., & Deakin, J. F. W. (1994). Receptive and expressive social communication in schizophrenia. *Psychopathology, 27*, 262–267.

Widiger, T. A., & Trull, T. J. (1993). Borderline and narcissistic personality disorders. In P. B. Sutker & H. E. Adams (Eds.), *Comprehensive handbook of psychopathology* (2nd ed., pp. 371–394). New York: Plenum Press.

Wierzbicki, M. (1984). Social skills deficits and subsequent depressed mood in students. *Personality and Social Psychology Bulletin, 10*, 605–610.

Wierzbicki, M., & McCabe, M. (1988). Social skills and subsequent depressive symptomatology in children. *Journal of Clinical Child Psychology, 3*, 203–208.

Wiggins, J. S. (1982). Circumplex models of interpersonal behavior in clinical psychology. In P. C. Kendall & J. N. Butcher (Eds.), *Handbook of research methods in clinical psychology* (pp. 183–221). New York: Wiley.

Wiggins, J. S. (1996). An informal history of the interpersonal circumplex tradition. *Journal of Personality Assessment, 66,* 217–233.

Williams, G. J., Chamove, A. S., & Millar, H. R. (1990). Eating disorders, perceived control, assertiveness and hostility. *British Journal of Clinical Psychology, 29,* 327–335.

Williams, J. G., Barlow, D. H., & Agras, W. S. (1972). Behavioral measurement of severe depression. *Archives of General Psychiatry, 27,* 330–333.

Wilsnack, S. C., Vogeltanz, N. D., Klassen, A. D., & Harris, R. (1997). Childhood sexual abuse and women's substance abuse: National survey findings. *Journal of Studies on Alcohol, 58,* 264–271.

Wilson, L. G., Rosenthal, N. E., & Dunner, D. L. (1982). The phenomenology of bipolar I manic–depressive illness. *Canadian Journal of Psychiatry, 27,* 150–154.

Windle, M., & Searles, J. S. (Eds.). (1990). *Children of alcoholics: Critical perspectives.* New York: Guilford Press.

Winton, E. C., Clark, D. M., & Edelmann, R. J. (1995). Social anxiety, fear of negative evaluation and the detection of negative emotion in others. *Behaviour Research and Therapy, 33,* 193–196.

Wittchen, H. U., Stein, B., & Kessler, R. (1999). Social fears and social phobia in a community sample of adolescents and young adults: Prevalence, risk factors, comorbidity. *Psychological Medicine, 29,* 309–323.

Wolin, S. J., Bennett, L. A., Noonan, D. L., & Teitelbaum, M. A. (1980). Disrupted family rituals. *Journal of Studies on Alcohol, 41,* 199–214.

Wonderlich, S. (1992). Relationship of family and personality factors in bulimia. In J. H. Crowther, D. L. Tennenbaum, S. E. Hobfoll, & M. A. P. Stephens (Eds.), *The etiology of bulimia nervosa: The individual and familial context* (pp. 103–126). Washington, DC: Hemisphere.

Wonderlich, S. A., & Swift, W. J. (1990a). Perceptions of parental relationships in the eating disorders: The relevance of depressed mood. *Journal of Abnormal Psychology, 99,* 353–360.

Wonderlich, S. A., & Swift, W. J. (1990b). Borderline versus other personality disorders in the eating disorders: Clinical description. *International Journal of Eating Disorders, 9,* 629–638.

Wonderlich, S., Ukestad, L., & Perzacki, R. (1994). Perceptions of nonshared childhood environment in bulimia nervosa. *Journal of the American Academy of Child and Adolescent Psychiatry, 33,* 740–747.

Woerner, P. I., & Guze, S. B. (1968). A family and marital study of hysteria. *British Journal of Psychiatry, 114,* 161–168.

Woody, S. R. (1996). Effects of focus of attention on anxiety levels and social performance of individuals with social phobia. *Journal of Abnormal Psychology, 105,* 61–69.

Worobey, J. (1999). Temperament and loving-styles in college women: Associations with eating attitudes. *Psychological Reports, 84,* 305–311.

Wright, D. M., & Heppner, P. P. (1991). Coping among nonclinical college-age children of alcoholics. *Journal of Counseling Psychology, 38,* 465–472.

Wuerker, A. M. (1994). Relational control patterns and expressed emotion in families of persons with schizophrenia and bipolar disorder. *Family Process, 33,* 389–407.

Wynne, L. C. (1968). Methodological and conceptual issues in the study of schizophrenics and their families. *Journal of Psychiatric Research, 6,* 185–199.

Wynne, L. C. (1981). Current concepts about schizophrenics and family relationships. *Journal of Nervous and Mental Disease, 169,* 82–89.

Wynne, L., Ryckoff, I., Day, J., & Hirsch, S. (1958). Pseudo-mutuality in the family relations of schizophrenics. *Psychiatry, 21,* 205–220.

Wynne, L., & Singer, M. (1963). Thought disorders and family relations of schizophrenics: II. A classification of forms of thinking. *Archives of General Psychiatry, 9,* 199–206.

Yama, M. F., Tovey, S. L., & Fogas, B. S. (1993). Childhood family environment and sexual abuse as predictors of anxiety and depression in adult women. *American Journal of Orthopsychiatry, 63,* 136–141.

Youngren, M. A., & Lewinsohn, P. M. (1980). The functional relation between depression and problematic interpersonal behavior. *Journal of Abnormal Psychology, 89,* 333–341.

Zahn-Waxler, C., Cummings, E. M., McKnew, D. ·H., & Radke-Yarrow, M. (1984). Altruism, aggression, and social interactions in young children with a manic–depressive parent. *Child Development, 55,* 112–122.

Zahn-Waxler, C., McKnew, D. H., Cummings, E. M., Davenport, Y. B., & Radke-Yarrow, M. (1984). Problem behaviors and peer interactions of young children with a manic–depressive parent. *American Journal of Psychiatry, 141,* 236–240.

Zakahi, W. R., & Duran, R. L. (1985). Loneliness, communication competence, and communication apprehension: Extension and replication. *Communication Quarterly, 33,* 50–60.

Zanarini, M. C., Gunderson, J. G., Marino, M. F., Schwartz, E. O., & Frankenburg, F. R. (1990). Psychiatric disorders in the families of borderline outpatients. In P. S. Links (Ed.), *Family environment and borderline personality disorder* (pp. 69–84). Washington, DC: American Psychiatric Press.

Ziegler-Driscoll, G. (1979). The similarities in families of drug dependents and alcoholics. In E. Kaufman & P. Kaufman (Eds.), *Family therapy of drug and alcohol abuse* (pp. 19–39). New York: Gardner Press.

Zimmer, D. (1983). Interaction patterns and communication skills in sexually distressed, maritally distressed, and normal couples: Two experimental studies. *Journal of Sex and Marital Therapy, 9,* 251–265.

Zoccolillo, M., & Cloninger, C. R. (1986). Somatization disorder: Psychologic symptoms, social disability, and diagnosis. *Comprehensive Psychiatry, 27,* 65–73.

Zuckerman, M. (1999). *Vulnerability to psychopathology.* Washington, DC: American Psychological Association.

Zuravin, S. J., & Fontanella, C. (1999). The relationship between child sexual abuse and major depression among low-income women: A function of growing up experiences? *Child Maltreatment, 4,* 3–12.

Index

Abuse
  alcoholism and, 169
  antisocial personality disorder and,
    130
  bipolar disorder and, 101
  dependent personality disorder
    and, 132
  role in the interpersonal paradigm,
    207
  social anxiety and, 57–58
  somatoform disorders and, 187
  substance use and, 174–176
  See also Sexual abuse
Achievement pressure, 127, 187
Affective style, 79–82, 103–104
Aggressiveness, 145, 162, 164–165
  See also Verbal aggression
Alcoholism
  See Substance use disorders
Antisocial personality disorder, 129–
    131
Assortative mating, 31, 166
Attachment
  alcoholism and, 169
  borderline personality disorder
    and, 120, 121
  depression and, 40
  role in the interpersonal paradigm,
    222
  sexual dysfunctions and, 200

  somatoform disorders and, 188–
    189
Attractiveness, histrionic personality
    disorder and, 127, 128

B

Bateson, Gregory, 66
Behaviorism, 3, 220–221
Biological paradigm, 5, 221–222
Biopsychosocial model, 222–223
Bipolar disorder
  affective style, 103–104
  childhood experiences, 100–102
  children of parents with, 109–110
  communication deviance, 104–105
  comorbidity with eating disorders,
    113
  comorbidity with personality disor-
    ders, 112, 133
  comorbidity with substance use
    disorders, 113, 180
  comparison with schizophrenia,
    97, 112–113
  conflict, 100, 106–107
  epidemiology, 97
  expressed emotion, 102–104, 108
  marriage, 106–108
  sexuality, 107
  social skills, 98–100
  social support, 104, 111

283

Bipolar disorder (*continued*)
  suicide, 108
  symptoms, 96–97
Borderline personality disorder, 119–123

C

Children
  alcoholism (COAs), 167–170
  bipolar disorder and, 100–102
  parents with bipolar disorder and, 109–110
  social anxiety and, 48, 54–55, 58
  somatoform disorders and, 186–187
  See also Abuse; Sexual abuse
Cognitive-behavioral theory, 4
Cognitive paradigm, 3, 4, 220
Communication deviance, 70, 71–75, 78–79, 104–105, 209
  See also Bipolar disorder; Schizophrenia
Conduct disorder, 129
Conflict
  alcoholism and, 166
  bipolar disorder and, 106–107, 110
  eating disorders and, 138, 149
  histrionic personality disorder and, 127
  personality disorders and, 115, 119, 124
  role in interpersonal paradigm, 212
  schizophrenia and, 79, 86
  sexual dysfunctions and, 196–199
  somatoform disorders and, 185, 186, 190
  substance use and, 173
Continuity hypothesis, 219
Coyne, James, 28–29, 204
Criticism
  eating disorders and, 139
  narcissistic personality disorder and, 124
  somatoform disorders and, 190

schizophrenia and parental, 76, 77, 82, 84
See also Affective style; Expressed emotion

D

Deception, 49
Decoding skills
  depression and, 23
  schizophrenia and, 88–90
  social anxiety and, 50
Dependent personality disorder, 131–133
Depression
  comorbidity with eating disorders, 153
  comorbidity with personality disorders, 133
  comorbidity with sexual dysfunctions, 200
  comorbidity with social anxiety, 60–61
  comorbidity with somatoform disorders, 184
  comorbidity with substance use, 179–180
  emotional contagion, 29–31
  epidemiology, 15
  loneliness, 40–42
  marriage, 34–37
  parenting, 37–38
  perfectionism, 33–34
  personal relationships, 32–34
  problem solving, 35, 37
  reassurance seeking, 29, 31–32
  rejection, 21, 28–30, 39, 42
  sexual abuse, 39–40
  social skills, 16–28, 26–28
  social support, 26, 33, 41
  symptoms, 15
Depressive realism, 18
Diathesis–stress models in
  bipolar disorder, 111
  depression, 27
  eating disorders, 152
  interpersonal paradigm, 216–217